# Complementary Therapies in Dental

*To Shirin, Leila and Zarrin*

# Complementary Therapies in Dental Practice

**Edited by Peter Varley**   BDS, FDSRCS, DDFHom

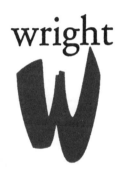
wright

Wright
An imprint of Butterworth-Heinemann
Linacre House, Jordan Hill, Oxford OX2 8DP
225 Wildwood Avenue, Woburn, MA 01801-2041
A division of Reed Educational and Professional Publishing Ltd

℞ A member of the Reed Elsevier plc group

OXFORD  BOSTON  JOHANNESBURG
MELBOURNE  NEW DELHI  SINGAPORE

First published 1998

©Reed Educational and Professional Publishing Ltd 1998

**British Library Cataloguing in Publication Data**

A catalogue record for this book is available from the British Library

**Library of Congress Cataloguing in Publication Data**

A catalogue record for this book is available from the Library of Congress

ISBN 0 7236 1033 9

Typeset by Keyword Typesetting Services Ltd, Wallington, Surrey, England
Printed and bound in Great Britain by Biddles Ltd, Guildford and King's Lynn

# Contents

# Contributor profiles

**Peter Varley** (Editor)   BDS, FDSRCS, DDFHom
Peter graduated as a dentist in Australia in 1975. He gained a Dental
Fellowship from the Royal College of Surgeons before establishing a dental
practice in Central London with three associate dentists, two hygienists, a
homoeopath, iridologist, acupuncturist, hypnotherapist and cranial osteopath.

He is a founder member and Chairman of the British Homoeopathic
Dental Association. He is a Dental Diplomate of the Faculty of
Homoeopathy and a member of the British Society of Occlusal Studies,
the Cranio Group, the British Medical and the British Dental
Acupuncture Societies. He is also a member of the British Dental
Association (BDA) and past member of the BDA Representative Board
and BDA Metropolitan Branch Council.

Peter has published a number of articles on dental homoeopathy and
complementary therapies and lectured throughout the UK. He has broadcast on London radio discussing homoeopathy.

Although he is one of the few dentists ever resident at the Royal London
Homoeopathic Hospital, his interests have always been broader. He has had
formal training in acupuncture, cranial osteopathy and nutrition and maintains a strong belief in the link between general and dental health.

*Chapter 1*
**Richard Fischer**   DDS, FAGD
Richard is in general dental practice near Washington DC. His practice has
developed a holistic approach to dentistry over many years, with an emphasis on homoeopathy and an interest in temporomandibular joint/cranial
function as well as the mercury and fluoride issues.

He graduated in 1973 and has been lecturing throughout the USA and
internationally since 1981. He has broadcast on national radio many times
and published a wealth of papers on dental homoeopathy.

In 1984 Richard was appointed Vice President of the National Board of
Homoeopathy in Dentistry as well as Course Director of Dental Seminars
for the centre. In 1995 he was elected President of the International
Academy of Oral Medicine and Toxicology. He is a Fellow of the
Academy of General Dentistry and the Academy of Stress and Chronic
Diseases. He has been awarded Certification by the American
Naturopathic Medical Board.

*Chapter 2*
**Ron Ehrlich**   BDS

Ron graduated in dentistry from Sydney Univerity in 1978. He runs a practice in the centre of Sydney promoting the concept of holistic dentistry, with a particular interest in the role of nutrition and exercise on general health.

He is interested in the biomechanics of the jaw and soft-tissue lesions as well as their relationship to the treatment of head, neck and jaw pain. Since 1990 he has carried out research at the Physiology Department, University of New South Wales investigating the effect of jaw muscles on other muscles of the body, collaborating with Mark Ninio, a leading Sydney podiatrist.

Ron has lectured internationally on nutrition and holistic dentistry. He is a member of the Australian Dental Association, the International Academy of Gnathology, the Australian College of Environmental and Nutritional Medicine, the International Association for the Study of Pain (IASP), the Australian Pain Society and the Australasian Society of Oral Medicine and Toxicology (ASOMAT).

*Chapter 3*
**Jonathan Howat**   DC(USA), DICS, FICS

Jonathan graduated as a chiropractor in the USA in 1970 and then returned to Rhodesia (Zimbabwe). He became President of the Rhodesian Chiropractic Association and later became the Chairman of the Zimbabwe Chiropractic Council. He moved to England in 1984 and became the Director of the Oxford Chiropractic Clinic, which specializes in Sacro-Occipital Technique and the Cranial Dental Sacral Complex.

He served on the Board of the Sacro-Occipital Research Society International (SORSI) and became President of SOTO (Sacral Occipital Technique Organization) International. In 1984 he formed SOTO Europe an organization affiliated to SORSI, which brought postgraduate education to the UK and Europe with the emphasis on increasing knowledge between dentists and chiropractors. He has lectured throughout the UK, Europe, South East Asia, Australia, USA and South Africa.

Jonathan is a Fellow of the International Craniopathic Society. He is Chairman of the Education Committee of SOTO Europe and an external lecturer on the Faculty of Anglo-European College of Chiropractic.

*Chapter 4*
**Richard Holding**   DO, MRO

Richard is an osteopath specializing in cranial osteopathy and one of the foremost proponents of kinesiology in this country. He graduated from the British School of Osteopathy in 1969 and taught under the auspices of the Sutherland Cranial Teaching Foundation for many years. He is a member of the International College of Applied Kinesiology and holds a Diploma from the International Academy of Nutrition.

Over the years he has evolved his blend of cranial osteopathy, clinical and applied kinesiology and traditional Chinese medicine into a highly effective system for the treatment of a wide range of illnesses and disorders.

Richard is a director of Ark International Training Seminars. He teaches extensively in the UK, USA and Europe as well as running a busy specialized practice in North London, concentrating on chronic disease.

*Chapter 5*
**Joseph Shafer**   DC(USA), DIBAK, CCSP
Joe graduated as a Doctor of Chiropractic in the USA in 1980. During 11 years working in Denmark he undertook postgraduate education in applied kinesiology, sports medicine and nutrition. He has Diplomate status in applied kinesiology and is a Certified chiropractic sports physician.

He was invited to assist 'Team Denmark', the national organization for the advancement of sport in treating athletes who did not respond to traditional therapeutic approaches. He works closely with dentists on temporomandibular joint and other related problems.

He is an Honorary Associate Professor at the Novokuznetsk School of Post-graduate Medicine in Russia. He is on the editorial board of several professional journals and is a member of a number of professional societies in Europe and the USA.

Joe has lectured to doctors, dentists, chiropractors and osteopaths in Italy, Holland, Scandinavia, Britain and Russia. Today much of his time is devoted to teaching and consulting work throughout Europe.

*Chapter 6*
**Simon Hayhoe**   MBBS, MRCS, LRCP, DA, FICAE
Simon is an anaesthetist with an acupuncture and hypnotherapy practice in Colchester (UK). He has a particular interest in dental anaesthesia and teaches on the Society for the Advancement of Anaesthesia in Dentistry (SAAD) sedation courses, lecturing on alternative methods of pain control.

He was a founder member of the British Medical Acupuncture Society (BMAS), and later a lecturer on both their medical and dental courses and Chairman of the Society.

Simon is Treasurer and British representative of the International Council for Medical Acupuncture and Related Techniques (ICMART) and has been awarded the ICMART diploma for service in the promotion of medical acupuncture. He is a Fellow of the International College of Acupuncture and Electro-Therapeutics and on the editorial board of their journal.

As Editor of *Acupuncture in Medicine*, the BMAS journal, Simon has sought to encourage doctors and dentists to accept acupuncture as a logical Western tool. He believes that acupuncture should become a normal medical treatment used routinely by doctors and dentists for appropriate problems.

*Chapter 7*
**Jack Levenson**   LDSRCS(Edin)
Jack is President of the British Society for Mercury Free Dentistry. He is also Dental Advisor and Executive Committee Member of the Environmental Medicine Foundation.

In 1969 he founded the Cavendish Medical Centre, Europe's first computerized medical screening centre. In 1985 he was responsible for the first major conference in this country on the dangers of mercury, called 'Hazards in Dentistry: The Mercury Debate'.

He was responsible for the dental sections of the Allergy and Environmental Medicine Departments at the Wellington and Lister Hospitals in London. He currently advises a number of similar clinics on the dental aspects of their work.

Jack lectures extensively on the subjects of mercury and safe amalgam removal, nutrition, allergies and other environmental factors which affect the health of the teeth and supporting structures. Currently he runs a practice confined to testing patients for mercury toxicity and advising both patients and dentists on protective procedures.

## *Chapter 8*
### Geoff Graham   BDS

Geoff graduated from Durham University (UK) in 1956 and started using hypnosis in his dental practice in 1960. He is a Founder Fellow (1969), Past President (1992–95) and Council Member (1969–present) of the British Society for Medical and Dental Hypnosis (BSMDH).

He is a Foreign Fellow of the American Society of Clinical Hypnosis, a Member of Honour of the Brazil Hypnotic Society and an Honorary Fellow of the Singapore Society of Clinical Hypnosis.

Geoff is a member of the International Society of Hypnosis and has lectured and conducted workshops throughout the world. He has written four books on hypnosis – two on formal hypnosis and two on neurolinguistic programming. They have been published internationally and will be part of the Russian teaching programme in psychotherapy.

## *Chapter 9*
### Angela Caine   LRAM, AGSM

Angela studied opera at the Guildhall School of Music. Her involvement with 'structure' began in 1988 when singing teachers and voice pathologists failed to solve her recurring loss of voice. Dental work done for cosmetic reasons then changed her tongue reference. These events made her aware of the connection between dentition and the voice.

She began a research programme that has involved dentists, orthodontists, chiropractors and osteopaths considering the voice as a function that should not be ignored during treatment.

Angela has lectured nationally on voice therapy and teaches music and the Alexander Technique for Southampton University and privately. She is on the database for the Performing Arts Medicine Trust, which takes care of the problems of professional musicians. She is also a member of the Cranio Group, an organization for the study of craniomandibular disorders. She works in Southampton with a chiropractor and a dentist treating voice problems through structural realignment.

## *Chapter 10*
### Stuart Ferraris   BChD, DGDP

Stuart graduated in South Africa in 1976. He travelled extensively before settling in North Wales where he has developed a successful holistic dental practice using a broad range of complementary therapies.

He is a member of the British Homoeopathic Dental Association, the British Medical Acupuncture Society, the British Society for Medical and Dental Hypnosis, the Foundation of Biological Medicine, the Natural Medicine Society plus many other dentally related societies, including the American Equilibration Society and the Cranio Group.

In 1992 Stuart was awarded the Diploma in General Dental Practice from the Royal College of Surgeons. He has appeared on television, published many articles on dental and natural health topics and lectured both nationally and internationally on running a holistic dental practice.

# Foreword

Modern therapies can be quite ineffectual when faced with chronic disease. They are often reduced to the provision of mere palliative, rather than curative treatment. Despite vast sums of money being spent on the NHS since 1948, the standard of health care in the UK has not substantially improved; demand has increased and the system has evolved as a sickness service.

In the BMA's booklet *Complementary Medicine – New approaches to Good Practice* published in 1993, complementary therapies are described as 'those which can work alongside and in conjunction with orthodox medical treatment.' There is clearly a wide diversity of these types of practice. They would include self-help therapies such as yoga and meditation; non-invasive therapies such as homoeopathy, hypnosis and nutrition; and interventive therapies such as acupuncture, osteopathy and chiropractic. All these therapies can be used as an additional and, therefore, complementary form of treatment. Many of the therapists will have received a basic training grounded in the orthodox medical sciences. They will be able to work and liaise with established health care professionals and communicate with their medical and dental colleagues in a common language.

There has been a long history of antagonism towards complementary medicine, but the rapidly increasing numbers of patients who are seeking help from such practitioners, has forced many European countries to review their current policies. In his address to the BMA in 1983, the Prince of Wales said that he feared that our preoccupation with modern medicine would divert our attention from 'those ancient, unconscious forces, lying beneath the surface, which will help to shape the psychological attitudes of modern man.' Whilst recognizing the importance of maintaining and improving professional standards, he believed that the art of healing should take account of the long neglected complementary therapies which 'in the right hands, can bring considerable relief, if not hope to an increasing number of people.'

In this book, Peter Varley has assembled contributions from a wide variety of skilled dentists and therapists who, whilst being acknowledged experts in many fields, have written individual chapters on their subjects. This will inform health professionals, who can then educate the public in the importance of a healthy lifestyle, explain the significance of our self-healing capacity and bring about the realization that health care is much more about health promotion than the alleviation of the symptoms of the disease.

The dental profession, who unlike their medical colleagues, see their patients on a regular basis, should be at the forefront of the holistic approach to health care. This book will be an excellent starting point and an invaluable reference.

Lord Colwyn   CBE, BDS, LDSRCS

# Preface

This book is aimed at the dentist with an interest in complementary medicine, but it is also for the complementary therapist with an interest in dentistry. It is not necessarily assumed that the reader attracted to the book has a detailed knowledge of complementary therapies and for this reason it may also be of interest to patients. Each chapter starts with general information on its discipline before progressing to more detail on the applications it may have in dentally related fields. The book cannot be considered to cover each discipline fully or to replace any of the larger texts in the field of complementary medicine. It should be used in conjunction with them.

The use of complementary therapies in dental practice is a new concept. There are many books on complementary medicine that occasionally touch on aspects of dentistry, but to have a single volume concentrating solely on dentistry with an overview of so many therapies is unique. I hope it is a vehicle to stimulate the dentist to enter uncharted waters, to introduce new ideas into their practice and to seek further reading in this constantly growing field.

In a book involving many authors it would be neither desirable nor practicable to impose complete uniformity of style. The character and presentation of each contributor is preserved as it would be if the contributors were taking part in a symposium or lecture course. Some points are repeated in various chapters. I feel this should be considered as positive reinforcement and have taken special care to include these repeats where a new point is also introduced or where a slightly different emphasis is made. At the end of each chapter there are references, a bibliography, a list of associations and details of relevant courses.

I would like to thank my wife for correcting spelling and teaching me to express myself clearly and to the staff at the Poland Street Dental Practice for their support and enthusiasm for complementary dentistry. I must thank all the contributors who are experts in their fields and have taught me so much of what I know in the world of complementary medicine. I particularly thank Stuart Ferraris for challenging and stimulating me over the years. Finally, I would like to thank the publishers for their confidence in me and their insight and help in creating this book.

P.D.V.

# Introduction

Peter Varley

*The doctor of the future will give no medicine, but will interest*
*his patients in the care of the human frame, in diet and in the*
*cause and prevention of disease.* Thomas A. Edison

Dentistry has traditionally been an orthodox profession. Yet unwittingly dentists have introduced into the very heart of their structure the one holistic mechanism that escapes most health professions – the six-monthly check-up. This unique opportunity to view people on a regular basis when healthy would be the holistic practitioner's dream. Most dentists waste the opportunity by looking only for disease.

Disease becomes apparent to the practitioner through the presence of signs and symptoms. When we adopt a holistic philosophy we have the means to reverse disease before the symptoms manifest themselves and to fine-tune the body so that health is maintained. Health is more than just the absence of disease. Health is a state of homeostasis; a balance of the spiritual, emotional, mental and physical aspects of the body. The holistic dentist, while recording the dental health of each patient, will also look at nutrition, check muscle and joint function, and assess stress and the effect of toxic materials on the immune system. They will be listening to the patient, thinking laterally and looking to other complementary practitioners for support. They will be the regular pivot to support the patient's health before disease manifests itself. They will be looking at the patient as a whole, not just their teeth.

Holistic practice embraces the concept of good practice. By their very nature complementary therapies require a thorough patient history, a detailed examination and an ability to listen. By providing these three criteria we are more than halfway to practising a holistic approach. The good orthodox dentist may follow these criteria, but stops short of using complementary therapies. He or she does a thorough temporomandibular joint examination, but fails to understand that the upper half of the joint is moving and that the muscles are attached to rhythmically moving bones. He or she also fails to understand that the bones may be locked in an unbalanced position and, if locked since childhood, growth may be compromised. They do not have the knowledge to treat these imbalances or the infrastructure to refer to the appropriate therapists. The purpose of this book is to provide some of that knowledge to dentists as well as stimulating the complementary practitioner to acquire an understanding of dentistry and to encourage both to work together.

To aquire knowledge takes commitment. The holistic dentist has usually spent countless hours in postgraduate education, many days away from the practice and frequent weekends away from the family. This creates financial and emotional stress. Once the knowledge is there and the systems are in place, they are rewarded with job satisfaction and the ability to provide a truly comprehensive treatment. The healthy, appreciative, reconstituted patient is the ultimate reward.

The use of complementary remedies is rising faster in Britain than in any other European country. In the UK a quarter of the population is using at least one form of complementary medicine at any given time.[1,2] The NHS is spending £1 million a year on complementary practitioners. Nearly half of general medical practices are estimated to have referred patients for alternative treatments. The first full-time NHS aromatherapist was recently appointed in Sheffield. Private medical insurers have responded to the rising demand. BUPA includes cover for acupuncture, chiropractic, homoeopathy and osteopathy in all of its policies, provided that referral is through a consultant. The economic impact of complementary medicine is enormous, with $12 billion being spent every year in the USA.[3] Now is the time for dentists to examine complementary medicine, embrace the concepts and integrate its disciplines into their profession.

The appeal of complementary therapies is related to the amount of time available, the use of touch, a non-invasive approach and a conviction in the methods used.[4] The arguments against complementary medicine are that it is unscientific, a placebo and a fringe activity. The scientific foundations of much in complementary medicine have not yet been substantiated, but research is changing this.[5,6] No successful treatment can in itself be unscientific. If it does work it is the job of science to discover why, which may involve rearranging some cherished dogmas.[7] In historical terms the application of scientific method to medicine is relatively young and not all orthodox disciplines have a sound scientific base. It has been estimated that about 85% of orthodox medical therapies are not supported by solid scientific evidence.[8]

When complementary medicine lacks a sound scientific basis its followers tend to substitute a philosophy. Philosophies, like religions, cannot be proven right or wrong and are usually unscientific by nature. However, one cannot say that a remedy associated with a philosophy is worthless. The history of medicine abounds with examples of effective therapies that were once used on the basis of a totally false rationale. Eventually the concepts are corrected and the effective therapy becomes part of established treatment.[9]

The success of complementary medicine can be puzzling to mainstream doctors. Its popularity is often said to be due to a placebo effect.[10] However, compared to a placebo some complementary remedies are very active, even to the extent that side-effects may be a problem.[11,12] In trials comparing remedy and placebo we must compare the response patterns over a given period.[13] We must assess how long a response lasts. Rabkin et al.[14] suggest that patients relapse after 10 days on placebo. Complementary therapies, if effective, will continue their effect over a longer term. Although complementary therapies may use the placebo effect to some extent, they do not carry a monopoly on this response. We cannot exclude orthodox treatments from using the placebo effect as well. Empathy and comfort can also be provided by mainstream doctors.

Since The Medical Act 1512 and the The Herbalists' Charter 1542 orthodox and complementary medicine have worked side by side. Even today the public have a choice between the medical doctor or the lay practitioner. This choice has allowed patients to attend to their medical needs without ever seeing a doctor. Yet when it comes to their dental needs the public have no choice. The dental profession has organized itself so that only they can practise dentistry. This has led to a certain degree of complacency by many dentists. It is not unusual for patients to report that their dentist routinely prescribes antibiotics, uses only mercury fillings and insists on taking X-rays. There are many members of the public to whom this is unacceptable. They feel trapped and express it through non-attendance or by seeking out one of the few holistic dentists available.

The development of complementary medicine is changing this situation. The Council for Complementary and Alternative Medicine has celebrated its tenth anniversary, having been formed in 1986 in direct response to the British Medical Association's highly critical review of complementary medicine.[15] Unlike five years ago, the question is no longer whether complementary medicine will be made available within mainstream health care; it has largely become a question of how such integration takes place. Although complementary therapies such as osteopathy and acupuncture are widely practised within the National Health Service, how these therapies are to be linked into the NHS on a national level is not yet clear. The Department of Health has agreed funding for pilot studies to assess how osteopathy and chiropractic should be made available on the NHS.

With the acceptance of complementary philosophy in mainstream medicine it is hoped that dentists will also embrace it. The dental profession must continue to question established thinking. Fundamental concepts in science, including medicine, have been changing. Physicists have been aware of it for some time, but those in the orthodox medical field have hardly started to take on board the implications of these changes. We are in the midst of a shift from Newtonian classical physics to Einstein's quantum energy. The medical model is still disease and substance orientated, rather than health and energy related. Complementary medicine is based on the quantum perspective that everything, including our bodies, is energy. Homoeopathy works at this level. Until orthodox medicine catches up with physics and considers the effects of energy meridians on the mental, emotional and physical elements of the human energy system, it will not be able to obtain or understand total health for its patients.[16]

It took the Flat Earth Society some time to realize and accept that Columbus did not actually fall off the end of the world; he was simply somewhere else and temporarily out of sight.[17] The edge of one person's world is no more than the beginning of another's. Our view tends to be entirely different depending on where we happen to be at a given moment in time. We hope that this book will contribute a little to changing that view.

# References

1 Fisher P, Ward A. Complementary Medicine in Europe. *Br Med J* 1994; **309:** 107–111.

2 A 1989 survey carried out for *The Times* by MORI revealed that 27% of the respondents had used non-orthodox medicine. This is a figure broadly in line with a 1991 Consumers Association survey which showed that 25% of their members used complementary therapies.

3 Eisenberg D M, Kessler R C, Foster C *et al.* Unconventional medicine in the United States. *N Eng J Med* 1993; **328:** 246–252.

4 Brewin T. Fraternizing with the fringe. *Br J Gen Pract* 1994; **44:** 243–244.

5 Ernst E. Is homoeopathy a placebo? *Br J Clin Pharmacol* 1990; **30:** 173–174.

6 Shekelle P G, Adams A H, Chassin M R *et al.* Spinal manipulations for low back pain. *Ann Intern Med* 1992; **117:** 590-598.

7 Earl Baldwin of Bewdley. Letters to the Editor. *The Times* 11 April, 1996.

8 Smith R. Where is the wisdom? *Br Med J* 1991; **303:** 798-799.

9 Goodwin J S, Goodwin J M. The tomato effect. Rejection of highly efficacious therapies. *J Am Med Assoc* 1984; **251:** 2387-2390.

10 Oh V M. The placebo effect: how can we use it better. *Br Med J* 1994; **309:** 69-70.

11 Soragna D, Montalbetti L, Bo P *et al.* Chiropractic complications. *Acta Neurol* 1993; **15:** 145–150.

12 D'Arcy P F. Adverse drug reactions and interactions with herbal medicines. *Adv Drug React Toxicol Rev* 1993; **12:** 147–162.

13 Quitkin F M, Rabkin J D, Markowitz M J *et al.* Use of pattern analysis to identify true drug response. *Arch Gen Psychiatry* 1987; **44:** 259–264.

14 Rabkin J G, McGrath P J, Stewart J W *et al.* The follow up of patients who improved during placebo washout. *J Clin Psychopharmacol* 1986; **6:** 274–278.

15 BMA Report. *Alternative Therapies.* London: BMA, Chameleon Press, 1986.

16 Beacon J. Electromagnetic stress in the home. *Positive Hlth* 1996; **16:** 34–36.

17 Lewis K. Editorial. *Dental Practice* 1996; **34(16):** 2.

# Homoeopathy

**Richard Fischer**

*The text of this chapter is based on a seminar presented in London by Dr Fischer to the British Homoeopathic Dental Association*

(Editor)

## Introduction

The dental profession is becoming increasingly aware of the indivisibility of dental health and overall health. The oral cavity is integrated with the rest of the body via the nerves, blood, lymphatic and glandular systems, acupuncture meridians, bones and joints and by the digestive tract which extends from the mouth to the anus.

Because of the mechanical nature of most dental procedures it can be convenient to forget that the mouth we are treating is connected to a vital human being. Yet the profound interrelationships between the mouth and the rest of the body have been recognized in the West for decades and by the Chinese for some fifty centuries.

When treating an oral health problem, the cause is often found locally, such as a broken tooth or lost filling. However, the cause can also be found outside the mouth. This is particularly true of the chronic maladies, such as periodontal disease. Examples include the bone resorption around the teeth of the diabetic patient,[1] and the gingival proliferation in the epileptic receiving Dilantin therapy.[2] The American Dental Association now recognizes the systemic contribution towards periodontal disease.[3] The dentist is sought for evaluation and treatment of these oral symptoms – even though they are more of a systemic disturbance.

Perhaps more common but less widely appreciated are those systemic maladies that result from oral sources, as described and documented by Dr Rheinhold Voll[4] and others.[5,6] Typical examples include the constipation of the temporomandibular joint (TMJ) patient due to an impaired chewing ability, the migraine headaches of a mercury-sensitive patient or the abdominal rash of the nickel-sensitive woman elicited when placing a nickel crown on her tooth. In these cases the patients traditionally seek the treatment of a physician because of the systemic nature of the symptoms – despite their oral origins.

Consider that only decades ago it was fairly common medical treatment for rheumatoid arthritis to extract all the patient's teeth. One cannot ignore the fact that what we do in our dental treatment can profoundly affect that individual's systemic health and vice versa. Once this concept is embraced, the role of homoeopathy in dentistry is much easier to appreciate.

Homoeopathy is a medical system that enjoys a long and rich heritage of scientific literature and a worldwide reputation for safe and effective therapeutics. Although its basic tenets go back to Paracelsus and Hippocrates, it was codified into a systematic medical science in 1789 by Dr Samuel Hahnemann, a German physician. Hahnemann had his primary text, called 'The Organon', published in 1810 and he based this science on three fundamental principles.

## Principles of homoeopathy

### Law of similars

The first principle of homoeopathy is the 'law of similars'. Any medicinal substance given in overdose produces its own unique set of signs and symptoms. When individuals become sick, they too develop their own unique set of physical, mental and emotional signs and symptoms – even two individuals with identical diagnoses will exhibit different symptom pictures.

Dana Ullman defines homoeopathic medicine as 'a natural pharmaceutical science in which the practitioner seeks to find a substance that would cause, in overdose, symptoms similar to those a sick person is experiencing. When the match is made, that substance is given in very small, safe doses, often with dramatic effects'.[7]

This law is embraced by allopathic medicine as well; for example, using Ritalin to treat hyperactivity in children (Ritalin is a drug which normally causes hyperactivity). Immunizations are based on the law of similars. Modern pharmacology has rephrased this principle into the Arndt–Schulz law: 'Every drug has a stimulating effect in small doses, while larger doses inhibit, and much larger doses kill.'

It must be recognized that symptoms are, in reality, manifestations of the organism's attempt to heal itself – to regain homeostasis. For example, when a person has a systemic infection, they will develop a fever. The fever is not the disease, but the body's attempt to rid itself of the infection via increased blood flow, cellular activity and interferon production. To treat the symptoms by reducing the fever will slow the body's healing response and can be counterproductive; for example, giving aspirin to a child with influenza can cause Reye's syndrome, a potentially fatal disease.

The homoeopathic approach is to respect the body's attempts to heal itself and gently support the fever. Suppressing the symptoms can allow the underlying disease to progress unchecked. It is analogous to cutting the wire to your car dashboard's warning light when it flashes that your engine is overheating.

## Minimum dose

The second principle is the minimum dose. Medicines given in material doses carry with them adverse side-effects. Hahnemann, in order to minimize these undesirable effects, attempted to determine the smallest dose of a medicine that would still be effective. In his research, he took various medicines of the era and serially diluted them to determine the minimum dose which would work.

He did this by taking one part of the medicinal substance and diluting it with 99 parts of distilled water or ethyl alcohol, and then vigorously shaking it to create a homogeneous solution. The resulting solution is termed a 1'C', or first centesimal potency (1 part in 100 parts solution). When one part of this solution is then diluted further with 99 parts of water or alcohol and shaken again, you have a 2C solution (1 part in 10 thousand parts solution). This process is continued to different strengths, usually 3C, 6C, 12C, 30C, 200C, 1000C (1M) and beyond.*

Here we arrive at homoeopathy's most controversial feature. According to Avogadro's law, by the time we get beyond the 12C potency there are, in all probability, no more molecules of the original medicine left. Although he predated Avogadro, Hahnemann was startled to observe clinically that the more a medicine had been potentized (i.e. diluted and shaken in this fashion) the longer it generally lasted, the deeper its curative effects, and the fewer the doses that were needed. These observations have now been verified by 200 years of clinical observation by homoeopaths throughout the world. 'Something' of the medicine remains in the potentized remedy, but what? Theories abound – the 'energy', or 'essence', or 'pattern', or 'vibration' of the medicine remains. The real explanation presumably lies somewhere in the realm of quantum physics. Those who wish a scholarly insight into this quandary should read Dr Colin Lessell's text, 'The Infinitesimal Dose'.[8]

## Single remedy

The last tenet of classical homoeopathy is the use of the single remedy. The actions of medicines are tested on healthy human subjects one medicine at a time. These tests are called 'provings'. This is vital and necessary for two reasons.

First, the subjects must be healthy to determine what reproducible and reliable symptoms are specific to the medicine being tested. If you test the medicine on someone who is sick, the information as to the true actions of the medicine would not be translatable to use on other people.

Second, we know that when medicines in material doses are used in combinations, we often get interactions which are unpredictable and dangerous. It would not only be impracticable, but impossible, to test

---

*In the decimal scale, at each stage the dilution is 1 in 10 rather than 1 in 100. In order to distinguish them from the centesimal scale preparations, decimal potencies are designated by the letter 'X' (e.g. 6X), or in some countries by the prefix 'D' (e.g. D6). So a D6 is identical to a 6X.

While a 6X is not identical to a 6C in actual dilutions, their potency can be considered to be approximately the same.

medicines in all the possible permutations to determine the infinite combination effects. Thus, all homoeopathic provings use only the one remedy being studied. The results of these provings form the basis of our materia medica. So to prescribe more than one remedy at a time necessarily conflicts with the law of similars, since we have no clinical data demonstrating what these medicines provoke in combination. While such combination remedies abound, most classical homoeopaths view their potential benefit as palliative.

## Homoeopathic prescribing

### Potency selection

In homoeopathic prescribing, remedy selection is imperative. However, in potency selection there are a number of different factors that one should take into consideration.

#### VITALITY OF THE PATIENT

The first factor is the vitality of the patient. In general, the higher their vitality, the higher the potency you can use. Most of the remedies for acute situations in a dental surgery would be used anywhere from 6C to 200C. If someone has high vitality, you may go up to 200C or even 1M, depending on the situation. Conversely, a 90-year-old fragile patient's vitality may be overpowered by a 1M potency and may then actually get worse after the remedy.

#### EMOTIONAL V. PHYSICAL

The second factor to consider is whether the symptoms are more emotionally or physically based. When more emotionally based (an anxiety state for example), they reflect a higher plane of pathology. Homoeopaths rank the emotional and spiritual levels at the highest plane of pathology. Below that is the mental, and then below that the physical. So the higher the plane of pathology, the higher the potency you may use.

#### ACUTE V. CHRONIC STATE

The third factor to consider in potency selection is the acuteness of the problem. Usually acute ailments with intense symptoms warrant higher potencies, because acute problems use up the energy of the medicine more quickly. Chronic ailments exhibiting a slower progression with less intensity usually warrant lower potencies.

#### CORRECT REMEDY

The fourth factor is your own certainty that you have the right remedy. The more certain you are, the higher the potency you might use. The more similar the patient is to the symptomatology of the remedy, the more sensitive or responsive they are going to be, so the higher the dilution you can give them.

The most common potencies to keep in the dental surgery are 6C, 30C and 200C of most of the remedies, and then gauge the potency to the situation. If you just use a few of these factors in your consideration, you will do well. Then if all else fails, if all you have is the 6C – then use the 6C. Homoeopaths will tell you that potency selection is generally the least important part of your prescription. If you have the correct remedy, the potency is usually going to work.

### Frequency of repetition

The more acute the condition, the more frequently you may need to repeat the remedy. If an hysterical child presents on emergency following an injury, one might give a dose of Aconite (for example) every 5 minutes until he or she is calm enough to proceed with your treatment.

For moderately acute conditions you may repeat the remedy every hour or two initially, and then less frequently as improvement begins. For more chronic conditions you may repeat the remedy two or three times daily. The most important rule of thumb is to have the patient discontinue the remedy when significant improvement occurs, otherwise aggravation or a proving may result.

## Specific conditions in dental practice

Below are some of the acute or specific conditions that occur in the dental surgery and how homoeopathy may be used to treat them.

### Anxiety

There are several very effective anxiety remedies. In order to practise dentistry, you have to get the patient into your office and into the chair. That is the first hurdle for a lot of our patients. Dentistry is not perceived as something pleasurable for most patients, and some of them have real phobias.

#### ACONITE

The anxiety remedy used most frequently is *Aconitum napellus*. The *Aconite* kind of fear is exhibited by sudden panic, dry mouth; the fidgety type of patient. For the dental patient it may be similar to when an adrenaline anaesthetic is injected into a blood vessel, a rush of adrenaline. The symptoms are heart palpitaitons, dry mouth, dilated pupils – the sensation of sudden shock. It is very short lasting and of very quick onset. *Aconite* works very well to manage this kind of fear. The usual potency is 200C.

CASE HISTORY

*I had a patient who was in his eighties and in very poor health. He had very severe heart problems which required a prophylactic antibiotic and nitroglycerin. He was a lovely gentleman. The first time he came to my office he had angina pains and palpitations, and this was just for the consultation. When he came and sat in the chair, he had already taken all of the nitroglycerin tablets that he was allowed for the day. I gave him one dose of Aconite 200, and within 2–3 minutes, the palpitations, the anxiety and all of that just subsided.*

*I referred him to a periodontist because he had some severe periodontal problems and he needed extensive crown and bridge work, and we got everything done very successfully. I know that Aconite helped him through that first consultation and made the patient and me feel confident enough to proceed with the required treatment. The periodontist was really quite nervous to do the surgery and probably could have used some Aconite himself. They both got through the surgery all right.*

### GELSEMIUM

The second most frequently used anxiety remedy after *Aconite* is *Gelsemium*. The *Gelsemium* patient – instead of the dry-mouth, wide-eyed jittery patient that *Aconite* presents – is the one that is drowsy, weak-kneed and trembling, and usually a bit nauseous or has nervous diarrhoea. This is the kind of fear you may have experienced walking into a final exam, when you are feeling unprepared.

In treating any of these anxiety states the 200C potency is used, assuming the vitality of the patient is there, because you are working at the emotional level.

### ARSENICUM

Another anxiety remedy is *Arsenicum album*. The anxiety in the *Arsenicum* patient is a little bit different from that of *Aconite*. This patient has chronic anxiety. They worry about a lot of things, especially their health, and they usually have type A personalities – very restless, irritable – and typically their symptoms are aggravated at night.

One of the keynotes of *Arsenicum* patients is that they are extremely chilly, and their chilliness is deep. You can put a warm sweater on them, yet they are still chilly. They are chilly to the bone and they suffer often from burning pains. *Arsenicum* is one of the great burning pain remedies (along with sulphur and phosphorus), but the peculiarity with *Arsenicum* is that the burning pains feel better from heat! This is a very unusual symptom. So when you find people with burning pains that feel better when you put heat on the affected part, that is a keynote for *Arsenicum*.

### COFFEA

Another successful remedy treating anxiety is *Coffea cruda* (homoeopathic coffee). *Coffea* has a peculiar anxiety picture; for instance, when you have consumed too much coffee, the phone rings next to you and you are startled off your chair. Similarly, *Coffea* patients are aggravated by any kind of sound, even music, which is a rare and strange symptom. *Coffea* patients will come into the dental surgery and if you have music piped in, they have to have it turned off. They just cannot stand the music. Not just because it is rock music; any kind of noise is going to drive them crazy. That is a keynote for *Coffea*.

The *Coffea* toothache is also unusual; it is worse from heat and better from cold. Pathologically, we think about that as a gangrenous pulp, where you actually have gas in the pulp chamber. The cold tends to shrink the gas inside the pulp, relieving the pressure. So the patient will put some ice-water in their mouth and it feels better; and as soon as the ice melts and the water warms up, the pain starts to build and build, resulting in an extreme neuralgic type of pain.

CASE HISTORY

*I remember the first time I saw a Coffea toothache; the patient literally came in with a jug full of ice-water and just kept holding the water in his mouth. After about a minute, when the water warmed up, he would have to take another mouthful to stop the pain. This is an unforgettable toothache once you have seen it. Coffea is also a remedy to consider with trigeminal neuralgias, particularly when accompanied by great nervous excitability and intolerance of pain.*

IGNATIA

A further anxiety remedy is *Ignatia*. The *Ignatia* patient may present with hysteria, and twitching of the muscles of the face and lips. *Ignatia* patients will be worse from cigarette smoke or coffee. *Ignatia* is a wonderful grief remedy for the patient who has lost a loved one or been jilted. Whenever you hear a patient report that they 'have never been well since' this sort of an emotional trauma, *Ignatia* is the first remedy that should come to mind.

There are other remedies like *Argentum*, but they are not so common. If you know these few remedies – particularly *Aconite*, *Gelsemium* and *Arsenicum* – you will be able to help most of your anxiety patients.

We also use *Rescue Remedy* (one of the Bach Flower Remedies) as well as hypnosis. These help wonderfully with anxious patients and, like homoeopathic medicines, are very user friendly.

With any anxious patient, once you know which anxiety state they go into, you should give them three or four doses of the appropriate remedy, usually a 200C potency, to take home with them. Instruct them that on the night before their dental visit (or whenever they start to worry about it) to take a dose. Usually that means one dose the night before, another dose the morning of, and another dose an hour before their appointment. You definitely want them to take the remedy ahead of time, to let it have a chance to work and to cover pre-appointment apprehension.

It is allowable to take more doses than recommended. If the patient feels the need for it and believes that he or she cannot take another dose, that alone can add to the anxiety. So give enough to get through the series of appointments.

There is some placebo affect with homoeopathy, just as there is with any therapy. In pharmacology we are taught that yellow pills work better than green pills, and green ones are more effective than blue pills, and so on. So pharmacology also uses the placebo affect. While we do not mind using the placebo affect (it can be a very powerful tool), we cannot rely on it. You always want the placebo affect working for you, not against you.

## Trauma

There are several common trauma remedies to discuss. We are thinking of the physical trauma here. Your patients have overcome the emotional trauma and they are in your surgery.

### ARNICA

For blunt trauma, bruises and soft-tissue injuries the primary remedy is *Arnica montana*. Most people who have used homoeopathic remedies probably started with *Arnica*. *Arnica* is for any kind of soft-tissue injuries – blunt injuries such as a tooth extraction, a crown preparation, haematomas, adjusting orthodontic wires, a blow to the jaw – anything of that nature. It has been said that if homoeopathy had nothing but *Arnica* to offer the world, it would be a priceless medical art. *Arnica* helps with the pain, swelling and bleeding due to any bruising type of injuries. Arnica also helps prevent infections in tissues similarly injured.

### HYPERICUM

*Hypericum* is also a wonderful remedy for trauma, but specifically for trauma to nerves, such as a deep filling that is close to the pulp, after root-canal therapy, for fractured incisors where you have a near exposure or exposure of the nerve, for paraesthesias following a mandibular third molar extraction. *Hypericum* is called the '*Arnica* for the nerves'. Any time you have a nerve injury, *Hypericum* is the first remedy you think about. Typically, in situations calling for *Hypericum*, the pain is excessive.

### STAPHYSAGRIA

Another trauma remedy with which I have had some wonderful success is *Staphysagria*. For those of you who do surgery, such as periodontal surgery, uncovering impacted wisdom teeth and apicectomies – any kind of an incision wound – *Staphysagria* is the remedy par excellence. This manages the pain in properly indicated cases better than morphine.

### CASE HISTORY

*I had a patient who was going into the hospital for major abdominal surgery (a hysterectomy). Because she had had very good results from some dental homoeopathic treatments we had given her, she asked: 'What can I do for the pain after the surgery?' She picked up some Staphysagria 200X and took it to the hospital and put it in a drawer. When she awakened after the surgery she was administered morphine, which did not touch the pain. She remembered she had the bottle of Staphysagria and within ten or fifteen minutes of taking the first dose the pain was quite manageable, and she got on fine. When she recounted this later, I thought that perhaps the morphine had just finally taken effect. However, she ran out of the Staphysagria while still on the morphine and the pain returned. So Staphysagria for that sort of thing is much more effective than morphine; just as stated in Kent's lectures.[9]*

#### MAGNESIA PHOSPHORICA

*Magnesia phosphorica* (*Mag phos*) is an excellent remedy for the dental surgery. It is used for muscle pains and muscle spasms. The keynotes with *Mag phos* are better from warmth, worse from cold, and better from pressure. A patient who has an acute TMJ flare-up and wants warmth, and holds a hand over the masseter muscle to provide some relief, needs *Mag phos*. This type of muscle spasm may result from an injury (such as an injection or a blow to the jaw), or simply may result from having a patient hold their mouth open during a prolonged dental visit. *Mag phos* is also a remedy for some facial neuralgias, particularly those aggravated by washing the face with cold water.

### Bone trauma

There are two excellent remedies for treating bone trauma, the first being *Ruta graveolens*.

#### RUTA GRAVEOLENS

If *Hypericum* is the '*Arnica* of the nerves' then *Ruta* is the '*Arnica* of the bones'. For any kind of periosteal injuries or bone surgery, contusions, apicectomies or when you are lifting a flap in periodontal surgery, exposing an impacted wisdom tooth – if the resulting pain is in the bone, think about *Ruta* as the remedy rather than *Arnica*.

Another indication for *Ruta* would be when orthodontic patients get their braces tightened or their spacers put in. The soreness resulting from spreading of the teeth usually responds to *Arnica*, but when *Arnica* does not work, *Ruta* usually will.

*Ruta* is also a good remedy following endodontic therapy where the file is overextended through the periodontal ligament into the alveolar bone. *Ruta* is the first remedy to think of for dry sockets. Sometimes a dry socket may initially call for *Belladonna*, if it has that acute, throbbing type of pain. However, *Ruta* is usually the remedy that is going to help bring the healing to completion.

With any of these pain remedies a dose every half-hour to an hour is recommended initially. That may be every 15 minutes for some people, or 3 times a day for someone else, depending on their tolerance and the level of pain.

The question arises regarding how to manage an impacted wisdom tooth extraction. *Arnica*, *Ruta* and *Staphysagria* have been mentioned as being of possible help. Typically, you will have an incision wound, bony injury and soft-tissue trauma. So which do you use? You should give your patients a small packet of each of those three remedies to take with them and instruct them like this: 'If the pain is in the incision wound when the anaesthetic wears off, use the *Staphysagria*; if it feels like it is down in the bone, use the *Ruta*; and if it is neither of those or if you are not too sure, use the *Arnica*.'

### SYMPHYTUM OFFICINALE

When discussing remedies for injured bones, *Symphytum officinale* must be mentioned. *Symphytum* is used more with actual fractures of bone. It not only helps heal fractures, but is useful in helping implants integrate successfully with the surrounding bone.

## Bleeding

### PHOSPHORUS

When we think of the great bleeding remedies, *Phosphorus* is certainly the most impressive; not only because it works so well, but because the bleeding with a *phosphorous* patient is so very red. This is indicated for bright red (arterial) blood flow.

### CASE HISTORY

*I had a patient come through town about 15 years ago. She had stopped by the pharmacy down the road, which happens to be a homoeopathic pharmacy, while she was driving to Florida from New England. She had bitten her tongue the day before and she could not get it to stop bleeding. The pharmacist looked at her tongue and sent her over to me. While she was out in the waiting room I took a look. Her tongue had a good bite into it and was oozing bright red blood. I gave her one dose of Phosphorus 200X to hold her until I could get her into the dental chair. Within minutes the bleeding had ceased with just that one dose. She got back in her car and drove the thousand miles to Florida with no further problems.*

### LACHESIS

When it is the dark, oozing venous kind of blood, *Lachesis* is the remedy of choice. It is the potentized venom from the bushmaster snake.

### CINCHONA

*Cinchona* (or *China*) is the remedy with which Hahnemann did his first proving. It is used for people suffering from excessive loss of blood or other body fluids. It is not a remedy that is going to stop the bleeding, like *Arnica* and *Phosphorus*, but if someone has lost quite a lot of blood and they feel the resulting weakness and fatigue, *Cinchona* will help them recover much more easily. It is a wonderful remedy for that purpose.

## Head injuries

Two remedies that aid in the recovery from head injuries are *Arnica* and *Nat sulph*.

### ARNICA

*Arnica* is indicated more if the symptoms are physically based – muscle soreness, a stiff neck or shoulders, strains, bruising, that kind of thing.

### NATRUM SULPHURICUM

The *Nat sulph* symptoms are really more neurologically or mentally based, as a result of the trauma – such as the inability to think clearly, melancholia, suicidal tendencies, or attacks of mania.

## Puncture wounds

Another injury common in dental practice is the puncture wound. In dentistry, this can result from the actual injections of local anaesthetics.

### APIS MELLIFICA

*Apis mellifica* is the honeybee, and when the honeybee stings you, it is a miniature injection. The pains with *Apis* are usually stinging or burning pains. If you have been stung by a bee, you remember how that feels. You usually see some oedema around the area, and it feels better with cold applications. The oedema is a watery kind of swelling, where the tissues just engorge with fluid. You will see these symptoms occasionally in a patient after an injection.

### LEDUM

*Ledum* is a good remedy for puncture wounds where the wound is cold to the touch and feels better from cold applications.

### HYPERICUM

With *Hypericum* it is more the nerve kind of pain. *Hypericum* is a good remedy to think of for traumatic neuritis and neuralgias. Typically, this pain is worse from cold. *Hypericum* is effective in treating paraesthesia of the lip, secondary to a mandibular block injection or a difficult mandibular third molar extraction.

## General anaesthesia

### PHOSPHORUS

For general anaesthesia or intravenous sedation the remedy that usually works most effectively in getting the patient out of that 'brain fog' when they are recovering from the anaesthetic is *Phosphorus*. Certainly, if there is any bright red bleeding, it is likely to help that as well. But it will also get the 'cobwebs' out of the brain, and help recovery from that drug-induced twilight zone.

## Bruxism

### TUBERCULINUM

George Vithoulkas, the master homoeopath from Greece, says the most commonly indicated remedy for night-time bruxing in children is *Tuberculinum*. It is not mentioned in Kent's 'Repertory'[10] under that rubric, so you have to add it in.

### CINA

Another one is *Cina*, not to be confused with *China* or *Cinchona*. But *Cina* is a remedy for tooth-grinding when the grinding is a result of intestinal parasites. You may see this more in children coming from third-world countries. You will read in some of the dental textbooks about grinding of the teeth being a result of intestinal parasites. It is not clear what the connection is physiologically, but *Cina* is the remedy to deal with that kind of grinding.

### BELLADONNA

Another remedy for grinding is *Belladonna*. The *Belladonna* patient who is grinding their teeth is usually suffering from a high fever. The *Belladonna* fever is a picture of a bright red face, a high fever where you can actually feel the heat by holding your hand over the head of the patient. When people have that high fever accompanied by grinding of the teeth, *Belladonna* will help the body overcome the fever and the bruxing.

### PODOPHYLLUM

*Podophyllum* is useful on occasions for night-time grinding in adults. It is also useful in the occasional case of diarrhoea accompanying eruption of the teeth.

## Teething

When the child is fractious and whining, wishing to be carried or petted, consider *Chamomilla*. Where there is excessive salivation or halitosis, consider *Mercurius solubilis*.

## Dry socket

A dry socket occurs following tooth extraction and breakdown of the blood clot. The use of *Phosphorus* prophylactically, to prevent excessive bleeding following extraction, can increase the likelihood of dry socket due to the lack of bleeding and subsequent poor clot formation that it may encourage.

Local treatment includes dressings soaked in a mixture of *Propolis* ∅ and *Plantago* ∅ (1 part tincture to 20 parts water) and the use of *Myrrh* mouthwashes (several drops in a glass of warm water). If there is throbbing pain, try *Belladonna*. Otherwise, *Ruta* is the prime remedy in the treatment of a dry socket, to be used at the outset of most cases. Where other remedies fail, consider *Hekla lava*. To assist in the expulsion of sequestra, give *Silica* 6C three times daily.

## Oral ulcers

My first reaction to oral ulcers is to treat them nutritionally. The treatment we use in our office is L-lysine, which is an amino acid. When people are under stress, or if they eat a lot of chocolate or nuts or other foods that are very high in an amino acid called arginine, these ulcers tend to manifest themselves.

We can control (not cure) them by administering L-lysine, which is usually available in 500 mg tablets. Two tablets per meal are used until the sores are gone, and for another week thereafter 1 tablet per meal.

Some patients get these ulcers recurrently. As soon as one batch goes away, another starts up. Nutritionally, keeping them on 1 tablet of lysine a day prevents 80% of recurrences and reduces the severity quite effectively.

Using the nutritional approach is easier, but it is only a palliative, not a cure. To treat them homoeopathically is preferable, but more difficult. You have to treat recurring ulcer patients constitutionally, as outbreaks are acute manifestations of a more chronic disturbance. An acute prescription may help in that particular instance, but it will recur if the underlying chronic terrain is not addressed.

### NATRUM MURIATICUM

Certain constitutional types are more prone to outbreaks of oral ulceration. *Natrum muriaticum*, for example, will often discourage those kinds of people from taking too much salt in the diet.

You may see patients who get these lesions when they brush their teeth with baking soda. That is often a *Nat mur* patient. The sodium in the baking soda has the same effect as the salt in the sensitive individual, causing these ulcerations. *Nat mur* patients are people who frequently crave salt, and because they eat a lot of salt are subject to kidney problems, oedemas, dry mucous membranes and excessive thirst. You should not give *Nat mur* for oral ulcers unless the patient fits the constitutional picture for this remedy. But if they do, then you would not need to use lysine, because the recurrences would be diminished or eliminated naturally.

### ALTERNATIVES

In 1994 I had the honour of speaking to the British Homoeopathic Dental Association in London. It was there that I learned of three other remedies for oral ulcers which I had never tried before.

***Propolis tincture***: applied topically to the ulcerated tissues, this takes the pain away within seconds. It can also be used as a mouthwash if the ulcers are at the back of the tongue or throat, where you cannot otherwise reach.

*Feverfew 30C*: hourly, beginning when the individual first senses they are about to suffer a breakout.

*Sulphur*: for the difficult or unresponsive case.

## Herpes labialis

This is one of the most common orofacial lesions. Predisposing factors may be fatigue following the influenza, a common cold (hence the name 'cold sore') or ultraviolet radiation. *Propolis* cream applied several times daily will relieve the pain and reduce the duration. *Nat mur* is one of the most successful remedies, especially in hot people. Other remedies to consider are *Rhus toxicodendron* or *Herpes simplex nosode*. A nutritional approach and the use of vitamin supplements is also helpful.

For the treatment of a predisposition to cold sores, constitutional therapy is indicated. The key remedies to be considered are *Natrum muriaticum*, *Sepia* and *Sulphur*. Long-term Zinc (15–30 mg daily) and Vitamin C (1–2 g daily) supplementation may also be helpful.

## Abscesses

### HEPAR SULPHURIS

*Hepar sulphuris calcareum* (*Hepar sulph*) is one of the most common remedies used in dental practice. The typical indication for *Hepar sulph* dentally is an early periapical abscess, where there may still be a little cold sensitivity in the tooth (or the patient may be chilly in general).

*Over the past 15 years we have avoided, in our practice, endodontic therapy in hundreds of patients (approximately 75% of those we have attempted) by using Hepar sulph (or other remedies) combined with injections of protamine zinc insulin (PZI) every couple of days for a week or two.*

*Why we think the PZI works is that it may help get more oxygen and blood into the area to assist the body's natural healing defences, and it seems to amplify the benefits of the homoeopathic treatment for this type of situation. Two to three units of PZI are injected into the mucobuccal fold adjacent to the tooth being treated. I caution the patient that this is an experimental treatment and get informed consent, for legal reasons.*

With Hepar sulph, potency selection for endodontic lesions may be particularly critical. Low potencies (6C or below) tend to promote drainage, and higher potencies tend to have the opposite effect; that is, they promote the shrinking of the abscess. If you have this type of swelling to treat and you want it to shrink, use at least the 12C or higher. The use of 30C or 200C is common. Unless the symptoms clearly dictate another remedy, in the periapical abscess cases, Hepar sulph is the remedy of choice.

### BELLADONNA

*Belladonna* is another remedy for early endodontic abscesses, if the symptoms fit. Where there is intense throbbing pain which comes on rather rapidly and is aggravated by any kind of touch or pressure or movement, try *Belladonna*.

With homoeopathy you can avoid root canal therapy in the majority of cases. What happens is that the apical third of the canal calcifies as a result of the body's inflammatory response, and attempts to wall off the infection. In other words, the body really attempts to do its own root canal therapy. We know that people were getting abscesses long before endodontists were invented. The body has a way of dealing with these things, and homoeopathic treatment can help support that physiological response.

If patients see an endodontist their success rate with root canals is about 98%, and the success rate with homoeopathic treatment is only about 75%. This approach perhaps should not be used if the tooth needs to have a crown. Here, the difference in the success rate is substantial enough not to want a patient to spend the money for a crown and then have to cut a hole through the crown later to perform root canal treatment. Instead, this approach is indicated more in cases where the tooth is structurally sound.

The whole issue of the advisability of retaining dead teeth in the mouth has been the subject of controversy for many decades. Dr George Meinig's book, *The Root Canal Cover-Up*,[11] is one of the more recent to question this practice. It is highly recommended to the reader who would like to learn more about this subject.

## SILICA

A remedy useful in the management of chronic periapical abscesses is *Silica*. It helps support the drainage of these abscesses, typically when there is a sinus draining into the buccal sulcus. It also helps the body throw off foreign bodies.

## CASE HISTORY

*I had an emergency patient come in some years ago who had a salivary stone in the sublingual gland. I could see just a little bit of the coarse stone sticking through the floor of the mouth. The tissue surrounding it was red and inflamed and extremely painful. I knew that Silica was a great remedy for getting splinters out or for getting other foreign bodies to be expelled from the body. So I gave her a few doses of Silica in the 6th potency. I asked her to return the next day because I expected she would have to see the oral surgeon to have it excised. She came back the next day with the stone in her hand. It measured over 1 inch (25 mm) long and had come out very uneventfully.*

## MERCURIUS SOLUBILUS

Another remedy which is often indicated in endodontic abscesses is *Mercurius solubilus vivus* (homoeopathic mercury). The toothache from a mercurius type of abscess is very sensitive to hot and cold and to chewing. It is usually a throbbing toothache and is worse at night, typically after midnight.

### Bacterial endocarditis

For the prevention of bacterial endocarditis when appropriate antibiotics are unavailable, or where the patient refuses to take them, consider *Pyrogen* 30 twice daily, for 1 day prior to and 7 days after the procedure.

### Homoeopathic dental kit

To cover all those conditions mentioned above it is useful to have a dental kit of acute remedies available in the surgery. A list of remedies that could be included in such a kit are listed in *Table 1.1.*

**Table 1.1   Recommended dental kit of acute remedies**

| | | |
|---|---|---|
| Aconitum napellus | Feverfew | Plantago tincture |
| Apis mellifica | Gelsemium sempervirens | Propolis tincture |
| Arnica montana | Hepar sulphuris | Pulsatilla |
| Arsenicum album | Ignatia | Pyrogen |
| Belladonna | Lachesis | Rescue Remedy |
| Calcarea carbonica | Ledum | Rhus toxicodendron |
| Calcarea fluorica | Magnesia phosphoricum | Ruta graveolens |
| Calcarea phosphorica | Mercurius corrosivus | Sepia |
| Calendula tincture | Mercurius solubilus | Silica |
| Carbo vegetabilis | Natrum muriaticum | Staphysagria |
| Chamomilla | Nitric acid | Sulphur |
| Cinchona | Nux vomica | Veratrum album |
| Coffea cruda | Phosphorus | Vervain |

## Chairside homoeopathic first aid kit

In addition to the general dental kit listed above it is wise to have a smaller emergency kit within arm's reach. The following are five remedies to keep as a chairside homoeopathic first aid kit.

#### RESCUE REMEDY

For those who are unfamiliar with *Rescue Remedy*, it is a Bach Flower Remedy with five different flower essences in a little brandy. The essences are Impatiens, Cherry Plum, Clematis, Rock Rose and Star of Bethlehem. A couple of drops on the tongue can be very sedating for patients.

#### CHAMOMILLA

*Chamomilla* takes care of almost any acute, untoward reaction from local anaesthetics, whether it be an allergic reaction, or an idiosyncratic reaction. It is also wonderful in helping wear off the local anaesthesia after the dental treatment is completed.

ACONITE

Aconite is used for angina, palpitations, panic, shock, and terrible fright during the middle of a procedure.

VERATRUM ALBUM

This is a remedy for someone who gets faint, cold and clammy, or just loses consciousness.

CARBO VEGETABILIS

They call *Carbo veg*, in homoeopathy, the 'corpse reviver' and almost literally it is that powerful. It is indicated for the patient with congestive heart failure, who can not get enough oxygen and wants to be fanned. *Carbo veg* is potentized charcoal and charcoal is wood that has been burned where there is not enough oxygen. Likewise, the *Carbo veg* patient cannot get enough oxygen into their blood and they will often get ashen grey in colour. Give them a dose of *Carbo veg* while you are waiting for the rescue squad and providing life support.

The question is often raised: 'If somebody is unconscious, how are you going to administer the remedy?' The answer is that you either dissolve it in water (if you have time) and wet their lips with it, or take a couple of tablets and just put them under the lip where they can dissolve. Remedies are also available as drops.

In addition to the homoeopathic emergency kit, the usual traditional emergency kit containing epinephrine, oxygen, smelling salts, etc., should be available immediately.

## Chronic dental prescribing

Now that we have looked at some of the homoeopathic treatments for the common acute dental problems, I would like to discuss the role of homoeopathy in the treatment of chronic dental and orofacial complaints. To evaluate and treat someone for a chronic dental problem (e.g. periodontal disease, chronic TMJ disorders or bruxism) one must exercise the same deliberation as when treating any other chronic condition. A thorough history and examination must be done. One must include not only the dental manifestations, but all levels of the patient's symptoms (physical, mental, emotional and spiritual) in the evaluation. 'How can a dentist evaluate one's mental condition?', you ask. Remember, the repertories and materia medicas are written in plain English, not in 'medicalese'. One need not be skilled in abnormal psychology to see that a patient is frightened, cheerful or angry. One need only observe and listen.

Dentists have particular expertise in evaluating a person's orofacial signs and symptoms (which comprise a significant portion of Kent's 'Repertory'[10] and this is the focus of our therapy. However, we are sometimes criticized for 'practising medicine without a licence', because through appropriate 'dental' therapy the patient's 'medical' condition improves. The introductory paragraphs show the error of such thinking. Homoeopathic remedies (like allopathic drugs) are not organ specific – they affect the entire person. When given penicillin for an infected wisdom tooth, the infected toenail responds as well. Likewise, it may not be our intention to witness a cure of sciatica or dyspepsia, but with the correct dental treatment such things do happen. As with the infected toenail, this does not imply that we are practising medicine. It is the individual's vital force that directs the evolution of cure, not the doctor.

## Myofascial pain dysfunction syndrome

Conventionally, the dentist treats this syndrome by balancing the bite on a clear plastic splint worn over the teeth. The bite may also be built up with bridges or dentures. The syndrome occurs when there is a disharmony between the balance of the bite and an increased stress level in the individual expressed through the muscles and joints of the jaw and face.

An intractable condition occurs when such a person may not respond to conventional treatment. The stress levels will not allow the patient to relax. This results in aching of the muscles themselves or damage to the related jaw joints. Addressing the stress levels through constitutional prescribing will improve the patient's response to conventional treatment.

Any patient suffering acute stress or depression following a major life event such as bereavement, divorce or redundancy may benefit from a constitutional assessment.

When general stress levels are low, but there is local inflammation of the fascia around the muscles, the periosteum of the bone or the cartilage of the joints, then a remedy such as *Bryonia* may be applicable, especially when the pain is worse with motion and better with rest. One may use *Ruta graveolens* when it is more joint related and better with movement.

A large portion of my practice has dealt with the care and treatment of people suffering from disorders of the TMJ (or jaw point). Because disorders of this joint cause such profound and diverse sequelae in the patient's overall health, they serve as a good vehicle to illustrate the indivisibility of oral and systemic health. The various signs and symptoms of TMJ disorders fully permeate a quarter of the pages of Kent's 'Repertory'.[10] They include headaches, earaches, grinding and popping noises in the joint, vertigo, pains in the neck, shoulders and back, indigestion, poor balance, unstable posture and many others.

CASE HISTORY

*A 20-year-old woman presented with a constant headache which had been present for 22 months. The headache worsened on her wakening in the morning and had begun 1 month after she had left home to attend college. There she related 'heading' a soccer ball during a game, after which she stayed up all night to study for an exam. She had been with a headache ever since!*

*She had difficulty eating because of chewing pains in the right temple. She also suffered from chronic constipation, insomnia and fatigue. She appeared pale, unsmiling and listless and she had not had her menses for seven months. Prior treatments had been of little help and included therapy by a neurologist, gynaecologist, psychiatrist, an allergist, internist, nutritionists, acupuncturist, chiropractors, dentists, a cranial osteo-path and a neurolinguistic programmer. She had a history of other head injuries. She was given* Arnica *in high potency.*

*Two months later she reported no significant change in her health. She was fitted with an orthopaedic appliance and put on an exercise programme to help alleviate her jaw muscle tension. Within days she began to sleep better, but over the next few months the headaches were still constant, although diminished. She still had no menses, was thirst-less and still constipated. She was given* Natrum muriaticum *1M.*

*Natrum muriaticum has headaches, worse in the morning, as part of the remedy picture. Also included are a great variety of menstrual complaints, constipation, diffi-culty sleeping and emaciation. It is the chronic of* Ignatia, *often, as Boericke says, 'having psychic causes of disease' (i.e. leaving home).*[12]

*When she returned a month later her appearance had dramatically improved. Her face was more animated, her dress more colourful and her voice more vibrant. She was sleeping well and her head and jaw pains had markedly lessened. Her cranial osteopath reported the first profound improvement in her cranial mechanism since he had begun treating her. Several days after the remedy was given she had her first menses in almost a year.*

## Periodontal disease

The patient with unexplained advanced periodontal disease, who does not respond to conventional treatment, may be suffering from mild immune deficiency. A detailed history is taken to discover which remedy applies to their phenotype. The aim of this remedy is to give their whole body a 'kick-start' to revitalize their immune response.

In addition to the conventional therapies of oral hygiene instruction, scaling, root planing and periodontal surgery, different constitutional reme-dies may be used for different patients with the same advanced periodontal disease. A few of these include:

- the weak, pale blonde with acne and catarrh – *Hepar Sulph;*
- the intransigent brunette – *Thuja;*
- the pale, retiring, hard-working waif – *Silica;*
- the pale, blue-eyed, shy blonde – *Pulsatilla;*
- the tall, fiery red-head – *Phosphorus;*
- the impulsive, irritable worrier – *Argent nit.*

The use of nutrient supplements and general dietary advice is another area that the homoeopathic dentist would be considering to support these patients.

*Mercurius* is one of the more important remedies in periodontal disease. When one reads the provings of Mercury in the materia medica, you will recognize the classical signs and symptoms of periodontal disease: 'Gums spongy, recede and bleed easily ... teeth loose, feel tender and elongated ... tongue yellow, flabby, teeth indented ... fetid odour from the mouth ... salivations greatly increased, bloody and viscid ...', etc. It is interesting to note here the similarity between the signs and symptoms of Mercury prov-ings (toxicity) and those of periodontal disease. It raises the question, if Mercury exposure can provoke all the signs and symptoms of periodontal disease, what impact is the Mercury escaping from amalgam fillings having on the incidence and progression of periodontal disease?

**The three constitutional types**

In taking a case history of a chronic dental patient, one can gain a great deal of information as to the patient's constitutional type by examining his or her oral and cranial structures. Here we must define 'constitutional' in its narrowest sense, based on the theory of constitutional typing by Nebel and Vannier and referred to by Professor Eizayaga as the 'genotypical' constitutional type. The constitution is the least changeable aspect of the person's totality; it is based largely on the structure and composition of one's tissues and skeletal framework and therefore is immutable and established long before birth.

Our skeletal and dental structures are composed of three calcium salts (or Calcareas) – the carbonate, phosphate and fluoride. Each of these salts impregnates our teeth and bones and thereby imparts to us distinctly different anatomical characteristics, different metabolic types as well as different disease propensities. Everyone belongs to one of these constitutional types: *Calcarea carbonica*, *Calcarea phosphorica* or *Calcarea fluorica*, depending upon which salt predominates in our make-up. To each of these constitutional types belongs a group of remedies or 'phenotypical' constitutional types. While it is common to see individuals who exhibit combinations of these three constitutional types (especially frequent is the phosphorica-fluorica mix type), one type will always predominate.

Nowhere are the anatomical differences among the *Calcareas* more dramatically illustrated than the dental apparatus. The dentist has a unique vantage for assessing a patient's constitutional type and can therefore can gain much insight into that individual's therapeutic needs. The information presented here is not in the homoeopathic materia medicas. Research by Tetau,[13] Royal[14,15] and Iliovici[16] has helped to consolidate the constitutional pictures described below.[17] (Although the masculine pronoun is used, these constitutional types are both male and female.)

CALCAREA CARBONICA

The *carbonica* type has broad shoulders, a broad forehead and large jaws. The teeth are very white and well aligned, but are slow to erupt with difficult teething. The fontanelles of his very large skull are slow to close and his head perspires easily. His tongue is dry, he does not like to talk and his teeth cannot endure any coldness – even cold air!

The *carbonica* resembles the oyster shell from which the remedy is made. He is resistant to change – 'a victim of inertia'. While slow to begin a project, once started he will continually plod ahead until the job is completed. While not terribly imaginative, he is logical and is good with mathematics (many mathematicians and accountants are carbonicas).

His long bones and spine are curved and his bones, joints and muscles are as rigid and inflexible as his opinions. He tends to develop hypertension, hypothyroidism, obesity and auto-intoxication due to his failure to remove toxins adequately from his body. The child exhibits delayed puberty and is frequently troubled by bed-wetting. He is chubby, his complexion has a chalky tint and he is prone to digestive complaints. The major remedies that are related to the *Calcarea carbonica* type aid in the elimination of

Table 1.2  Anatomical and orofacial keynotes (including TMJ)

|  | Calcarea carbonica | Calcarea phosphorica | Calcarea fluorica |
|---|---|---|---|
| Skeleton | Resistant | Fragile | Irregular, exostoses |
| Hand | Strong and thick | Long and narrow | Small, soft and pliable |
| Perspiration | Localized to head and neck | All over | Very little (skin dry) |
| Athletic type | Good endurance (fullback) | Lacks endurance but has brilliant bursts of energy (quarterback) | Not well coordinated (team mascot) |
| Orofacial | Large, broad head, open fontanelles | Elongated head, open fontanelles | Asymmetrical head |
| Jaws and arches | Large elliptical | Narrow elongated elliptical | V-shaped, irregular |
| Vault (palate) | Low | Gothic | Narrow and very deep |
| Tooth eruption | Delayed and difficult dentition | Early but painful teething | Teeth erupt out of normal sequence |
| Teeth | White with broad stocky crowns. Upper incisors flat and square. Sensitive to cold | Yellow and long. Upper incisors rectangular with curved facial surfaces | Grey-white teeth. Gum-boils, sensitive to pressure and eating, looseness of teeth |
| Occlusion (bite) | Teeth well aligned | Often malposition in anterior teeth | Irregularly set into arches with saggital forward or backward malposition |
| Temporomandibular Joint | Strong and tight | Fine and slack | Hyper-stretch |

the body's toxins: *Sulphur, Hepar sulph, Graphites, Silicea, Carbo veg* and *Lycopodium*.

CALCAREA PHOSPHORICA

The *phosphorica* type is mentally precocious and develops early. He is tall, with long arms and legs and his back is stooped. The skull is long (front to back) and narrow, as are the jaws. The forehead is elevated and the nose is strong. The teeth are oval and have a yellow cast to them. The palate is narrow with a gothic (high) vault.

He is very imaginative and artistic and does not tolerate manual labour or any regularity in his lifestyle. Because he cannot stay with any task for very long, he seldom masters anything – despite being a perfectionist at heart. He has long eyelashes, his hair is fine and his skin delicate. When he perspires, he does so all over. He tends toward hyperthyroidism, palpitations and tuberculosis.

The major remedies that are related to the phosphorica constitutional type are *Natrum mur, Ferrum, Kali carb, Iodum, Arsenicum album, Phosphorus* and *Stannum*.

### CALCAREA FLUORICA

The *fluorica* type is the picture of instability, both mentally and physically. The bones are deformed and the muscles and ligaments are very lax, producing an S-shaped posture. The arms hyperextend at the elbows. The dental arch and the alignment of the teeth are irregular. The upper jaw protrudes, the feet are abnormally small and the hair is hard and brittle.

He dislikes exercise and has little physical endurance. He cannot concentrate on anything for long periods of time and seldom perspires at all. His temperament is unstable, he has little control over his reactions, and he will say whatever is on his mind. All of his symptoms are worse at night, but he feels better when in the mountains. He tends toward arteriosclerosis, arthritis and hypertension.

The major remedies that relate to the *fluorica* constitutional type are: *Mercurius, Aurum metallicum, Argenticum nitricum, Kali bichromicum, Platina, Nitricum acidum, Baryta carbonica* and *Syphyilinum*.

*Table 1.2* summarizes the characteristics of the three *calcarea* groups.

## Conclusion

This chapter presents a brief overview of the role of homoeopathy in dentistry as it relates to acute and chronic prescribing and to the three basic constitutional types. Correct homoeopathic prescribing for dental maladies will frequently provoke salutary systemic effects. This should not threaten or alarm us. It is simply a reflection of the natural law of cure and illustrates the fact that the dental apparatus is an indivisible component of the integrated whole person. It cannot be otherwise; and for this we should all be grateful – doctor and patient alike.

## References

1 Stafne W B. *Roentgenographic Diagnosis*, 3rd edn. p 82. Philadelphia: W B Saunders, 1969.
2 Kerr D A, Ash M, Millard H D. *Oral Diagnosis*, 3rd edn. St Louis: C V Mosby Company, 1970.
3 Clark N G, Carey S E. Etiology of chronic periodontal disease: an alternative perspective, *J Am Dent Assoc*, May, 1985; **110:** 689-691.
4 Voll R. *Interrelations of Odontons and Tonsils to Organs, Field Disturbances and Tissue System*. D311 Velzen, West Germany: M.L. Publishers, 1976.
5 Adler E. *Neural Focal Dentistry – Illness Caused by Interference Fields in the Trigeminal*. Houston: Multidiscipline Research Foundation, 1984.
6 Char J. *Electric Acupuncture for Dentistry*. Pearl City, Hawaii: Nutri-Kinetic Dynamics Inc, 1980.
7 Ullman D. *Homoeopathy and Medicine for the 21st Century*. Berkeley, California: North Atlantic Books, 1988.
8 Lessell C B. *The Infinitesimal Dose: The Scientific Roots of Homoeopathy*. Saffron Walden: C W Daniel, 1994.
9 Kent J T. *Lectures on Homoeopathic Materia Medica*. New Dehli: Jain Publishing, 1984.
10 Kent J T. *Repertory of the Homoeopathic Materia Medica*. 6th edn. Box 2524 Karol Bagh, New Delhi, 110005: Indian Books and Periodicals Syndicate, 1987.
11 Meinig G E. *The Root Canal Cover-Up*. Ojai, CA: Bion Publishing, 1993.

12 Boericke W. *Materia Medica with Repertory*, 9th edn. New Delhi: Jain Publishing Ltd, 1987.
13 Tetau M. Homoeopathy, holistic medicine: terraine, constitutions, temperament. *J Ultra Molecular Med* 1983; **1(3)**: 22-25.
14 Royal F F. Understanding homoeopathic constitutions, Part I. *J Ultra Molecular Med* 1983. **1(2)**: 14-20.
15 Royal F F. Understanding homoeopathic constitutions, Part II. *J Ultra Molecular Med* 1983. **1(3)**: 16-20.
16 Iliovici E. A new concept in essential homoeopathic mineral compositions. *J Ultra Molecular Med* 1983. **1(3)**: 12-15.
17 Fischer R D. Homoeopathy with a dental accent. *Homoeopathy Today* 1984. **4(9)**: 4.

# Bibliography

*Anthroposophic Dental Practice*, Association of Anthroposophic Dentists, Stuttgart, Germany, 1985 (avail: Raphael Pharmacy, Fair Oaks, CA).

Banerjee P. *Dentistry (in Homoeopathy)*, 3rd edn. Howrah-1, West Bengal: Shiva & Co Medical Publisher, 1992.

Carter J G, Carter W. *Herbal Dentistry*. Chapel Hill, NC: University of N. Carolina, 1990.

Central Council for Research in Homoeopathy, *Review and Revision of Kent's Repertory in Relation to Other Works - Chapter 'Teeth' - Additions from Boericke's Repertory*. New Delhi: Central Council for Research in Homoeopathy, 1988.

de Prevost J. *A Homoeopathic Approach to Dentistry and Oral Biology*. Sainte-Foy-les-Lyon, France: Bioron, 1986.

Foster J. (translator) *Toothache and Its Cure with Homeopathy*. New Delhi: B. Jain Publishers Pvt Ltd, 1990.

Lessell C B. *A Textbook of Dental Homoeopathy*. Saffron Walden: C W Daniel, 1995.

Lessell C B. *The Dental Prescriber*. London: The British Homoeopathic Dental Association, 1983.

Palsule S. G. *Dentistry and Homeopathy*. New Delhi: B. Jain Publishers Pvt Ltd, 1991.

Singh H. *Dental Caries and Pyorrhoea with Their Homeopathic Treatment*. New Delhi: Indian Books and Periodicals Syndicate, 1982.

Sivaraman, *Your Tooth Troubles Cured with Homoeopathic Medicines*, Jain Publishing Ltd, 1993.

Stockton F W. *A New Approach to Oral and Dental Disease*. Watsonville, CA: Freedom Press.

Vakil P. *Tongue That Does Not Lie*. Bombay: Vakil Homoeopathic Prakashans, 1988.

Verspoor R, Morin R. *Homoeopathy: A Modern Approach to the Practice of Dentistry and the Restoration of Health*, Ottawa: North American Research Centre for Homoeopathy in Dentistry, 1993.

# Associations

British Homoeopathic Dental Association
2b Franklin Road
Watford, Herts. WD1 1QD
UK
Tel: 01923 233336
Fax: 01923 233336

Faculty of Homoeopathy
2 Powis Place
Great Ormond Street
London WC1N 3HT
UK
Tel: 0171 837 9469
Fax: 0171 278 7900

British Homoeopathic Association
27a Devonshire Street
London W1N 1RJ
UK.
Tel: 0171 935 2163
Fax: 0171 935 2163

National Center for Homoeopathy
801 North Fairfax Street, Suite 306
Alexandria, VA 22314
USA
Tel: 001 703 548 7790
Fax: 001 703 548 7792

The UK Homoeopathic Medical Association
6 Livingstone Road
Gravesend, Kent DA12 5DZ
UK
Tel: 01474 560336
Fax: 01474 560336

International Foundation for Homoeopathy
PO Box 7
Seattle, Washington 98020-0007
USA
Tel: 001 206 776 4147
Fax: 001 206 776 1499

Ainsworth's Homoeopathic Pharmacy
36 New Cavendish Street
London W1M 7LH.
UK
Tel: 0171 935 5330
Fax: 0171 486 4313

American Institute of Homoeopathy
23200 Edmonds Way, Suite A
Edmonds
Washington 98026
USA
Tel: 001 206 542 5595 (No fax)

## Courses

Courses are held in London and Glasgow.

The Foundation Course, Parts 1–5. A 5-day introductory course for doctors, veterinary surgeons, dentists, pharmacists, nurses, midwives, podiatrists and paramedical disciplines.

The Intermediate Course, Parts 6–10. A 5-day course for doctors, dentists and veterinary surgeons. Three days are multidisciplinary and, for dentists, 2 days specialize in dental homoeopathy. This course is in preparation for the Diploma in Dental Homoeopathy Examination held once a year by the Faculty.

Details can be obtained from:

The Academic Department
Royal London Homoeopathic Hospital
Great Ormond Street
London WC1N 3HT
UK
Tel: 0171 837 8833
Fax: 0171 837 7229

The Academic Department
Glasgow Homoeopathic Hospital
1000 Great Western Road
Glasgow G12 0NR
UK
Tel: 0141 337 1824
Fax: 0141 337 2276

# Nutrition

**Ron Ehrlich**

## Introduction

A useful observation as to what constitutes a balanced diet for humans is the empirical evidence of centuries of application. Dr Weston Price,[1] Dr Sir Robert McCarrison, Arnold DeVries and others have travelled extensively, studying the living and eating habits of native tribes around the world known for their excellent health and freedom from disease. They have all concluded that the eating habits of these people are largely responsible for their superior health. Dr Melvin Page has coined the phrase 'Ancestral Diet' defining this as 'the foods that your ancestors ate over the past 1000–2000 years'.

Consider how long it has taken to reach this point in our evolution; how our internal biochemical systems have adapted in order to maintain homeostasis. Then consider the enormous changes that have occurred over the last 100 years. We have strayed so far from our ancestral diet it is remarkable that more of us do not suffer ill health. Degenerative diseases plague Western culture, even though it enjoys such a high standard of living. Perhaps we all suffer from degenerative diseases to some extent and perhaps the lesson that we have yet to learn is just how good, good health feels.

Nutrition is a new science and there is still discussion among 'experts' about which foods we should eat and in which combinations for maximum benefit. There are many theories about diet and many of these are frequently revised.

Dentists are well placed to provide nutritional advice. They should not only be involved in a biomechanical perspective when looking at optimal function of the masticatory system. The mouth is the first part of the digestive process and dentists are perfectly placed to advise what should be consumed and monitor it through their regular contact with their patients. The potential to improve the individual's health and that of society as a whole is enormous.

The subject of nutrition is central to any discussion on individual and community health. The number of books written on the subject, together with the various diets and supplements that are offered, are bewildering to both practitioners and patients alike.

Very little independent research is done on nutrition; most is in some way funded by the food, chemical, drug and vitamin industries. This adds to the confusion. It is now possible to find scientific research to support almost any position.

Nutrition is a complex issue that must deal with many factors. These include:

- Soil quality – soil degradation and leaching of nutrients is endemic in the modern agricultural business.
- Use of fertilizers and pesticides – there is widespread and ever increasing use to increase yield.
- Agricultural diversity – there is a lack of diversity in much of modern agriculture.
- Food distribution, storage and processing – from fields to markets to processing and packaging, transportation, distribution and storage. The road from growing to eating is a long and tortuous one with food often unrecognizable on the plate and stripped of the potential to optimally nourish.
- Air and water quality – heavy metal pollution, greenhouse gases, rising salt levels and the availability of quality water are all affecting our health.
- Dietary habits – cultural and social pressures constantly challenge our decisions to eat what we know is good for us.
- Commercialism – a political and social issue so large and diverse that it affects every aspect of food production and consumption.
- Consumerism – in this fast world, image and convenience often dictate which food or drink we should have, bypassing any health priority.
- The widespread use of antibiotics – while saving lives, antibiotics have been abused in both food production and medicine. They not only raise the expectation of the 'quick fix', but also affect our natural digestive bacterial population that are so central to maintaining a proper balance.
- The use of other prescription and recreational drugs – alcohol, tobacco and the long-term use of prescription and non-prescription drugs compromise our health and mask the real barriers to achieving optimal health.

Evidence indicates that the bulk of illness in modern society is the result of a multitude of food and dietary modifications interacting metabolically with stress and lack of exercise.[2]

It has become apparent that many of the now prevalent degenerative diseases are not caused by simple bacterial or viral infection, but rather by a combination of variables which produce a significant breakdown in the efficiency of the reparative and defensive mechanisms of the human body. If this breakdown continues for a number of years, it causes significant deterioration of function which allows disease to develop.[3]

The main function of our digestive system is to absorb adequate nutrients to support the body's systems in maintaining a state of equilibrium or homeostasis. Examples of homeostasis include the body's self-regulation of hormone and acid-base levels, the composition of bodily fluids, cell growth and body temperature.

Nutrition is defined by the British Society of Nutritional Medicine as: 'The sum of the processes involved in taking in nutrients, assimilating and utilising them.'

The main nutrients known to be essential for humans are:

- amino acids ( protein);
- carbohydrates;
- essential fatty acids;
- vitamins;
- minerals;
- water, fibre and oxygen.

Four factors influence nutritional status:

- the quality and variety of the food we eat;
- the quantity of the food we eat;
- the efficiency of digestion, absorption and utilization;
- biochemical individuality.

# The basics of good nutrition

What we eat directly affects the normal functioning of our bodies. However, what we eat is often dictated to us by industrial and commercial expediency, with little regard to our long-term health and quality of life.

Our diets tend to be high in fat, salt, protein and simple carbohydrates and consequently the incidence of degenerative diseases such as high blood pressure, heart disease, arthritis, diabetes and chronic pain are very high in western society.

The advisability of the use of vitamin and mineral supplements also causes much confusion and it is important to realize that recommended dietary allowance (RDA) more often refers to the prevention of dietary deficiency disease rather than the achievement of optimal health. This explains the sometimes tenfold difference between the RDA and a therapeutic dose.

## Fats

### TRIGYLCERIDES AND FATTY ACIDS

Triglycerides comprise about 95% of the lipids in food and in our bodies. They are the storage form of fat when we eat calories in excess of our energy needs. Burning up the stored fat allows us to live without food for periods of time.

All triglycerides have a similar structure, being composed of three fatty acids attached to a glycerol molecule. Glycerol is a short-chain carbohydrate molecule that is soluble in water, and when triglycerides are metabolized the glycerol can be converted to glucose. Fatty acids differ in their length and degree of saturation. They are commonly composed of a chain of 16–18 carbon molecules with attached hydrogen molecules. The number of hydrogen molecules determines the saturation of the fat. When each carbon has its maximum number of hydrogen molecules attached, the fat is said to be saturated; that is, filled to capacity with hydrogen.

Each time we sit down to a meal we are involved, either passively or actively, in psychosocial and political decision-making. Within that context the decision most commonly made results in the current US diet deriving 42% of its total calories from fat, most commonly saturated fats.[4]

All fats are composed of varying amounts of saturated, monounsaturated and polyunsaturated 'fatty acids'. No naturally occurring fat has just one or two of these types of fatty acids: all are made up of a combination of the three types.

A major concern of the modern processed diet is the high level of saturated and hydrogenated polyunsaturated fats. Hydrogenation is a chemical process that attempts to overcome the stability and spoilage of unsaturated fats. There has been much speculation about the stability of polyunsaturated oils which react readily with other elements, particularly oxygen, to form damaging 'free radicals' and thus may render cells more susceptible to cancer.

Many diseases are linked to a high-fat diet, including arteriosclerosis, hypertension and certain cancers, most notably colon, rectal and breast cancers.[5] Excessive fat has also been implicated in aggravating type II late onset diabetes because it appears to hamper the ability of insulin to transport glucose and it promotes obesity, which is a risk factor for diabetes.

### SATURATED FATTY ACIDS

Foods high in saturated fatty acids are mostly animal products such as butter, whole milk, cheese, egg yolks, beef, pork and lamb. Coconut and palm oil are also very high in saturated fatty acids and are commonly used in many processed foods.

There are no known benefits from eating saturated fats, but there are clearly established health problems associated with eating them.

### UNSATURATED FATTY ACIDS

There are two varieties, monounsaturated and polyunsaturated. If two adjoining carbon atoms are attached by a double bond, there is room for a pair of hydrogen atoms, and the fatty acid is said to be monounsaturated. When more than one area of the carbon chain can accept additional hydrogen atoms, the fat is said to be polyunsaturated.

#### Monounsaturated fatty acids

Foods high in monounsaturated fatty acids include olive, peanut, canola (rapeseed), and avocado oils.

#### Polyunsaturated fatty acids

Foods high in polyunsaturated fatty acids include vegetable oils such as corn, safflower, sunflower, soybean, cottonseed and sesame oils. Much has been made of the term 'polyunsaturated' and the fact that it is 'cholesterol free', but there are three points worth mentioning.

First, a high intake of polyunsaturated fats has direct links to obesity which carries a high health risk. Too much fat (particularly polyunsaturated fats) may increase gallstone formation.[6]

Second, the chemical stability of polyunsaturated oils is questionable, with the possibility of forming free radicals rendering cells and tissues more susceptible to ageing and cancer.

Third, there are no population groups which have a good health record while consuming a diet high in polyunsaturated vegetable oils.

#### ESSENTIAL FATTY ACIDS

This term refers to linoleic acid (omega-6 family) and linolenic acid (omega-3 family) which are called 'essential' because they are vital for health, yet cannot be made by the body. They assure growth in children, maintaining the integrity of cell membranes and producing prostaglandins.[2] Linoleic acid and linolenic acid are found in generous quantities in whole grains, beans, peas and vegetables. Omega-3 fatty acids are found in fish, particularly mackerel, trout, halibut and herring. However, fish may be contaminated with a variety of potentially toxic or carcinogenic pollutants.[7]

#### CHOLESTEROL

Cholesterol is a vital part of all animal cell membranes and is a precursor to many hormones and to vitamin D. It is a waxy substance that cannot dissolve in water; neither can it dissolve in blood, which is mostly water. Cholesterol has to get to the cells, where it may be needed, so a fleet of special water-soluble carriers called lipoproteins – molecules of fat linked with protein – are used to transport cholesterol and other water-insoluble products like triglycerides throughout the blood stream. Low-density lipoproteins (LDL-cholesterol) will end up in the arterial walls if the serum level is elevated. Some of it will finish up in the cells of the arterial walls where it triggers the growth of atherosclerotic plaque. Should the LDL-cholesterol level remain high, this plaque will block blood flow and trigger a heart attack or stroke.

By contrast, high-density lipoproteins (HDL) appear to act as scavengers that seek out excessive cholesterol and take it away from the tissues and arteries back to the liver where it can be used for bile acids. HDL levels are determined primarily by genetic factors and the only safe way to increase them is to stop smoking, maintain a healthy weight and to exercise. Saturated fat in all its forms is the single most potent dietary influence on total and LDL cholesterol levels.

The ratio of LDL to HDL gives a greater indication of the risk of coronary disease than the total cholesterol. A ratio of 1:1 would suggest a low risk, whereas a ratio of 5:1 would represent a high risk.

There are two different ways that serum cholesterol levels are elevated. First, through the intake of dietary cholesterol. Various reports suggest this accounts for only 5–10% of the body's total cholesterol. Second, through the internal manufacture of cholesterol by the body in response to the intake of saturated fats.

It is important to realize that only a small proportion of our total cholesterol comes through dietary intake, whereas the vast majority is manufactured by the body. Unfortunately this point has been overlooked or trivialized by claims of many fatty foods being 'cholesterol free' while still being high in fat and destined for the body conversion to cholesterol.

The fact is that we do not need to eat any cholesterol because our cells can make all that we need. Studies have shown that with a marked reduction of the blood cholesterol, coronary heart disease can be slowed, stopped or even made to regress.[8] A programme consisting of a low-fat, low-sodium, low-cholesterol, high-fibre eating plan; moderate exercise, lifestyle management and cessation of smoking, not only can halt but can actually reverse atherosclerotic effects of coronary heart disease.[9]

The cholesterol-free status of monounsaturated fatty acids has been overstated. Recent studies have shown that while substituting these oils for saturated fats may well reduce LDL 'bad' cholesterol, it will not reduce HDL 'good' cholesterol which still contributes to a high-fat diet, leading to obesity and all its problems.[10]

Recommended foods that decrease cholesterol include: fruit, vegetables, beans, peas, oats, barley and sweet potatoes. Note that even though polyunsaturated fats may lower cholesterol levels, high-fat diets are linked with obesity and a greater risk of certain cancers.

## Carbohydrates

Our bodies are best suited to the plant and fruit-based diets of early humans. Our long digestive tracts, the structure of our teeth, the enzyme content of our saliva, the fact that we have hands and not claws, our metabolic make-up, our kidneys – all unchanged for thousands of years – demonstrate this.

Carbohydrates are made up of sugar molecules and are considered the best food for the human body. It is here that the confusion begins, as carbohydrates are often associated with high-calorie diets and weight gain. In order to understand the importance of carbohydrates we must understand the difference between simple, complex, refined and unrefined carbohydrates.

### SIMPLE CARBOHYDRATES

Simple carbohydrates are those found in table sugar and fruit. They are either monosaccharides or disaccharides (which means they consist of either one or two sugar molecules).

### COMPLEX CARBOHYDRATES

Complex carbohydrates, which include starches found in vegetables, legumes and grains, are composed of hundreds to thousands of sugar (glucose) molecules chained together.

### UNREFINED CARBOHYDRATES

Unrefined carbohydrates include whole food, such as whole unprocessed fruits, vegetables, grains and legumes. All unrefined carbohydrates, both simple and complex, provide us with energy, fibre and very important nutrients. Unrefined carbohydrates will give longer lasting fuel as well as protein, minerals, trace elements, essential fatty acids and generous amounts of vitamins. With their high-fibre content, unrefined carbohydrates will satisfy the appetite as well as providing the benefits to digestion by absorbing water and making stools larger and softer. They enhance movement of digested food through the digestive tract more quickly, allowing food less time to stagnate and deposit chemical impurities and cancer-promoting compounds on the intestinal wall. Fibre has also been shown to reduce serum levels of LDL-cholesterol and total cholesterol.[11] Fibre also helps to stabilize insulin and blood sugar levels.[12]

REFINED CARBOHYDRATES

Refined carbohydrates are most commonly sugars, which go under a variety of names including glucose, fructose, sucrose, maltose, corn syrup, maple syrup and molasses. They have negligible nutritional value and provide what is often called empty calories, because of the ease with which they make energy available to the body. They tend to trigger higher insulin levels and increase serum triglycerides. The body deals with excessive amounts of rapidly absorbed sugars by converting them into fat in the liver, resulting in increased serum triglycerides and total cholesterol. They also decrease the HDL (good scavenging) cholesterol and so increase the risk of cardiovascular disease.

We will discuss the effects of refined carbohydrates on dental health later in this chapter.


## Proteins and amino acids

Protein is a crucial component of every living cell and of many of the chemicals needed for life. Our blood vessels, bones, skin, nerves, muscles, cartilage, lymph and hair all contain protein, as do our enzymes, antibodies and some of our hormones. We could not digest food without proteins and many other vital bodily functions depend on it. These functions include blood clotting, delivery of oxygen and nutrients to our body's cells as well as defence against deadly bacteria.

The building blocks of protein are amino acids. The human body can manufacture all but eight of the 20 amino acids. These eight *essential* amino acids are isoleucine, leucine, lysine, methionine, phenylalanine, threonine, tryptophan and valine. There are two *semi-essential* amino acids called arginine and histidine. The remaining 10 are alanine, aspartic acid, cysteine, cystine, glutamic acid, glycine, hydroxyproline, proline, serine and tyrosine.

Ideally protein should come from non-fat dairy products, lean meat, lean poultry, fish, grains, vegetables and legumes. As recently as 1900 most of the western world derived nearly 70% of its protein from plant, not animal sources. This is not the case today, with meats, poultry, fish, eggs and cheese being consumed in large amounts.

While protein is an essential part of our diet we do not need too much of it. Recommended daily allowance is 44 g for the average woman and 56 g (2 oz) for the average man, while some authorities feel 1g/kg body weight is a reasonable guide. The problem with protein is twofold. First, our dietary intake of protein is unnecessarily high; second, our major source of that protein tends to be high in fats, often in combination with sugar and/or salt.

Amino acids are made up of a weakly acid molecule in conjunction with a strongly basic amino molecule group. When the acid portions are removed from the amino acids, the basic amines become messengers in the nervous system. When the amine portions are removed, the remaining 'acid' can be used for fuel, detoxification or in many other processes throughout the body. The amino acids play innumerable roles in human health and disease.

Amino acids have a complex interaction with the four families of essential nutrients: the inorganic (minerals and trace elements), the fats (linolenic and linoleic acids), the vitamins and the proteins. As all amino acids are absorbed and metabolized in a similar fashion, there is great competition particularly with other amino acids in the same group. The 20 amino acids are listed below in their various groups:

- **aromatic amino acids** – phenylalanine, tyrosine, tryptophan;
- **sulphur amino acids** – cysteine, methionine, cystine;
- **urea cycle amino acids** – arginine;
- **glutamate amino acids** – glutamic acid, proline, aspartic acid, hydroxy-proline;
- **threonine amino acids** – threonine, glycine, serine, alanine;
- **branched chain amino acids** – leucine, isoleucine and valine;
- **amino acids with important metabolites** – lysine, histidine.

Braverman and Pfeiffer[13] propose that two principles of medicine should be:

- to imitate the body's natural healing mechanism;
- if a drug can do the job of medical healing, a nutrient can do the same job.

*Table 2.1* below outlines drug–nutrient interactions.

**Table 2.1 Drug–nutrient interactions**

| Drug | Nutrient with similar action | Nutrient with antagonistic action |
| --- | --- | --- |
| Antidepressant | Tyrosine, tryptophan, methionine | Glycine, histidine |
| Anti-heart failure | Tyrosine, taurine, carnithine | Niacin, tryptophan |
| Anticoagulants, e.g. aspirin | Vitamin E, max EPA | — |
| Anticonvulsants | Glycine, GABA, taurine, alanine, tryptophan | Aspartic acid |
| Anabolic steroids | Leucine, isoleucine, valine, alanine | Glutamic acid, Aspartic acid |
| Antivirals | Lysine, zinc | Arginine |
| Antitoxins | Glycine, cysteine | — |

## Vitamins

Vitamins are substances needed in extremely small amounts to bring about certain chemical changes or reactions in our bodies. Generally speaking, vitamins cannot be made by the body but must be obtained from food. There are two broad categories of vitamin:

- **fat soluble** – A (retinol and beta-carotene), D, E, F (essential fatty acids), K.
- **water soluble** – C, B complex ($B_1$, $B_2$, $B_3$, $B_5$, $B_6$, $B_{12}$, biotin, choline, inositol).

Much debate surrounds these components of our diet which are so essential in maintaining optimal health. Confusion arises when one compares RDAs with therapeutic doses, the levels required to achieve optimal health. The difference between these two levels can often be tenfold and the distinction between them needs to be clearly understood.

The question as to whether supplements are necessary or not, highlights some of the issues challenging our understanding of nutrition and health. In an ideal world supplements would be unnecessary where soil quality is good, where food is eaten fresh and whole, where there is no environmental or chemical pollution, where a well-balanced diet is eaten and where our lives have minimal stress. Clearly this is not the case for the vast majority of the population; in fact the opposite would be true.

It is also important, in determining the need for supplementation, that we have a clearer idea of what we understand by optimal health, not merely defining it as a lack of apparent disease.

## Minerals

Minerals are also an essential part of our diet, helping regulate fluid balance, growth and development, muscle and nerve function as well as many other biochemical processes. The most practical way of thinking of them is to divide them into the following.

### MACRO-MINERALS

Macro-minerals include calcium, phosphorus, magnesium, sodium, potassium and chlorine. These are bulk elements that are required in quantities of several hundred milligrams per day. They are involved in structural functions (bones and cells) as well as metabolic ones. Calcium metabolism is discussed later in this chapter.

### TRACE ELEMENTS

Trace elements include iron, zinc, copper, manganese, iodine, chromium, selenium, molybdenum, cobalt and sulphur. These are required in very small quantities (a few milligrams per day or less). They have subtle but vitally important effects on the metabolism.

Research trace elements include vanadium, nickel, tin, lithium and a few other very rare elements which, although not shown to be essential, do seem to have an influence on the working of the body.[14]

### SALT (SODIUM)

Salt is the most widely used seasoning. In many cultures, particularly western ones, salt is overused and may contribute to such problems as hypertension, fluid retention, electrolyte imbalance and difficult pregnancies. Most salt is sodium chloride, though potassium chloride is also used, as are other salt substitutes.

A natural, ancestral diet contains less than 1 g/day of sodium and elevated blood pressure was rare. Nowadays, 6–12 g/day of salt are consumed by people eating processed and snack foods or as salt added in cooking and food preparation. Salt is 40% sodium and 60% chloride, therefore 5 g of salt (about 1 teaspoon) contains approximately 2 g of sodium.

## Water

Water is an essential part of life. Our bodies comprise at least 60% water. However, even if our water supply is free of deadly bacteria, such as cholera and typhoid, it may still contain many potentially harmful contaminants such as lead, mercury, aluminium, cadmium, nitrates, chlorine, fluoride, pesticides, industrial chemicals, bacteria, viruses and parasites.

We lose water daily through skin, urine, bowels and lungs. Drinking water requirement varies according to the water content of the food we eat, the climate we live in and the amount of physical activity we do. Water is best consumed at several intervals throughout the day – one or two glasses on waking and also about an hour before each meal. Water should not be drunk with or just after meals as it can dilute digestive juices and reduce food digestion and nutrient assimilation.[15] Water is also best consumed at room temperature.

### FLUORIDATION

Fluoridation is another controversy. The first criticism of adding fluoride to the water supply, which has been occurring throughout the Western world over the last 50 years, is that it is impossible accurately to determine dosage, as people consume varying amounts of water. The obvious adverse effect of fluoride is irregular, mottled enamel, but there are also reports of hip fracture, cancer, joint and ligament calcification. Again, studies and clinical observation vary as to the degree of this problem.

The positive effect of fluoridation is the reduction of tooth decay. In my practice in Sydney, Australia, which has had fluoridation since 1968, the reduction of tooth decay is certainly impressive. However, research continues to challenge this connection and confuse both patient and open-minded practitioner alike, which shows that non-fluoridated areas have shown similar reduction in rates of decay. This may be from the daily topical application of fluoride during brushing, which is thought to have a greater preventive effect against decay than the ingestion of fluoride in the water.

My own feeling is that the fluoride issue is typical of the way western medicine approaches a problem. Rather than dealing with the cause, in this case very obviously being diet (high frequency of sugar intake), it looks for an additive to mask the problem. Not only will excellent dietary practices reduce our rate of decay and periodontal disease, but they will also have profound effects on our general health. This is the most basic premise of holistic dental practice philosophy.

## Nutrition and general health

In determining how we should use nutrition, one must consider whether we are eating to maintain optimal health or whether we are trying to overcome a particular health problem.

### Therapeutic *v.* prophylactic nutrition

One should consider the difference between therapeutic and prophylactic nutrition. Therapeutic nutrition is applied to individuals who have specific, biomedically related problems. Prophylactic nutrition is for day-to-day living and designed to provide nutrients within a range of variability to meet the individual's need to maintain optimal health.

### Maintaining optimal health

This may be summarized by following these basic principles. The food we eat should be:

- whole fresh food, e.g. whole grains, brown rice;
- complex carbohydrates, i.e. fruits, vegetables;
- low fat, **not** just cholesterol free;
- free of artificial colouring, preservatives, salt or sugar;
- preferably eaten raw.

Such a diet enhances our immune system, thereby reducing our susceptibility to disease and helping us to achieve optimal health.

*Table 2.2* outlines a list of common foods to avoid *and* include when following a diet for optimal health, while *Tables 2.3–2.5* outline natural sources of the major vitamins and minerals that can be derived from a natural balanced diet.

IMMUNITY-ENHANCING NUTRIENTS AND THEIR BEST SOURCES (EXCLUDING RED MEAT AND DAIRY PRODUCTS) (*see Table 2.3 on page 37*)

### Treating a health problem

When treating a health problem we must first eliminate those foods to which the patient is intolerant and then provide, if necessary, therapeutic doses of any supplements that are lacking.

**Table 2.2 A diet for optimal health**

| Foods to avoid | Foods to include |
| --- | --- |
| White bread | Stoneground, wholemeal bread |
| Shop-bought cakes and biscuits | Home-made, low-fat, sugar-free cakes |
| Marmalade and jam | Sugar-free jams and fruit spreads |
| Sugar | Malt extract, honey, black molasses |
| | (*if taken frequently may cause decay*) |
| Salt | Herbs, mild spices, seeds |
| Malt vinegar | Cider or wine vinegar |
| Salted butter, margarine, lard, cooking oils | Ghee, cold-pressed sunflower oil, olive oil |
| White rice, refined cereals and packaged breakfast foods | Whole grains and cereals, including brown rice, barley, rye, maize, oats, buckwheat |
| Red meat | White deep-sea fish. |
| | Beans, peas, lentils; nuts and seeds; tofu |
| Battery poultry and eggs | Free-range chicken or turkey; up to 4 free-range eggs per week |
| Cow's milk and cheese | Soy milk, yoghurt (Sheep or goat) |
| Frozen or tinned vegetables and fruit; commercial desserts and ice cream | Fresh, organic vegetables and fruit, sundried fruit; home-made, sugar-free desserts |
| Coffee, tea, cocoa, Coca-Cola, soft drinks | Herb and fruit teas, bancha tea; fresh vegetable and fruit teas |
| Tap water | Filtered tap water, spring water, preferably not refrigerated |

The best way to assess those foods to which the patient is intolerant is to carry out the basic diet experiment.[16] The main value of the diet experiment is that it helps you learn what is best for your body. The theoretical thinking behind the diet experiment is that we are all unique biochemically and what is good for most people may not be good for you personally. We will discuss the basic diet experiment in detail later in the chapter.

## Nutrition and oral health

Optimal nutrition for oral health is no different from nutrition for achieving optimal general health. Oral health must include consideration of the following structures:

- teeth;
- gingivae;
- supporting structures of the periodontal ligament;
- underlying alveolar bone ( the bone supporting the teeth);
- arch form of the upper and lower jaws;
- relationship of upper and lower jaws (occlusion);
- temporomandibular joints;
- posture of the head and neck;
- muscles of mastication, including the muscles of the head and neck;
- general body health to support the above.

One must consider whether we are eating to maintain optimal health or whether we are trying to overcome a particular health problem.

**Table 2.3 Immunity-enhancing nutrients and their best sources (excluding red meats and dairy products)**

| Vitamin A (retinol) | Vitamin B₂ (riboflavin) | Vitamin B₅ (pantothenic acid) | Vitamin B₆ (pyridoxine) |
|---|---|---|---|
| VEGETABLES | VEGETABLES | VEGETABLES | VEGETABLES |
| Sweet potatoes | Spinach | Broccoli | Soy beans |
| Carrots | Broccoli | Cabbage | Lentils |
| Spinach | Asparagus | Cauliflower | Potatoes |
| Pumpkin | Mushrooms | Mushrooms | Tomatoes |
| Turnip greens | Watercress | Peas | Corn |
| Broccoli | Soy beans | Legumes | Spinach |
| Asparagus | | | |
| Lettuce (iceberg) | FRUIT | FRUIT | FRUIT |
| Tomatoes | Avocados | Elderberries | Cantaloupe |
| Chicory | Peaches | | Bananas |
| Watercress | Prunes | NUTS AND SEEDS | Avocados |
| | | Peanuts | |
| FRUIT | NUTS AND SEEDS | Sesame seeds | NUTS |
| Watermelon | Almonds | | Walnuts |
| Cantaloupe | Cashew nuts | CEREALS | |
| Apricots | | Wheatgerm and bran | CEREALS |
| Peaches | CEREALS | Most wholegrains | Brown rice |
| Nectarines | Wheatgerm | | Wheatgerm and bran |
| Prunes | Barley | FISH | |
| | | Salmon | FISH |
| OTHER | FISH | | Salmon |
| Eggs | Most | OTHER | Tuna |
| | | Brewer's yeast | |
| | OTHER | Molasses | OTHER |
| | Brewer's yeast | Royal jelly | Brewer's yeast |
| | Molasses | Eggs | Molasses |
| | Eggs | Chicken | Eggs |

| | | *RDA (av. adult)* | |
|---|---|---|---|
| 4000–5000 iu | 1.2–1.7 mg | 10 mg | 1.75–2.2 mg |

The basics of sound nutrition incorporate a diet low in fat, high in unrefined complex carbohydrates, a small amount of animal protein, and avoiding refined carbohydrates, salt, and preservatives. We have now strayed so far from our ancestral diet that degenerative diseases plague our society and the majority of people endure less than optimal health.

Calcium metabolism is an excellent example of nutrition's significant and far reaching effect on our general and oral health. So many health problems relate to the deposition of calcium where we do not want it (e.g. atherosclerosis, arthritic joints, kidney stones and gallstones) and the loss of calcium from where we do want it (e.g. teeth, bones, nerve and muscle function).

Conditions which relate to suboptimal calcium metabolism are widespread in the community. It is important to realize that calcium metabolism is inexorably linked to phosphate intake. Calcium binds to phosphate in the ratio of 1 calcium to 2 phosphates. The body will always try to maintain a balance in serum calcium, the calcium measurable in the blood. On a low calcium diet the serum calcium will return to within normal limits, at the

**Table 2.4 Immunity-enhancing nutrients and their best sources (excluding red meats and dairy products)**

| Folic acid | Vitamin C | Vitamin E | Calcium | Copper |
|---|---|---|---|---|
| VEGETABLES | VEGETABLES | VEGETABLES | VEGETABLES | VEGETABLES |
| Asparagus | Green peppers | Soy beans | Turnip greens | Beans |
| Spinach | Broccoli | Cold-pressed | Spinach | Peas |
| Broccoli | Spinach | oils | Broccoli | Lentils |
| Pumpkin | Cabbage | Broccoli | Beans | |
| Carrots | Watercress | Brussels | Carrots | FRUIT |
| Beans | Tomatoes | sprouts | Garlic | Prunes |
| Lentils | Cauliflower | Spinach | Kelp | Raisins |
| | Potatoes | | Watercress | Cherries |
| FRUIT | Parsley | NUTS AND SEEDS | | |
| Melon | Turnip greens | Pecans | FRUIT | CEREALS |
| Apricots | | Walnuts | Prunes | Wholewheat |
| Avocados | FRUITS | Most seeds | Oranges | |
| | Oranges | | Rhubarb | OTHER |
| NUTS | Strawberries | CEREALS | Dates | Seafood |
| Walnuts | Lemons | Wheatgerm | Figs | Molasses |
| Hazelnuts | Grapefruit | Bran | | |
| Almonds | Rose hips | Wholegrains | NUTS AND SEEDS | |
| | Kumquats | | Peanuts | |
| CEREALS | Kiwi fruit | OTHER | Walnuts | |
| Wholewheat | Pineapple | Eggs | Amonds | |
| Rye flour | Guava | | | |
| | | | FISH | |
| OTHER | | | Sardines | |
| Egg yolks | | | Salmon | |
| | | RDA (av. adult) | | |
| 400 μm | 60 mg | 30 iu | 800–1200 mg | 2–5 mg |

expense of bone density, 3–4 weeks after calcium intake levels have been reduced.

Phosphates levels are high in the typical Western diet. Red meat contains phosphates in the ratio of 38 phosphates to 1 calcium. Carbonated soft drinks are extremely high in phosphates as they are used to buffer the acidity. Consumption of carbonated soft drinks has increased dramatically in the last 30 years. High protein intake, particularly derived from animal source, is high in phosphates. Phosphates bind to calcium. Bones and teeth are forms of calcium phosphate. If, however, serum phosphate levels are high, calcium is leached from bone to bind to the phosphates.

When considering the impact that our diet has on our health it is important to realize that oral health is no exception and reflects the impact that poor nutrition has on our health in general. In the 1930s Dr Weston Price[1] travelled the world living with and studying isolated peoples and their diets, and conducting testing to determine the deterioration that occurred (physical, social and psychological) after they adopted a modern Western diet. Many millions of dollars are now funding medical research to find the cause of several diseases that Price so conclusively demonstrated were the result of nutritional deficiency.[17]

Price studied and compared isolated and modernized communities in Switzerland, Wales, Alaska, South Pacific islands in Melanesia and

**Table 2.5 Immunity-enhancing nutrients and their best sources (excluding red meats and dairy products)**

| Iron | Magnesium | Potassium | Selenium | Zinc |
|------|-----------|-----------|----------|------|
| VEGETABLES | VEGETABLES | VEGETABLES | VEGETABLES | VEGETABLES |
| Spinach | Spinach | Cabbage | Onions | Corn |
| Beans | Broccoli | Kale | Garlic | Beetroot |
| Asparagus | Corn | Spinach | Tomatoes | Peas |
| Peas | Kelp | Mint | Broccoli | Carrots |
| Brussels sprouts | Legumes | Potatoes | Asparagus | Spinach |
| Turnip | | Watercress | Legumes | Mushrooms |
| | FRUIT | Legumes | | Soy beans |
| FRUIT | Figs | | CEREALS | |
| Prunes | Lemons | FRUIT | Wheatgerm | FRUIT |
| Apricots | Grapefruit | Oranges | Whole grains | Cherries |
| Peaches | Apples | Lemons | | Pears |
| Raisins | | Grapefruit | NUTS | |
| Strawberries | NUTS AND SEEDS | Bananas | Most | NUTS AND SEEDS |
| | Almonds | Raisins | | Most nuts |
| NUTS AND SEEDS | Sesame seeds | | FISH | Pumpkin seeds |
| Most nuts | Sunflower seeds | SEEDS | Tuna | |
| Sesame seeds | | Sunflower | | CEREALS |
| Sunflower seeds | CEREAL GRAINS | | OTHER | Wheatgerm |
| | Wholegrains | CEREALS | Brewer's yeast | |
| CEREALS | | Wholegrains | | FISH |
| Whole grains | OTHER | | | Herring |
| | Honey | FISH | | |
| OTHER | | Haddock | | OTHER |
| Molasses | | | | Eggs |
| Egg yolks | | | | |
| | | *RDA (av. adult)* | | |
| 10–18 mg | 300–400 mg | 900 mg | 50–200 mcg | 15 mg |

Polynesia, African tribes, Australian Aborigines and New Zealand Maoris. What he found was that on their natural ancestral diet the incidence of dental decay affected a very small proportion of the population, whereas a modern diet high in refined carbohydrate increased the incidence of tooth decay dramatically. *Table 2.6* summarizes his findings.

Not only did Price link tooth decay to poor nutrition, but also showed that in a natural ancestral diet jaws are well formed without significant

**Table 2.6 Summary of Price's findings on the effect on tooth decay, comparing isolated and modernized communities**

| Community | Community isolated (decay rate per 100 teeth examined) | Community modernized (decay rate per 100 teeth examined) |
|-----------|--------------------------------------------------------|----------------------------------------------------------|
| Switzerland | 2.3 | 20.2 |
| New Caledonia | 0.14 | 26 |
| Fiji | 0.42 | 30.1 |
| Polynesia | 0.6 | 33.4 |
| African tribes | 0–0.6 | 12.1 |
| N.Z. Maori | 0.76 | 95 |

crowding, yet within one generation of eating a modernized diet dental crowding and malocclusion were widespread.

## Tooth decay

The relationship between diet and decay is well established, with the frequency of consumption of refined carbohydrate (sugar) being a critical factor. Most attention has focused on the intake of sucrose and its relationship to the incidence of decay. Diet may affect caries either by:[18]

- altering the structure and resistance of the tooth during its development and immediately after eruption;
- changing the environment and influencing bacterial attack through sugar intake.

More recently Leonora, Tieche and Steinman[19-21] have suggested that rather than being just a local effect of sugar on tooth structure, there is also a systemic effect. There is a fluid flow through the tooth. In people resistant to dental decay it is from the pulp through the dentine and then through the enamel.

The direction of flow is under the control of the hypothalamus. This produces a parotid hormone-releasing factor which causes the parotid gland to produce a parotid hormone, which controls the direction of fluid flow in the tooth. With adequate parotid hormone, the fluid flows from inside the tooth out. With the ingestion of sugar, the flow is reversed possibly resulting in decay.

However, any refined carbohydrate which results in the formation of acid will contribute to the decay process. Other factors also contributing to the decay process include:

- Frequency of sugar – a diet with small or large amounts of sugar taken at frequent intervals leads to a high decay rate. A small or large amount of sugar taken only once or twice a day does not cause decay. It is the frequency not the quantity that is the problem. Low-frequency intake gives time for the decay area to recalcify to the extent that no clinical decay will appear.
- Saliva – increased flow rate increases the pH (reducing acidity) through the production of bicarbonate ions, which will neutralize the acid being formed from sugar. Increased saliva by volume will also dilute any acid formed.

## Periodontal disease

Periodontal disease refers to inflammation of the gingivae (gums) which if allowed to persist may result in the inflammation of the periodontal ligament and the possible destruction of the underlying bone. It has been suggested that the factors associated with periodontal disease can broadly be divided into two categories.

**1. Extrinsic (local) factors**
- bacterial – plaque, calculus, enzymes, decomposition products and food debris;
- mechanical – calculus, food impaction, poor restorations and malocclusion;
- parafunction – bruxism, clenching.

**2. Intrinsic (systemic) factors**
- endocrine dysfunctions – puberty, pregnancy, postmenopausal;
- metabolic – diabetes, leukaemia;
- psychosomatic or emotional disorders;
- drugs and metallic poisons;
- nutritional deficiency.

Diet, beyond refined carbohydrate intake, is rarely mentioned in the major dental textbooks as a factor in gum disease apart from scant references to bleeding gums in scurvy caused by lack of vitamin C. This is disappointing but hardly surprising, given the low priority that diet seems to play in the treatment of other disease states within the practice of medicine.

Price[1] demonstrated a clear relationship between diet and the increase in dental decay and the incidence of crowding and malocclusion. Classically, gum disease is thought of as an imbalance in host–parasite relationship. There are of course two sides to this equation, with the majority of treatment centring on the removal of plaque (the parasite) to treat gum problems. Needless to say it would be dental heresy to suggest that plaque control is not the most appropriate course of treatment. There is however the host to consider.

Diet is the most logical way of optimizing our health, improving the quality of our tissues on a cellular level, their ability to regenerate and repair, and generally bolstering our immune system. The diet that provides for excellent health of the gums is no different from that which provides for our optimal general health. Broadly speaking, our diet should follow five basic principles:

- whole food, unrefined complex carbohydrates;
- variety;
- low in fat;
- fresh food, free of artificial colouring, flavouring, preservatives, sugar and salt;
- preferably eaten raw.

Cheraskin[22] reported on studies of children who were undergoing orthodontic treatment, comparing gingival inflammation, tooth mobility, labial debris (plaque) and the changes in gingival inflammation. One group were given supplements of multivitamin/trace minerals, whereas the other were given a placebo.

The evidence suggests a greater tendency to either hyper- or hypoglycaemia in those subjects responding unfavourably to orthodontic treatment. This study gives a strong indication of the importance of the individual's biochemistry on periodontal health and specifically on the use of supplements to bolster the individual's response.

Of particular importance for periodontal health is vitamin C because of its necessity in maintaining collagen as an essential part of cell walls. The role of coenzyme Q10 (ubiquinone) in periodontal treatment has received some attention recently. Coenzyme Q10 is a substance involved in electron transport in mitochondria, the power packs of cells. It has some chemical characteristics similar to vitamin E and is found in a wide range of food. Some research has been done recently on this subject suggesting that topical application of coenzyme Q10 improves adult periodontitis not only as a sole treatment but also in combination with plaque control.[23] A more traditional view questions the experimental technique and conclusions of some of the research.[24]

### MOUTH ULCERS, INCLUDING COLD SORES

These are both a common problem for many people. They run their course in 7–10 days but can be painful and interfere with normal eating. They are often related to being run-down and tired and may indicate deficiencies in the B group vitamins and zinc. Apart from rinsing with warm salt water to prevent infection, tincture of propolis or calendula are excellent ways of promoting healing. Supplementation with B group, particularly B6 together with zinc and magnesium, may also be useful in preventing the occurrence.

### HALITOSIS (BAD BREATH)

Apart from the obvious of poor oral hygiene, bad breath can be caused by any deficiency of the digestive apparatus. Decayed teeth, diseased gums or tonsils and retained food particles that become putrefied are all involved in causing bad breath.

Bad breath may also originate from further down the digestive tract through poor digestion. Failure of the detoxifying system to perform its function allows build-up of body toxins, impairing the absorption and assimilation of food. The liver–kidney–adrenal axis normally meshes the digestive function and the excretion mechanism to maintain health and well-being.

Digestion may also contribute through putrefaction of proteins in the stomach and small intestine. This takes place when there is a deficiency of hydrochloric acid and other digestive secretions, especially those of the pancreas. The intestinal flora become abnormal with a build-up of putrefactive bacteria. Improper bowel activity becomes a part of the picture and the total depressive effect on the body produces a stress condition and the adrenals become involved. Stress and fatigue add to the burden.

Apart from the basic oral hygiene techniques of brushing and flossing, the therapeutic diet mentioned above with the use of digestive enzymes and 'friendly' bacterial supplementation is effective in restoring optimum digestion and the elimination of bad breath.

# Nutritional support for mercury toxicity

The mercury issue will be discussed elsewhere in this book; however, I will make some points concerning mercury toxicity and nutrition. Fifty per cent of the amalgam filling material is mercury. Mercury is toxic. It escapes from the filling and is stored in the organs, primarily the kidney, liver and brain.[25,26] Mercury from the fillings has been shown by the World Health Organisation to be the greatest contributor of mercury load to the body. Essentially there are two separate issues:

- Should amalgam be used at all? My view is that it should not be and were it discovered today and subjected to the same testing as new materials, it would certainly be banned.
- Should all amalgam fillings be removed? My view is that removal should be undertaken cautiously and that more research needs to be conducted examining the health benefits of amalgam removal done under strict protocol.

For those embarking on amalgam removal and undergoing a subsequent detoxification programme, the suggested nutritional protocols are outlined below.

## Pretreatment

Supplementation should be commenced 2 weeks prior to the first appointment and continued for 2–3 months after the last appointment. The purpose of supplementation is as follows:

- to condition the cell membrane so that toxic metals may be more easily removed from the internal parts of the cell as well as from the cell surface;
- to break the binding of proteins from protein–mercury compounds;
- to release mercury from these compounds;
- to provide a transportation link (usually to sulphur) to carry mercury off for excretion.

The greatest exposure to mercury occurs when the material is placed and when it is removed. Removal needs to be done carefully under rubber dam and supported by certain nutritional supplements.[27] It is not suggested that all the supplements mentioned below are taken by all patients. There are a range of supplements that could be considered, depending on the patient's health when amalgam removal is undertaken.

- Glutathione: one 50 mg tablet or capsule 3 times/day on an empty stomach.
- Methionine: one 200–500 mg tablet 3 times/day. Methionine is the precursor for the manufacture of cysteine in the body and the extra supplementation of this critical sulphur-amino acid should increase available cysteine.
- N-Acetyl-L-cysteine (NAC): if further cysteine is required.
- Methylsulphonylmethane (MSM): 500–2000 mg/day. This provides a bioavailable source of sulphur which is essential in the formation of disulphide bonds and the proper conformation of body proteins.

- Vitamin $B_6$: one 50 mg tablet/day is needed in the metabolic process that converts methionine to cysteine and then into glutathionine. B6 is also useful in reducing swelling and pain after routine dental procedures.
- Vitamin C: one 500 mg tablet with each meal. Vitamin C can affect the response to dental anaesthesia, dissipating its effect more quickly than desired. Therefore, do not take vitamin C 12 h before dental treatment, should this be a problem.
- Zinc: one 15–30 mg tablet after evening meal. Zinc is absolutely critical, given its role in DNA synthesis, for the growth and development of rapidly dividing mucosal epithelial cells and as a co-factor for many of the liver detoxification enzymes. Deficiencies of zinc will induce dysfunction of gut, liver and immune system.
- Magnesium: one tablet per day, providing 100 mg of elemental magnesium after the evening meal or at bed time.
- Vitamin $B_1$: one 50 mg tablet with each meal. $B_1$ is also effective in reducing pain associated with routine dental operative procedures.
- Vitamin E: 100–400 iu/day. However, should blood pressure rise, then start on a lower dose of 50-100 iu/day for the first 30 days. Products of oxidation such as lipid peroxides, which can be caused by mercury, are converted to harmless products by vitamin E and glutathione peroxides (a selenium-containing enzyme derived from glutathione and selenium).
- Selenium: one 50 $\mu$g (not mg) or liquid equivalent of sodium selenite. Vitamin C precipitates selenium, making it unavailable for absorption, so the two supplements should be taken 2 h apart. Also, care should be taken that the selenium in tablet form is often yeast based, which may be a problem to those patients with a history of candida (thrush).
- Acidophilus capsules, powder or liquid: to help restore gut flora affected by the widespread use of antibiotics in medicine and agriculture.
- B complex: 15–25 mg of each of the various B vitamins. Some research suggests that $B_{12}$ can help methylate mercury, which is a more toxic form of mercury; therefore, eliminate excessive $B_{12}$ during the replacement procedure.
- Garlic products contain high levels of sulphur and selenium.

**Post-treatment**

After the removal of the amalgam fillings, the protocol below can be followed:

- increase glutathione to 2 capsules 3 times per day for a total of 6 capsules or 300 mg;
- increase vitamin C to 1000 mg with each meal and 1000 mg after the evening meal;
- add pantothenic acid ($B_5$) one 100 mg tablet with breakfast and the evening meal;
- add an amino acid complex.

Post-treatment supplementation should continue for at least 2–3 months after the last amalgam filling has been removed.

**Detoxification**

The body's ability to rid itself of a toxic substance such as mercury is dependent upon:

- mobilization of that substance which is bound in the cells of tissues and organs;
- proper liver function;
- excretion through the kidneys via the urine and elimination in the stool via the bile.

In the liver, detoxification includes two general phases:

- phase I – cytochrome enzymes (including P450) act to oxidize, reduce or hydrolyse. Some of these can then be excreted;
- phase II – conjugation enzymes convert toxins to water-soluble form for excretion or elimination.

Each of these phases may be reduced or enhanced in activity, depending upon the availability of critical rate-limiting nutrients. The importance of optimal gut barrier function is critical to our health in general, but absolutely vital when embarking on a detoxification programme, particularly on patients whose health is compromised. The importance of an optimal diet already mentioned in this chapter cannot be overstated. There is a strong interrelationship between diet and stress affecting gut barrier failure and the liver's ability to effectively detoxify the body.[28] The two major causes of gut barrier failure are diet and stress.

DIET

A poor diet can cause irritation and/or inflammation of the mucosal epithelial cells, leading to increased permeability, decreased enzyme and lysosomal activity, atrophy and malabsorption. This results in:

- malnutrition deficiencies;
- food and chemical allergy/intolerance – reactions to foods and chemicals can induce mucosal dysfunction and permeability via the release of inflammatory mediators such as histamine and prostaglandins (the importance of which will be emphasized below in the section on chronic pain) or by direct toxic effects such as alcohol, antibiotics, nitrites and non-steroidal anti-inflammatory drugs (NSAIDs).
- microbial imbalance – loss of mucosal defences such as gastric acidity, beneficial intestinal flora and IgA antibody levels creates an environment favourable for pathogenic organisms.

STRESS

Emotional, physical, chemical, allergic, infectious or environmental stress results in increased production of stress hormones (catecholamines) which reduce blood flow, resulting in a decrease in oxygenated blood being supplied to intestinal organs (stomach, pancreas, liver and gut mucosa). This causes impaired function, with symptoms such as bloating, reflux, indigestion, cramping, wind, colic or diarrhoea.

The impaired gut barrier function results in large reactive food antigens and microbial toxins entering the liver where they are filtered, detoxified and eliminated. If, however, the phagocytic Kupffer cells and detoxifying enzyme systems of the liver are already overloaded, detoxification will be impaired.

Mercury has a special affinity for enzymes with a suphhydryl protein component. These enzymes are involved in intracellular respiration, free radical scavenging and detoxification. Mercury disrupts communication systems by uncoupling the energetic and information processing machinery. Neurological, immunological, hormone and enzyme-dependent essential cell functions are affected. The use of supplements listed above, particularly the sulphur-containing amino acids, attempts to support the detoxification process by binding to the mercury.

### Chelating agents

Several drugs have been used to aid in the removal of mercury from the body, bearing in mind that mercury is essentially bound up in the cells of organs.

- DMPS (2,3-dimercapto-1-propanesulphonic acid) – marketed as Dimaval.
- DMSA (2,3-dimercaptosuccinic acid) – marketed as Kelmer, it has a major difference from DMPS in that DMSA accelerates mercury elimination from the brain, but DMPS had no effect. Mercury levels in the blood, liver and kidneys decreased more effectively with DMSA.[29]

Two excellent studies have been done which demonstrate the problem of mercury as being one of retention toxicity and the effectiveness of DMPS as a chelating agent.[30] Table 2.7, from Godfrey and Campbell,[31] demonstrates the difference between mercury levels before and after using DMPS.

To remove mercury from the tissues the chelator must bind it more strongly than any substance already present in the body. In addition, the

**Table 2.7 Mercury levels pre- and post-DMPS use**

| Subjects | Time | Urine Hg ($\mu g/l$) |
|---|---|---|
| Patients with history, symptoms and signs suggestive of Hg toxicity $n = 80$ | pre-DMPS<br>post-DMPS | 5.4<br>314.3 |
| Dental personnel $n = 10$ | pre-DMPS<br>post-DMPS | 10.2<br>330.0 |
| Treated patients $n = 10$ | pre-DMPS<br>post-DMPS | 1.4<br>10.7 |
| Control group $n = 10$ | pre-DMPS<br>post-DMPS | 1.8<br>39.1 |

chelator must not remove metals from the enzymes which require them to function properly.

Daunderer[32] treated 800 amalgam/mercury toxic patients. Some still exhibited symptoms years after amalgam removal. There was a subsequent amelioration of their symptomatology after the use of DMPS.

*Note*: Both DMSA and DMPS will also remove zinc. Zinc deficiency should be corrected prior to starting any chelation treatments and zinc should be supplemented during treatment. Alternative chelation agents which may be used are:

- D-Penicillamine – not widely used, but is effective as intermittent therapy. Side-effects include autoimmune symptoms and essential nutritional mineral depletion.[33]
- EDTA – often used for heavy metal detoxification and effective in particular for lead. EDTA binds only weakly to mercury and will remove it from the cell surface and blood, but not from inside the cell.

Homoeopathic remedies are also frequently used to support the body following amalgam removal and are dealt with in Chapter 1.

## Nutritional support for temporomandibular dysfunction (TMD)

A significant proportion of the population suffer from chronic pain of the head and neck. Pain is defined 'as an unpleasant emotional experience caused by the activation of the nociceptive system'.[34] Ninety percent of head and neck pain is musculoskeletal in origin and it is postulated that this occurs as a result of soft tissue lesions.[35] Soft-tissue lesions are defined as a tear or damage to the muscle, fascia, tendon, ligament or periosteal attachment of the muscle to the bone. The nociceptive system is activated by either mechanical stresses (compression, torsion or twisting) or chemical mediators (lactic acid, bradykinins, prostaglandins and histamine). These chemical mediators are produced by the body.

The jaw, while rarely the primary cause of head and neck pain, is frequently a predisposing factor preventing the soft-tissue lesions, which commonly occur in the posterior cervical region, from healing through the synergistic activity of the muscles of mastication and the trapezius and sternocleidomastoid muscles.[36,37] As dentists we must not only be aware of how to support the jaw with occlusal therapy, but must also be aware of the bigger picture and advise our patients how to optimize their health and healing capabilities.

The problem of food allergies is important in the treatment of chronic pain of musculoskeletal origin. Pain is contingent on activation of the nociceptive system. One of the most potent chemical mediators of the nociceptive system is histamine. Food allergies or intolerances can result in the production of histamine and this may be a basic point that is frequently overlooked. Allergies or intolerances will also affect the absorption and utilization of essential nutrients. The basic diet experiment involves food that is simple and wholesome. Incorporating a simple elimination diet under the guidance of a nutritionist may identify an underlying problem which is often overlooked.

There are two programmes to consider in the nutritional support of TMD:

- to facilitate healing of the soft-tissue lesions;
- to minimize exposure to histamine by reducing the exposure to food sensitivities.

## Healing through nutrition

In order to facilitate healing, optimal nutrition is an excellent starting point, particularly in conjunction with structural work on soft tissues. The priority at this stage is to improve the function of the gut barrier. The two factors that influence gut barrier are diet and stress. Improvement in function of the gut barrier can be initiated by the basic diet experiment. The use of the basic diet experiment is an excellent therapeutic approach to provide the foundation for optimal health and healing.[16]

### A BASIC DIET EXPERIMENT

The purpose of the 10-day basic diet experiment is to test whether the patient's body is 'intolerant' to any of the 11 food groups: foods which may cause the patient to be constantly tired, tense or irritable, to have headaches or to be overweight because some of these foods may cause the patient's body to retain water.

### Foods to eat

The patient can eat any of the foods listed below unless they are restricted by their doctor or they are allergic to them:

- fresh fruits and vegetables (except corn – used as an additive) which may be eaten raw, boiled, steamed or baked; fresh frozen foods are allowed;
- poultry and seafood – boiled, baked or grilled with lemon and/or butter;
- salads with lemon juice or vinegar with olive oil dressing;
- purified water, herbal teas and unsweetened fruit juices – apple, carrot, grapefruit, orange, pineapple, tomato, or V8;
- sea salt, spices, rice, beans and nuts (except soy beans and peanuts – these are used in a lot of processed foods).

### Foods to avoid

For at least 10 days the patient should not eat from any of the following 11 food groups, so they can use 'food sensitivity testing instructions' (see below) to determine their personal biocompatability to each of these food groups:

1. Wheat and wheat flour products.
2. Corn and corn sweeteners.
3. Milk and dairy products (butter OK).

4. Peanuts and peanut products.
5. Beef, lamb and veal.
6. Pork and high-fat meats.
7. Soybean products.
8. Eggs.
9. Coffee and decaffeinated coffee.
10. Chocolate and cocoa products.
11. Sugar and refined sugar products.

### Other instructions

- read labels carefully and avoid food that contains sugar, salt, food additives, colourings or preservatives;
- no alcohol or beer, except that one glass of wine per day is allowed;
- do *not* start or modify any exercise programme;
- if a smoker, do *not* stop until after the diet test;
- stop taking vitamin supplements except HCl (hydrochloric acid).

**Warning**: Patients may have headaches and fatigue during the first 5 days of the diet experiment. These and other withdrawal symptoms strongly indicate that they suffer from 'food sensitivities'.

### Food sensitivity

To minimize the patient's exposure to histamine in the tissues it is necessary to test for food sensitivities.

#### FOOD SENSITIVITY TESTING INSTRUCTIONS

After completing the 10-day basic diet experiment, the patient will be able to test for body and brain sensitivities to the 11 foods groups restricted during the diet test.

Accurate food sensitivity testing requires that, during the 10-day restriction period, the patient should be unconditional about not eating from any of the 11 food groups they are asked to eliminate from their current diet. For example, the patient may be sensitive to wheat, sugar and coffee. If they stop using coffee and sugar for 10 days, their food sensitivity to wheat may continue to cause them to have headaches, to be tired, to retain water or whatever their individual reactions are to incompatible foods. At the end of the 10 days, you might falsely conclude that they are not sensitive to either coffee or sugar; after all, there was not any noticeable change in their symptoms.

It is highly likely that they will experience cravings or withdrawal symptoms, particularly in the first 5–7 days. It is best to start the 10-day elimination period on the last day of their work week, since any withdrawal symptoms they may have will usually be worst on days 2 and 3, their days off.

It is very helpful for them to keep a 'food and weight log' during and after the basic diet experiment. For example, they can record their morning weight at the start of the 10-day elimination period to determine if they have lost any weight by the end of the initial 10-day test. In addition to their weight, they should record what foods they eat at each meal and how they feel after eating those foods, especially when they start formal food sensitivity testing. This log is also useful to record their withdrawal symptoms, since many people do not remember what their sufferings were after they get well.

There are three ways to tell whether they may need to do formal food sensitivity testing to determine which specific foods their body is sensitive to:

- if during the sixth to tenth days of the basic diet experiment they feel much better than before the 10-day elimination period;
- if they had withdrawals during the first 5 days of the diet experiment. Please appreciate that the more severe their withdrawals are, the more important it is for them to do formal food sensitivity testing;
- if they lost 2.7–4.5 kg (6–10 lb) during the 10-day test, it is very important to do food sensitivity testing to determine which of those 11 food groups are causing their body to retain water.

When they are ready to start testing specific foods, they should make a list of the foods they want to test. It is best to test the foods they believe are compatible for them and then test the foods they believe their body is sensitive to. It is also wise to test those foods to which they may be sensitive on a day off work, since it is highly probable that they will have a return of their original symptom, i.e. they may get a headache.

In general, they may test one food per day, eating as much of that food as they would normally have eaten any day prior to doing the 10-day elimination period. After eating that food:

- they should notice any symptoms that occur within the first few hours after eating that food;
- they should weigh themselves the morning after eating the food being tested to see if they gained more than about 1 kg (2 lb). If they gain more than that amount the morning after reintroducing any food into their diet, that food is probably causing their body to retain water.

If, after reintroducing a food into their diet they do not notice adverse effects, they test another food the next day. However, if they have a negative reaction to any food, they need to stop food testing until their symptoms cease, which may be up to 5 days later; i.e. they need to resume the basic diet experiment.

Finally, it is important to understand that they are not being asked to permanently eliminate the 11 food groups restricted during the initial 10-day test. Many foods eliminated in the diet experiment are healthy foods for most people, but they are also foods to which some people are sensitive. They only need to permanently eliminate from their diet those food groups which directly provoke physical or mental symptoms, as proven by the formal testing.

They may also identify foods their body can tolerate in moderation, but to which their body or mind reacts negatively if they consume too much of that food. For example, most people seem to tolerate sugar in moderation, but develop problems if they constantly eat a lot of refined white sugar.

In summary, the main value of the basic diet experiment is that it helps patients learn what is best for their individual body. The theoretical thinking behind the basic diet experiment is that we are all unique biochemically and that what is good for most people may not be good for the patient personally.

### Supplementation

The use of vitamin supplements can be helpful in supporting deficiencies and promoting health. It is important to distinguish whether supplements are taken prophylactically to prevent disease or therapeutically to deal with a health problem.

If undertaking the basic diet experiment, no supplements should be taken for the period of elimination and subsequent food testing, except for the digestive aid hydrochloric acid.

My own preference is to optimize our food intake to provide the correct balance of essential nutrients, rather than to take supplements. However, if supplements are to be taken, particularly with regard to chronic head, neck or jaw pain, the following can play a significant role in re-establishing a balance and facilitate healing:

- Calcium and magnesium are essential for proper muscle function and should be in the proportion of 2:1, requiring 800–1200 mg of calcium to 400–600 mg of magnesium per day. Apart from the obvious importance of calcium to formation and maintenance of healthy bone, calcium is also important for proper muscle contraction, nerve transmission, cell division and some enzyme systems.
- Magnesium is considered the anti-stress mineral. It functions to relax skeletal muscle as well as smooth muscle of blood vessels and the gastrointestinal tract. Magnesium also helps in the release of energy by transferring the key phosphate molecule to adenosine triphosphate (ATP), the body's key energy source generated by the cytochrome system. Lack of magnesium will amplify the adrenal gland's response to stressful stimuli by increasing the output of stress hormones (catecholamines).
- B group vitamins are useful in providing energy by helping convert carbohydrate to glucose. Excessive refined sugar intake depletes the body of B group vitamins. They are also helpful in fat and protein/amino acid synthesis. However in the early stages of treating chronic pain patients, $B_5$ (pantothenic acid) should be restricted as it can stimulate the adrenal glands, increasing stress hormone output, thereby adversely affecting digestion.
- Digestive enzymes and hydrochloric acid will also aid in digestion, particularly the digestion and absorption of proteins.
- The optimizing of digestion and detoxification of the liver as discussed above.
- To repair and maintain the tensile strength of cartilage, muscle fascia, tendons, ligaments and periosteum it is necessary to increase collagen, elastin and proteoglycan synthesis. The availability of essential amino acids, lysine, proline and cystine, forms the basis of the growing collagen polypeptide chain. This chain is further hydroxylated in the presence of

ferrous iron, ascorbate. $B_6$, $B_5$, magnesium, manganese and silica all act as essential enzymatic co-factors.
- D-Phenylalanine has been shown to be helpful in reducing pain.[38]


## Conclusion

Nutrition is critical to our general health and the basics of what constitutes good nutrition have been discussed. This can be summarized by ensuring our diet is:

- wholesome – whole, unrefined food;
- high in complex carbohydrates;
- low in fat, sugar and salt;
- low in animal protein;
- free of colouring, artificial flavouring or preservatives;
- preferably eaten raw.

Also discussed were some of the problems that make following these guidelines so difficult. These may be due to poor quality soil, air or water, to poor quality food production, transport, processing, storage and marketing, or our dietary and cultural habits. In an ideal world where stressors are minimal, be it environmental, emotional, nutritional or postural, and we are eating an excellent quality and quantity diet, there would be no need for supplementation.

Dentistry deals with aspects of health which range from the basics of tooth decay and health of the gums to nutritional support associated with mercury toxicity and chelation therapy. The dentist's involvement in jaw dysfunction which is an integral part of chronic head and neck pain raises the issue of nutritional support to facilitate healing of muscle lesions and joint structure.

Central to any philosophy of health and treatment must be that the body has a tremendous capacity to heal itself and a natural desire to restore balance and maintain homeostasis. Optimal nutrition must provide us with the building blocks for all the body's system to reach its full potential.

Dentists are well placed to provide ongoing nutritional advice and support. They see their patients on a regular basis, monitoring their oral health which often reflects underlying health problems, particularly if dentists know what they are looking for. They are after all helping to maintain the first part of the digestive tract, so it seems perfectly reasonable to monitor what is consumed.

The way to achieving excellent health appears deceptively simple:

- fresh and wholesome diet free of chemicals and preservatives;
- regular and gentle exercise;
- quality time to relax on a daily basis.

Nutrition is not only a complex issue but a challenging discipline. The rewards however are great.

Good health!

# References

1 Price W. *Nutrition and Physical Degeneration*, 50th ann edn. New Canaan, Conn: Keats, 1989.

2 Rubin D, Felix C, Shrader C. *The Omega 3 Phenomenon*. London: Sidgwick & Jackson Publishers, 1988.

3 Bland J. *Your Health Under Siege*. Wellingborough: Thorsons Publishers Ltd, 1985.

4 Pritikin R. *The Pritikin Program*. New York: Simon & Schuster, 1990.

5 Diehl H, Mannerberg D. Hypertension, hyperlipidaemia, angina and coronary heart disease. *In* Trowell H C, Burkitt D P (eds). *Western Diseases: Their Emergence and Prevention*. Cambridge, MA: Harvard University Press, 1981.

6 National Research Council. *Diet and Health: Implications for Reducing Chronic Disease Risk*. Washington DC: National Academy Press, 1989.

7 Lefferts L V. Good fish bad fish. *Nutrition Action Health Letter* 1988; **15:** 5–7.

8 Blankenhorn D H, Nessim S A, Johnson R L et al. Beneficial effects of combined cholestipol–niacin therapy on coronary atherosclerosis and coronary venous bypass graphs. *J Am Med Assoc* 1987; **257:** 3233–3240.

9 Ornish D M et al. Can lifestyle changes reverse atherosclerosis? *Circulation, Supplement* (Abstracts from the 61st Scientific Sessions, American Heart Association) 1988; **14:** 11.

10 Grundy S et al. Comparison of monosaturated fatty acids and carbohydrates for reducing raised levels of cholesterol plasma in man. *Am J Clin Nutr* 1988; **47:** 965–969.

11 Anderson J W, Story L, Sieling B et al. Hypocholesterolemic effects of oat-bran or bean intake for hypercholesterolaemic men. *Am J Clin Nutr* 1984; **40:** 1146–1155.

12 Anderson J W, Gustafson N J, Bryant C A et al. Dietary fibre and diabetes: a comprehensive review and practical application. *J Am Dietetic Assoc* 1987; **87:** 1189–1197.

13 Braverman E R, Pfeiffer C C. *The Healing Nutrients Within: Facts, Findings and New Research on Amino Acids*. New Canaan, Conn: Keats Publishing, 1987.

14 Davies S, Stewart A. *Nutritional Medicine*. London: Pan Books, 1987.

15 Haas E M. *Staying Healthy with Nutrition*. Berkeley, CA: Celestial Arts Publishing, 1992.

16 Eversaul G. *Dental Kinesiology*. Las Vegas: privately published, 1977.

17 Fonder A C. *The Dental Physician*. Rock Falls, Illinois: Medical-Dental Arts, 1985.

18 Jenkins G N. *Physiology and Biochemistry of the Mouth*, 4th edn. Oxford: Blackwell Scientific Publications, 1978.

19 Leonora J, Tieche J M, Steinman R R. The effect of dietary factors on intradentinal dye penetration in the rat. *Arch-Oral-Biol* 1992; **37(9):** 733–741.

20 Leonora J, Tiech J M, Steinman R R. Further evidence for a hypothalamus, parotid gland, endocrine axis in the rat. *Arch-Oral-Biol* 1993; **38(10):** 911–916.

21 Leonora J, Tieche J M, Steinman R R. High-sucrose diet inhibits basal secretion of intradentinal dye penetration-stimulating hormone in pigs. *J Appl Physiol* 1994; **76(1):** 218–222.

22 Cheraskin E. The hidden nutrient connection. *In* Hosl E, Zaccrisson B U, Baldauf A (eds). *Orthodontics and Periodontics*. Illinois: Quintessence Books, 1985.

23 Hanioka T, Tanaka M, Ojima M et al. Effect of topical application of coenzyme Q10 on adult periodontitis. *Mol Aspects Med* 1994; **15 Suppl:** 241–248.

24 Watts T L. Coenzyme Q10 and periodontal treatment: is there any beneficial effect? *Br Dent J* 1995 March 25; **178(6):** 209–213.

25 Hahn L J, Kloiber R, Vimy M J et al. Dental 'silver' tooth fillings: a source of mercury exposure revealed by whole-body image scan and tissue analysis. *FASEB J* 1989; **3:** 2641–2646.

26 Hahn L J, Kloiber R, Vimy M J et al. Whole body imaging of the distribution of mercury released from dental fillings into monkey tissues. *FASEB J* 1990; **4:** 3256–3260.

27 Ziff S, Ziff M F, Hanson M. *Dental Mercury Detox*. Orlando, Fl: Bioprobe Publisher, 1993.

28 Dietch E A. The role of intestinal barrier failure and bacterial translocation in the development of systemic infection and multiple organ failure. *Arch Surg* 1990; **125:** 403–404.

29 Aposhian H V. DMSA and DMPS – water-soluble antidotes for heavy metal poisoning. *Ann Rev Pharmacol Toxicol* 1983; **23:** 193–215.
30 Aposhian H V, Bruce D C, Alter W *et al.* Urinary mercury after administration of 2,3-dimercaptopropane-1-sulphonic acid; correlation with dental amalgam source. *FASEB J* April 1992; **6(7):** 2472–2476.
31 Godfrey M, Campbell N. Confirmation of mercury retention and toxicity using DMPS. *J Advance Med* Spring 1994; **7(1):** 19–30.
32 Daunderer M. Mobilisation test for environmental metal poisonings. *Forum des Praktischen und Allgemdn-Arztes* 1989; **28(3):** 88. English translation in the *Bioprobe Newsletter* November 1989; **5(6):** 5–10.
33 Jaffe R. Chelation therapy for acute and chronic metal intoxication. Conference Paper, American Academy of Biological Dentistry, 1994.
34 Headache Classification Committee of the International Headache Society. Classification and diagnostic criteria for headache disorders, cranial neuralgias and facial pain. *Cephalgia* 1988; **8 Suppl 7:** 1–96.
35 Kraus H. Muscular aspects of oral dysfunction. *In* Gelb H (ed). *Clinical Management of Head, Neck and TMJ Pain and Dysfunction.* Philadelphia: W B Saunders Co, 1977.
36 Ehrlich R, Garlick D, Ninio M. The effect of jaw clenching on two neck and two trunk muscles. Unpublished, submitted Sep 1997.
37 Clark G T, Browne P A, Nakano M *et al.* Co-activation of sterno-cleido-mastoid muscles during maximum clenching. *J Dent Res* 1993; **72(11):** 1499–1502.
38 Budd K. Use of D-phenylalanine, an encephalinase inhibitor, in the treatment of intractable pain. *In* Bonica J *et al.* (eds). *Advances in Pain Research and Therapy*, Vol 5. New York: Raven Press, 1983.

# Bibliography

Bland J. *The 20-Day Rejuvenation Diet Program.* New Canaan, Conn: Keats, 1997.
Bland J. *Your Health Under Siege.* Wellingborough: Thorsons Publishers Ltd, 1985.
Davies S, Stewart A. *Nutritional Medicine.* London: Pan Books, 1987.
Haas E M. *Staying Healthy with Nutrition.* Berkeley, CA: Celestial Arts Publishing, 1992.
Pritikin R. *The Pritikin Program.* New York: Simon & Schuster, 1990.

# Associations

The British College of Nutritional Medicine
East Bank, New Church Road
Smithills
Greater Manchester BL1 5QP
UK
Tel: 01884 255059
Fax: 01884 255059

Institute of Optimum Nutrition (ION)
Blades Court
Deodar Road
London SW15 2NJ
UK
Tel: 0181 877 9993
Fax: 0181 877 9980

The Howell Institute of Nutrition
Research House
Fraser Road
Greenford
Middlesex UB6 7DX
UK
Tel: 0181 810 5644
Fax: 0181 810 5645

Australian College of Nutritional and
Environmental Medicine (ACNEM)
13 Hilton Street
Beaumaris
Victoria 3193
Australia
Tel: 00 613 9589 6088
Fax: 00 613 9589 5158

Dental Health Foundation – Australia
The University of Sydney
NSW 2006
Australia
Tel: 00 612 9660 8808
Fax: 00 612 9351 4734

## Courses

Details of general courses in nutrition can be obtained from the above associations. There are no courses as yet limited to nutrition in dentistry.

# Chiropractic

**Jonathan Howat**

## Introduction

From outward appearances the chiropractic and dental professions do not appear to overlap in their respective fields. On closer scrutiny and in a more functional application, the two professions are interlinked. Consequently, over the last decade, a greater collaboration has developed between the professions in reaching a satisfactory conclusion to many related problems.

The term chiropractic is derived from the Greek words *cheiro* (hand) and *praktikos* (to practise). Chiropractic was founded in 1895 by Dr Daniel David Palmer, a Canadian living in Davenport, Iowa, USA. It is now the largest natural healing profession in the world. It uses the inherent recuperative powers of the body for the maintenance of health through the normal balance of the nervous system and the spinal, muscular and skeletal structures.

The brain and spinal cord form the central nervous system, which controls and regulates the functions of the body. It is protected by the cranium of the skull and the spinal column, made up of vertebrae interspersed by discs. Trauma such as birth injuries, sports accidents and even minor falls can cause individual vertebra of the spine to misalign or subluxate. This can irritate the spinal nerve roots and inhibit the flow of nerve impulses. A spinal subluxation occurs when a vertebra moves out of its juxtaposition, occludes the intervertebral foramen, impinges a nerve root and interferes with normal nerve transmission. The biomechanical change at the spinal nerve root level can affect the function of the autonomic and peripheral nervous systems, producing many varied and far-reaching symptoms at either a musculoskeletal, neuromuscular or visceral level.

### Examination

The chiropractor takes a comprehensive case history, then carries out a physical examination. This includes orthopaedic and neurological tests, cranial nerve examination, postural analysis, assessment of spinal vertebral ranges of motion, biomechanical indicators and assessment of temporomandibular joint dysfunction. X-rays are taken when indicated to establish changes in structural and biomechanical stability and pathology.

With the information obtained, the chiropractor will embark on a regimen of treatment designed to return the patient to a point of biomechanical and neurological stability. General chiropractic treatment is in the form of spinal adjustments made to realign the vertebrae, correcting subluxations, balancing the pelvis and thereby restoring normal nerve function. Chiropractic care is gentle and natural; it responds to the body's needs and does not include drugs or surgery.

## Education

Education is administered by the Council for Chiropractic Education (CCE). This is an international body that controls and regulates the academic training of chiropractors throughout the world. The council ensures that all chiropractic colleges maintain a consistent level of performance, with a common syllabus and curriculum and a consistency within the classroom, technique rooms, scientific facilities, laboratories and clinics. Therefore, no matter where a chiropractor has graduated, the academic programme is uniform. If chiropractors graduate from CCE recognized colleges and have fulfilled the national or state requirements of the country in which they are practising, they have no problem in registering with the relevant national professional association.

The chiropractic curriculum consists of basic science subjects such as anatomy, physiology, biochemistry, microbiology and physics. Medical subjects such as gynaecology, obstetrics, paediatrics, embryology, pathology, radiology, anatomy, toxicology, pharmacology and clinical first aid are also included.

Chiropractic courses include palpation, adjustive techniques, postural assessment, spinal biomechanics, extremity techniques, rehabilitation of sports injuries, neurological and orthopaedic evaluation, ethics and jurisprudence, and administration of chiropractic offices. On an undergraduate basis, an introduction to several chiropractic techniques, both active and passive, is established in an attempt to ensure that graduate chiropractors have a variety of techniques at their disposal.

## Clinical techniques

Chiropractic has many techniques which can be applied in order to correct subluxations and reinstate neurological function. Over the years these techniques have originated through clinical research by individuals who have adapted procedures to help stabilize and balance the spine and pelvis.

Some techniques are osseously related, with adjustments made specifically to the vertebrae and pelvis, some are active using specific adjusting thrusts to the vertebrae, while others are passive allowing the body to rebalance and stabilize itself under more subtle forces. There are also techniques which incorporate all aspects of physiology including the nervous, lymphatic, vascular, meningeal and cerebrospinal fluid systems. These various techniques have evolved from clinical experience and research as well as the fundamental recognition that the body works as a whole but is dependent on the integral parts to function at a homeostatic level.

Listed below are some of the more popular techniques used in chiropractic.

### APPLIED KINESIOLOGY (AK)

Developed by Dr George Goodheart of Detroit, USA. It is a diagnostic and treatment system that tests muscles to determine areas of neurological malfunction, their causes and methods of correction and balancing.

### GONSTEAD TECHNIQUE

This system uses full spine X-rays to determine levels of spinal subluxation confirmed by nervoscope reading and palpation. It was developed by Dr Clarence Gonstead of Wisconsin, USA.

### ACTIVATOR

An activator is a hand-held instrument developed by Dr W. C. Lee and Dr A. W. Fuhr which applies a direct, accurate and specific thrust with high velocity, reinstating a bone into its correct juxtaposition.

### PETTIBON TECHNIQUE

This technique is named after its developer Dr Burl Pettibon of Vancouver. It is used to reduce abnormal curvatures and angles of the spine.

### COX TECHNIQUE

This is a method of reducing disc protrusions of the lower back. Developed by Dr James Cox of Fort Wayne, USA.

### GROSTIC TECHNIQUE

This is a very specialized technique of aligning the head and neck, reducing distortion in the vital upper neck area, where the spinal cord is most vulnerable to subluxation.

### SPINAL COLUMN STRESSOLOGY

Spinal column stressology was designed by Dr Lowell Ward of California, USA to locate areas of spinal and meningeal fixation due to stress of all types and help reduce destructive postural stress habit patterns.

### SACRO-OCCIPITAL TECHNIQUE (SOT)

The sacro-occipital technique was founded and developed by Dr Major Bertram DeJarnette in Nebraska, USA in the early 1930s. It concerns itself primarily with the dural meningeal system and the production, circulation and absorption of cerebrospinal fluid. It takes its name from the fundamental requirement of a balance between the sacrum and occiput. Without this balance the sacro-occipital pump mechanism becomes destabilized, affecting the flow of cerebrospinal fluid. This is essential to the normal function of the central nervous system.

SOT is a diagnostic technique and passive in its application. It is viewed as the ideal technique for paediatric and geriatric patients and complements other osseous adjustive techniques encompassing a wide range of uses. The cranial component of SOT may require a multidisciplinary approach due to the large influence that dental occlusion has on the balance of the skull.

ASSOCIATED TECHNIQUES

Apart from chiropractic techniques there are many other additional areas the patient may need to address in order to help the body re-establish itself as a normal functional organism. These include nutrition, exercise, hot and cold therapy, microcurrent therapy and rehabilitative supports. A close liaison with other professional disciplines may be needed with certain techniques to enhance the chiropractic adjustment. For example, it might require podiatrists to stabilize the arch of the foot, nutritionists to oversee or plan a balanced diet and dentists to stabilize the temporomandibular joint with the use of splint therapy or to establish upper or lower arch expansion with orthopaedic appliances, followed by orthodontic appliances.

## The scientific basis of chiropractic

This is discussed in detail in 'The Essential Principles of Chiropractic' by Virgil Strange.[1] Homeostasis is defined as the ability of the organism to maintain a physiological equilibrium regardless of the variations in the environment. *Gray's Anatomy* defines the nervous system as 'the system that controls and regulates the activities of all the other systems in the body and enables them to co-ordinate their activities for the benefit of the organism as a whole'. The nervous system is housed and protected by the skeletal system in a normal structural and functional relationship.

Chiropractic rationale developed from long-standing clinical and physical observations that distorted skeletal relationships cause nervous system dysfunction. It is based on the following three facts:

- homeostasis enables the organism to remain vital and function within its environment;
- the nervous system controls and regulates homeostasis;
- instability of the skeletal structure impairs the function of the nervous system.

Chiropractic is able to hypothesize that skeletal disrelationships, particularly in the spinal structures, can result in the loss of nervous system integrity and thus a loss of homeostasis and health to the body.

### Dural meningeal system

The brain and spinal cord are protected and supported by the dural meningeal system which includes the pia mater, arachnoid mater and dura mater, the three coverings of the brain and spinal cord. The duramater in the cranium is made up of two layers.

The first, or endosteal, layer which covers the internal surface of the cranium, exits through the sutures and becomes continuous with the periosteum of the outer covering of the cranium.

The second, or meningeal, layer covers the surface of the brain. It forms the intracranial dural support mechanism, also known as the reciprocal tension membrane system. This separates the various hemispheres of the brain and supports the brain. It also forms the entire venous sinus system which drains the brain and spinal cord of cerebrospinal fluid.

The intracranial dural membranes consist of the falx cerebri, the falx cerebellum, the tentorium cerebelli and the diaphragma sellae. These membranes act as baffles within the cranium supporting the two cerebral hemispheres, and separating them from the cerebellum (*Figure 3.1*). No matter what position the cranium is in, the brain is at all times supported and stabilized.

The anchor points for the reciprocal tension membranes are:

- the crista galli of the ethmoid bone – the anchor point for the falx cerebri;
- the petrous portion of the temporal bones – the anchor point for the tentorium cerebelli;
- the internal occipital protuberance and the foramen magnum – the anchor points for the falx cerebellum;
- the anterior and posterior clinoid processes of the sphenoid bone – the anchor points for the diaphragma sellae.

From the foramen magnum the dural meningeal system consists of the spinal dura which is firmly anchored at the foramen magnum, the ring of the

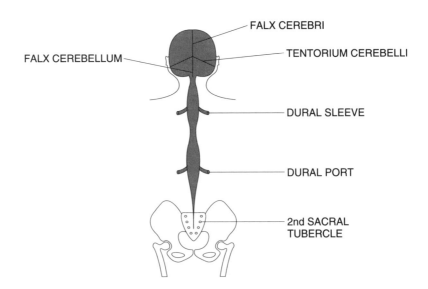

**Figure 3.1** Normal dural meningeal system

atlas, the body of axis and, according to some anatomical authorities, to the body of the third cervical vertebra. From there the dural tube descends and, apart from some rudimentary attachments at each vertebral level, has no further firm attachments until the second sacral tubercle where the dural meningeal system is firmly adhered. Each spinal nerve root exits through the intervertebral foramen covered in a dural sleeve – a continuation of the dural meninges – terminating at the dural port, which then becomes continuous with the epineurium of the nerve.

## Skeletal system

The skeletal system which protects the central nervous system consists of the 22 bones of the skull, 24 spinal vertebrae (7 cervical, 12 thoracic and 5 lumbar), the sacrum (5 fused segments) and the coccyx (5 fused segments). The sacrum is supported bilaterally within the pelvis by the ilia forming the sacroiliac joints. These joints are unique within the skeletal structures as being one of the few joints supported entirely by ligaments without any muscular attachments directly across the joint. This characteristic suggests that the sacroiliac joint is not able to be protected voluntarily, and is therefore a safety valve for disrelationships within the pelvic-sacral and sacrolumbar junctions.

When the structural stability of the pelvis is disrupted, the areas of concern are the sacroiliac joints and the lumbar-sacral junction – L5/S1. The sacroiliac joint is made up of an auricular boot which consists of dry hyaline cartilage surrounded by a synovial membrane containing synovial fluid. The superior and inferior interosseous ligaments support the sacroiliac joint above and below the auricular boot articulation.

The pivot point of the sacrum within the sacroiliac junction occurs at the level of the second sacral tubercle – the same level at which the dural meningeal system anchors.

## Ventricular system

This consists of two lateral ventricles, the third ventricle and the fourth ventricle. Cerebrospinal fluid is generated in the choroid plexuses of the ventricles and flows from the two lateral ventricles into the third ventricle and from the third ventricle through the aqueduct of Sylvius into the fourth ventricle. The cerebrospinal fluid then exits through the lateral apertures of Luschka and the medial aperture of Magendi. It circulates down the spine in a helical movement towards the sacrum. It then circulates upwards again and through the foramen magnum into the subarachnoid space and the cisterns of the brain. It continues up towards the arachnoid granulations where it is absorbed into the superior sagittal sinus and drained from the brain through the venous sinus system.

The smooth circulatory movement of cerebrospinal fluid around the brain and spinal cord is motivated by a combination of the cardiovascular system, diaphragmatic respiration and what is known as the primary respiratory mechanism (PRM). PRM is established *in utero* and thought to be produced by the glia cells and in particular the oligodendroglia cells. This circulation is imperative for the maintenance of homeostasis.

### The Lovett–Brother relationship

A biomechanical state, namely the Lovett–Brother relationship, describes the skeletal reciprocity between paired bones of the cranium, pelvis and spine. Atlas and L5 will move in an equal and opposite direction to each other in order to maintain a balanced vertical position against gravity; likewise axis and L4, C3 and L3, C4 and L2, etc. reciprocate with one another. Similarly the ilia will reciprocate with the temporal bones and the occiput with the sacrum.

This paired reciprocal relationship between cranial and skeletal bones is important when assessing biomechanical faults within the system and how they can be rectified to balance homeostasis. For example, changes in the position of the ilia will change the positions of the temporal bones. These changes will, in turn, affect the tension on the tentorium cerebelli (which anchors to the petrous portion of the temporal bone). In turn the straight sinus becomes distorted and has a detrimental effect on the venous sinus drainage of the brain, resulting in an adverse effect on homeostasis.

### Physiological adaptive range

The physiological adaptive range as referred to by Dr Gerald Smith in his book 'Cranial Dental Sacral Complex',[2] begins with the optimum health and high tolerance factor that the body has at birth. Injuries and traumas from birth and thereafter require the body to compensate over many years while the tolerance decreases without any symptomatic effect. At some stage tolerance reaches a minimum capacity when the body will not be able to adapt any further. This is the limit of physiological adaptive range and results in an established condition producing a myriad of symptoms.

### Diaphragmatic respiration

Observations shown on magnetic resonance imaging (MRI) scan indicate that the ventricles of the brain expand during inhalation and contract on the exhalation stage of respiration. It has also been demonstrated by MRI and computed tomography (CT) scan that on inhalation the diaphragm depresses, forcing the abdominal organs downward onto the pelvic floor, flaring the ilia into external rotation and decreasing the lumbar lordosis. This, in turn, causes compression on the sacral bulb (the lower part of the dural meningeal system).

The compression on the sacral bulb forces cerebrospinal fluid up in a helical motion towards the foramen magnum, through the various cisterna and the arachnoid granulations. The cerebrospinal fluid is then absorbed into the superior sagittal sinus from where it is taken by the blood stream back to the heart for recirculation.

On the same inhalation phase the ventricles of the brain expand and fill up with cerebrospinal fluid. This is produced and secreted by the choroid plexuses of the ventricles.

The expansion of the brain on inhalation also has the effect of causing compression on the cisterns, forcing cerebrospinal fluid up toward the superior sagittal sinus before reabsorption takes place. The effect of an increased brain dimension during inhalation also means that the dural meningeal system expands in the cranium. This results in the effect of a shortening of the spinal cord while the sacral apex moves anteriorly. There is also increased tension on the intracranial reciprocal tension membranes, the dentate ligaments and the ligamentum nuchae.

On the exhalation phase of respiration the ventricles compress, forcing cerebrospinal fluid from the lateral ventricles, through the other ventricles and foramena downward in a helical movement towards the sacral bulb. As air leaves the lungs, the diaphragm returns to its peak rest position, the abdominal organs move upward, the lumbar lordosis returns to the lumbar spine, the ilia become internally rotated and the sacral apex moves posteriorly while the sacral bulb becomes enlarged.

The effect of the sacro-occipital pump in the exhalation phase means that, as the ventricles compress, the cisterns expand drawing cerebrospinal fluid into the cisterns before being compressed on the next phase of inhalation. The reciprocal tension membranes relax as do the dentate ligaments and the ligamentum nuchae. The spinal cord elongates as there is less tension in the intracranial dural meningeal system.

**Cranial sacral pump**

In the 1930s, Dr Major DeJarnette, the founder of the Sacro-Occipital Technique showed that there was a reciprocal function producing motion between the occiput and the sacrum. Provided that the pelvis is balanced and in a symmetrical position, diaphragmatic respiration will provide an anterior/posterior apical movement of the sacrum while the occiput and frontal bone move away and towards one another, expanding and contracting the coronal, lambdoid and sagittal sutures of the brain.

On the inhalation phase, the sutural system is expanded which allows micromotion between the cranial plates, producing bilateral symmetric motion between the parietal bones, temporal bones, frontal bone and the occiput. The sphenoid bone acts as the interlink: the sphenobasilar synchrondosis of the occiput forming the posterior pivot of the cranium, the pterygoid plate of the sphenoid and the maxillary tuberosity of the maxillae bone forming the anterior pivot of the cranium. The posterior pivot is highly influenced by pelvic instability while the anterior pivot is affected by dental malocclusion.

# Chiropractic considerations

The chiropractic attitude is to enhance the body's tolerance by stabilizing the skeletal structures. This improves neurological integrity and thus homeostasis. It allows the body to adapt and compensate, providing an asymptomatic environment and a quality of life.

### Skeletal dysfunction – bilateral sacroIliac fixation

Trauma during the birth process or in the ensuing years can lead to distortion and rotation of the pelvis. This bilaterally locks the sacroiliac joints, producing an oblique or diagonal distortion of the sacrum which in turn twists the dural meningeal system affecting the spinal dura and the intracranial reciprocal tension membranes. The torquing effect of the dural meningeal system affects cerebrospinal fluid flow, creating a hydrostatic pressure change around the spinal cord, spinal nerve roots and the brain. This affects not only the production and circulation of cerebrospinal fluid, but also the absorption and drainage of cerebrospinal fluid through the venous sinus system. The resultant change in biochemical status at these levels changes neurological integrity and hence homeostasis.

The biomechanical effects of a rotational pelvis means that one ilia moves posteriorly and the reciprocal ilia moves anteriorly. This affects the position of the acetabula, producing a relative discrepancy in the length of the legs. This discrepancy is a physiological adaptation and not a physical leg length discrepancy (*Figure 3.2*).

This bilateral sacroiliac lock means that one ilia is externally rotated and the other internally rotated, both in a predisposed fixed position. The Lovett–Brother relationship produces a biomechanical adaptation and compensation in the cranium. This predisposes a fixed position of each temporal bone into internal rotation and external rotation opposing their pelvic counterparts. Both glenoid fossae are now out of synchronization, affecting the translation of the mandible, producing a malocclusion (crossbite, premature contact or loss of vertical). Posturally this patient when observed in a standing position will move in an anterior to posterior direction in an attempt to enhance motion of cerebrospinal fluid already inhibited by the torque of the dural meningeal system.

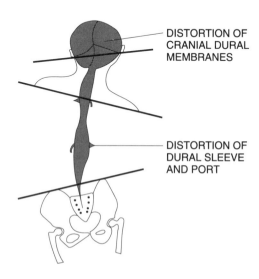

DISTORTION OF
CRANIAL DURAL
MEMBRANES

DISTORTION OF
DURAL SLEEVE
AND PORT

**Figure 3.2** Bilateral sacroiliac fixation

## Sacroiliac lesion

The relatively long or short leg discrepancy over a period of time puts tremendous pressure on the superior and inferior interosseous ligaments at the sacroiliac joint. This may reach a point where the physiological adaptive range of the joint exceeds its ability to compensate. The interosseous ligaments, particularly on the short leg side of the pelvis, will start to stretch, changing the cohesive nature of this highly proprioceptive nerve bed within the sacroiliac joint. As the interosseous ligaments stretch, they may on occasions tear due to severe trauma. The synovial membrane ruptures and the dry hyaline cartilage becomes moist as a result of the presence of synovial fluid.

The resulting subluxation means that the weight-bearing joint is now unable to support the body against a gravitational pull. As a result the body's defence mechanism goes into action in an effort to stabilize and support the structure and protect the central nervous system. When this patient is observed on a postural distortion analyser, the movement will be from side to side in a lateral sway. This is due to the unilateral slip of the sacrum on the ilium where the sacroiliac joint has lost its structural integrity (*Figure 3.3*).

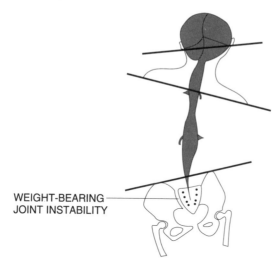

WEIGHT-BEARING
JOINT INSTABILITY

**Figure 3.3** Unilateral sacroiliac lesion

## The sacroiliac and temporomandibular joint

The sacroiliac joint and the temporomandibular joint are the two most highly proprioceptive joints in the body and compensate and adapt for one another all the time. It is well documented that man swallows in excess of 2000 times a day. Each swallow produces an occlusal contact, creating light pressure on the teeth. The swallowing mechanism is nature's way of balancing the cranium and all its components. Provided that the bite is bilaterally symmetrical with posterior support, full dentition, no incisal interference and a normal vertical, then the swallow will balance all the cranial components.

However, if the swallow is asymmetric or does not fulfil the above criteria, the entire cranium will become unbalanced and over a long period craniofacial distortions will result and affect the cranial physiology and hence temporomandibular joint and sacroiliac balance.

### The latissimus dorsi muscle

This muscle arises from the external lip of the crest of the ilium and the spinous processes of the sacral, lumbar and lower six thoracic vertebrae. It attaches to the transverse process of T6, travels across the inferior border of the scapula and inserts into the bottom of the intertubercular groove of the humerus. The latissimus dorsi contracts in an effort to support the side of the sacroiliac lesion, elevating the involved hip-bone but at the same time unavoidably depressing the pectoral girdle and humerus, stretching the brachial nerve distribution into the shoulder and arm (*Figure 3.4*).

Over a period of time this constant muscle spasm gives rise to bursitis of the glenohumeral joint, producing the likes of frozen shoulder, tennis elbow and, indirectly, carpel tunnel syndrome. The irritation on the brachial nerve plexus can give rise to paraesthesia as far down as the fingertips.

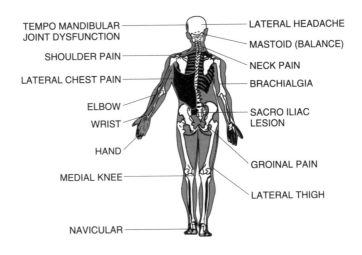

**Figure 3.4** Areas of complication involved in sacroiliac lesion

### The trapezius and sternocleidomastoid muscles

To counteract the spasm of the latissimus dorsi the opposing trapezius and sternocleidomastoid muscles contract, creating a pull on the occiput and on the temporal bone. This distorts the glenoid fossa of the temporal bone and changes the relationship of the condyle of the mandible within the glenoid fossa. This will lead to a changed relationship of the occlusion between the maxillae and mandible, creating a dental malocclusion.

The continued sternocleidomastoid muscle spasm pulls on the mastoid bone and disrupts the internal acoustic meatus. This may affect cranial nerves VII and VIII and can disrupt the cochlear vestibular mechanism, affecting hearing and balance. The opposite temporalis muscle now reacts in a defensive mechanism.

### The temporalis muscle

The anterior portion of the temporalis muscle is described as being highly proprioceptive, particularly as far as the body's position is concerned within its centre of gravity. Because of the sacroiliac lesion and the body's inability to support itself against gravity, the anterior temporalis goes into spasm and transfers this spasm through to the medial and posterior branches of the temporalis.

The temporalis muscle and its fascia cover the lateral sutures of the skull, including the frontal, parietal, occipital, temporal and sphenoidal sutures. The effect of spasm on the temporalis creates a fascial pull through the periosteum, jamming the sutures and creating torsion and tension on the endosteal dura. This action closes the jaws and causes a retrusion of the mandible in the glenoid fossae – once again changing the occlusion between the maxillae and mandible and reinforcing a dental malocclusion.

### The pterygoid muscles

Due to the changed position of the condyle of the mandible, the lateral and medial pterygoid muscles contract, creating a distorted effect on the sphenoid bone (the pterygoid muscles attach to the pterygoid plates of the sphenoid bone). A retrusion of the mandible also changes the centre of gravity of the skull, producing a forward head position. This disturbs the lordosis of the mid-cervical spine and the long-term effects can cause degenerative joint disease at the levels of C3/C4 and C5.

### Sub-pelvic muscles

As far as related muscular contractions below the pelvis are concerned, the sacroiliac lesion will disturb Poupart's ligament or the inguinal ligament, creating groinal pain and disturbance of the pelvic floor. Further contraction of the gracilus and sartorius muscles into their insertion points on the medial aspect of the knee and medial meniscus affect the position of the knee: The tensor fasciae latae derotates the opposite knee, the medial and lateral colateral ligaments of the knee change the weight-bearing vectors of the thigh and lower limb. This disturbs the relationship of the knee, the ankle and the arch of the foot.

Should this be compounded over many years it results in a breakdown of biomechanics from the feet, knees, hips, pelvis, spine, pectoral girdle and cranium. Once the sacroiliac lesion is correctly defined, diagnosed and stabilized, the treatment will bring structural stability back to all the aforementioned areas. This will allow function to resume, neurological integrity to re-establish and homeostasis to be maintained.

### Lumbar 5/sacral 1 discogenic syndrome

The inability of the sacroiliac lesions to support the body against gravity puts a tremendous strain on the paravertebral muscles surrounding the lumbar-sacral junction. The constant effort by the superior and inferior interosseous ligaments in trying to maintain the sacroiliac joint throws a greater emphasis of compensation and adaptation onto the lumbar-sacral disc area. As the physiological adaptive range breaks down and the sacroiliac joint becomes weaker, the stress into the lumbar-sacral disc will produce a disc prolapse. Herniation and then rupture may follow. This produces a severe sciatic neuritis which, depending on the type of lesion produced at the lumbar-sacral junction, will dictate whether the treatment is conservative or requires invasive surgery (*Figure 3.5*).

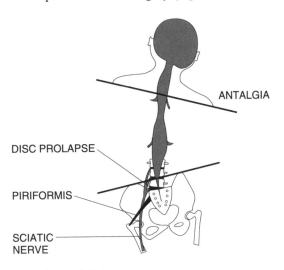

**Figure 3.5** Lumbosacral discogenic lesion

At this point there is a total breakdown in the dural meningeal system. When the patient is observed on a postural analyser they will show very little movement and more of an antalgic muscular spasm either towards or away from the side of sciatic involvement, depending on the type of disc lesion. Although the problem appears to be at the lumbosacral junction, it may be a temporomandibular joint dysfunction being adapted for at this junction over a long period of time and being consistently reinforced by the swallow and chew mechanism. This should be classified as a non-traumatic lesion with an insidious onset not necessarily provoked by anything more than a repetitive malocclusion.

### Ascending stress major

The discussion so far has taken into account primary chiropractic considerations whereby the major lesion has been at the sacroiliac or lumbar-sacral joints and will destabilize the pelvic girdle. Dr Jean Pierre Meersseman, a well-known chiropractic exponent on craniodental dysfunction, defines this as an ascending stress major. This is because the primary structural instability at the pelvis will ascend, producing compensation and adaptation throughout the system and resulting in a temporomandibular joint dysfunction or a dental malocclusion.

**Sutures**

Work done by Retzlaff and Mitchell[3] discusses the histological formation of the suture which consists of five layers. The first layer is a zone of connective tissue which bridges the suture and is designated the sutural ligament. The next layer consists of osteogenic cells and both these layers appear to be continuous with that of the periosteum of the skull bones. This periosteal layer and sutural ligament is found on both sides of both the outer and inner surfaces of the suture. The central space is made up of connective tissue, blood vessels and nerve fibres which is totally consistent with the morphology and histology of a normal joint.

# Cranial considerations

### The anterior and posterior pivots

The sphenoid bone is the central bone of the cranium and pivots posteriorly at the sphenobasilar synchondrosis with the occiput and anteriorly at the pterygoid plate with the maxillary tuberosity of the maxillae. These points are commonly known as the posterior and anterior pivots respectively (*Figure 3.6*).

Distortion at either the anterior or posterior pivot will create distortive changes within the cranium at the reciprocal tension membranes, affecting the cerebral hemispheres, cerebellum and the brain stem. Trauma at birth,

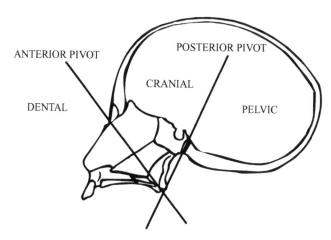

**Figure 3.6** Anterior and posterior pivots of the cranium

often produced by a forceps delivery, can create damage to the greater wings of the sphenoid, inducing torsion and affecting the anterior and posterior pivots. Similarly, a ventouse delivery will have an effect on the superior sagittal suture, affecting the superior sagittal sinus and the entire venous sinus system. This will disturb the homeostasis of the cranial reciprocal tension membranes. Further changes to the cranium become evident later on in life through sports injuries, motor vehicle accidents, whiplashes, falls, bumps and jolts.

### POSTERIOR PIVOT

The posterior pivot, the sphenobasilar synchondrosis, can be directly influenced by a pelvic distortion affecting the occiput, and the occiput in turn affecting the sphenobasilar synchondrosis. The lesion at the sphenobasilar synchondrosis could be a cranial inferior or superior vertical strain, a side-bending torsion or a torquing effect of the sphenobasilar junction (see Chapter 4 for more detail on these terms). All of these will have direct implications on the brain stem and the reciprocal tension membranes.

### ANTERIOR PIVOT

The anterior pivot will be influenced by a dental malocclusion. This can produce a side-bending torsion, creating a shearing of the maxillary tuberosity against the pterygoid plate or a torquing effect at the anterior pivot. Due to the position of the pituitary in the body of the sphenoid bone, distortions of this bone will affect the pituitary, particularly at the anterior and posterior clinoids where the diaphragma sellae supports the hypophyseal stalk of the pituitary gland. As the pituitary is the master controlling endocrine gland, structural changes of the sphenoid bone will bring about pathophysiology of the pituitary, thereby affecting the endocrine system.

When assessing cranial considerations the craniopath has to consider the maxillary/mandible relationship, the occlusion of the teeth and the effect the maxillae is having on the maxillosphenoid junction at the anterior pivot. He also needs to ensure that the pelvic girdle and thus the posterior pivot is balanced structurally.

## The cranial nerves

It is interesting to note that embryologically the ethmoid bone, the body and lesser wings of the sphenoid, the basilar and condylar area of the occiput and the petrous portion of the temporal bone are all generated in cartilage and then become bone. The frontal squama, the parietals, the greater wings of the sphenoid, the temporal squama and the occipital squama are generated in membrane and act as membrane throughout life.

The optic canal (cranial nerve II) and the superior orbital fissure (nerves III and IV and ophthalmic division of nerves V and VI) lie in the cartilaginous part of the sphenoid bone. The foramen rotundum (maxillary branch of V) and the foramen ovale (mandibular branch of V) lie in the membranous part of the sphenoid bone. The internal acoustic meatus (nerves VII and VIII) lies in the cartilaginous petrous portion of the temporal bone. The jugular foramen (nerves IX, X and XI) lies in the cartilaginous basilar area of the occiput, and the hypoglossal canal (nerve XII) lies in the cartilaginous condylar portion of the occiput.

All 12 pairs of cranial nerves exit through apertures formed in bone at the base of the skull. Change in the anterior and posterior pivot will distort or occlude these apertures, affecting cranial nerve function. The symptomatic manifestations as a result of cranial nerve disturbance at any or all of these apertures produce neurological imbalance, loss of nerve integrity and breakdown of homeostasis.

### Intra-oral corrections

Cranial faults affecting anterior and posterior pivots through the sphenoid bone can be corrected by the chiropractic craniopath using intra-oral contacts. These may be at either the hard palate, the maxillae or at the pterygoid plates of the sphenoid bone. This will affect the anterior pivots, the posterior pivots, the internal and external rotation of the temporal bone, the occiput and frontal bones. These corrections can only be done once the dental and pelvic components have been structurally balanced and neutralized.

Eighty per cent of the central nervous system is found in the cranium and the body will at all times create a protective and defensive environment to ensure preservation of this structure. Both compensation and adaptation will take place, either in the pelvis or in the occlusion, so as to afford maximum protection to the brain. Any attempt to make cranial corrections prior to stabilizing the pelvis and occlusion will result in a lot of unnecessary neurological reaction.

# Dental considerations

### Malocclusion

Changes in the relation between the maxillae and mandible can be brought on early in life, by pelvic or cranial distortions creating side-bending, torsion and vertical strain of the posterior pivot, i.e. the sphenobasilar synchondrosis. Early temporomandibular joint dysfunctions may be brought about by the fetal position prior to the birth process, impacting the jaw on one side and distracting it on the other. Processes such as thumb-sucking may change the occlusion, and early crossbites, if seen, may be easily rectified.

### Class II – divisions 1 and 2

The concern from a chiropractic craniopathic standpoint occurs towards puberty in the Class II – Div 1/Div 2 children, where the maxillary arch is shaped like an inverted 'V'. This is due to bilaterally internally rotated maxillae which have the effect of overcrowding the upper and lower jaws. The orthodox treatment for this situation is the removal of two upper first bicuspids and/or two lower first bicuspids followed by fixed appliances on both upper and lower jaws. Also possible is the attachment of headgear in order to retrude maxillary growth and allow an aesthetic effect on the Class

II – Div 1 scenario. A Class II – Div 2 mouth is already in a position to retrude the mandible as the upper incisors are already distalized. The long-term effects of this are devastating for the recipient as the changes made are permanent.

The problems that ensue are as follows. Retrusion of the mandible in the glenoid fossae creates irritation on the retrodiscal tissue. This affects the proprioceptive nerve bed and forces the temporal bones into bilateral external rotation. This affects the internal acoustic meatus which influences cranial nerves VII and VIII, ultimately affecting the vestibular cochlear mechanism which results in vertigo, tinnitus and loss of equilibrium.

The tentorium cerebellum then becomes locked in an external mode, affecting the posterior clinoid processes and the diaphragma sellae. This in turn affects the hypophyseal stalk of the pituitary gland and hence the endocrine secretions of the anterior pituitary which produces all the master control level hormones. The effect on the tentorium cerebelli also affects the straight sinus and ultimately the venous drainage system of the brain, affecting cerebrospinal fluid hydrostatic balance.

### SPINAL LORDOSIS AND LOCKING OF THE CRANIAL SUTURES

Continued incisal interference and forced retrusion of the mandible will eventually cause a forward head tilt. This changes the lordosis of the cervical spine, bringing in an anterior curve at the level of C3, C4 and C5 which may result in degenerative changes at those levels.

The anterior head position of the skull results in the anterior portion of the temporalis muscle (highly proprioceptive against gravity) going into spasm. This may create a muscle spasm through the entire temporalis muscle. The temporalis muscle covers all the sutures of the lateral part of the skull. Spasm of this muscle will lock these sutures. The cranial plates will lose their mobility and as a result respiration of the cranium becomes inhibited and so does homeostasis.

In this regard it is also useful to note that, in embryological development, cells from the neural tube area control the brain, the spinal cord, the central nervous system, half of the pituitary gland as well as the premaxillae and four maxillary incisors. In a normal occlusion the incisors should not come into contact at any point on swallowing or mastication.

### HYPO-ADRENIA

A clinical observation that the author has made involves mainly females in their late teens to early twenties who have been diagnosed as having myalgic encephalomyelitis (ME). Many have had either two or four bicuspid extractions. When the pituitary gland is aggravated, the production of ACTH occurs stimulating the adrenal glands. Over a period of time continued overuse of the adrenal glands will produce a condition of hypo-adrenia, resulting in a loss of immune system function and a breakdown in tolerance and resistance.

Glandular fever may ensue, followed by fluctuating pyrexia, hormonal changes, erratic and painful menses, malaise, memory and concentration loss, speech distortion, leg and arm pains, headaches, visual changes, blood sugar and metabolic rate fluctuation. Coupled with the pathophysio-logical stress are the social, academic and financial changes in the girl's life. These include end-of-school examinations, leaving home, a new environment at university or workplace and new social demands with the opposite sex. At this time a poor diet is often supplemented with junk food and the introduction of tobacco and alcohol.

Until recently this demoralizing condition of ME was blamed on a psychosomatic cause with a drop-out, failure attitude. It is now recognized as having a true pathophysiological aetiology. The observations mentioned are not usually discussed, as the symptomatic picture does not totally unravel for 6–8 years after the extractions and fixed appliances have taken place.

ARCH EXPANSION

The alternative approach to Class II – Div 1/Div 2 type children is to expand the upper and lower arches well before puberty. This would culminate in fixed upper and lower arch appliances and then an upper removable retainer for about 6 months.

In this way the integrity of the system is maintained. No teeth are removed, the occlusion is maintained, the mandible is allowed to protrude without any damage to the reticular disc or retrodiscal tissue area. Head posture is maintained so that cervical lordosis is also maintained. There is no interference to the reciprocal tension membranes, the venous sinus drainage, the diaphragma sellae or the tentorium cerebelli. The growth hormone that is produced at puberty is allowed to function without inhibition, which it certainly is not in the case of pubescent extraction of the upper and lower bicuspids.

WISDOM TEETH EXTRACTION

As the children who had two or four bicuspid extractions become adults and reach their mid to late twenties, the wisdom teeth appear and they too need to be extracted because of the underdevelopment of the maxillae and mandible and the artificial jamming of the teeth on the upper and lower jaw. The result is that by the time these people are 30 years of age, 25% of their natural dentition has been removed artificially and without any just cause, bar that of pure aesthetics.

The tragedy when dealing with this type of dental major, is that the entire procedure has to be reversed as these patients become overclosed and lose their vertical dimension. The treatment required is expansion of the upper and lower arch, protruding the mandible, erupting the posterior teeth to increase the vertical and using bridgework or implants to negate the loss of the premolar dentition (*Figure 3.7*).

## Loss of posterior support

Loss of dentition anywhere in the posterior jaw means that all the mastication will take place on the opposite side. This, over a period of time, will create an imbalance and impaction of one temporomandibular joint and distraction of the other. This will, in due course, affect vertical dimension

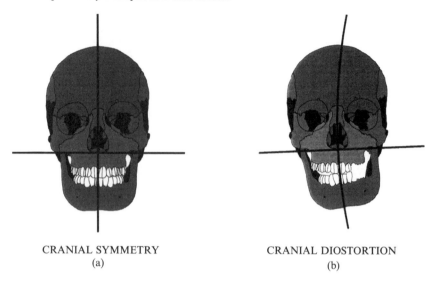

CRANIAL SYMMETRY                    CRANIAL DIOSTORTION
(a)                                (b)

**Figure 3.7** (a) Normal bite and (b) Abnormal bite

as well as causing spasm of the lateral and mesial pterygoid muscles, creating a possible malocclusion.

As a result of these changes, one tooth will contact prematurely and over a period of time cause damage to the cusps that contact one another. This, in turn, may cause either a tooth to crack or become loosened in the alveolus, resulting in possible extraction. A loss of dentition requires rehabilitative measures either in the form of crown and bridgework or implants.

Loss of posterior support may occur as a result of tooth loss. The teeth on either side of the space collapse towards one another, creating a loss of vertical and overclosing, causing damage to the retrodiscal tissue area and a jamming of the temporal bone which, again, forces a malocclusion. These types of malocclusion will affect the anterior pivot at the maxillae-sphenoid junction. As this is a major area of cause, it needs to be addressed prior to any changes made to the cranial vault (*Figures 3.8* and *3.9*).

**Descending stress major**

The malocclusions described affect the anterior pivot which in turn affects the sphenoid, then the sphenobasilar synchondrosis and, because of the torsion on the posterior pivot, it ultimately affects the occipital-sacral pump mechanism. Once the sacrum is disturbed and becomes distorted, the ilia on both sides will distort and produce a bilateral sacroiliac fixation which will ultimately degenerate into a sacroiliac lesion followed by a discogenic breakdown at the lumbar-sacral junction. Dr J. P. Meersseman defines the malocclusion, unstable occlusion or temporomandibular joint dysfunction as a primary descending stress major.

The treatment plan, as far as the dental malocclusion is concerned, has to be assessed for incisal interference, loss of dentition, premature contact and

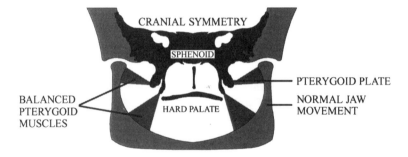

**Figure 3.8** Normal bite

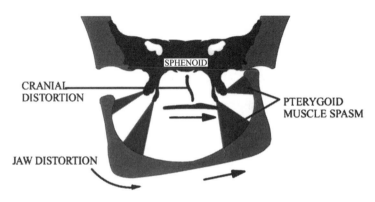

**Figure 3.9** Abnormal bite

loss of vertical on the merits of what will create a normal occlusal contact between the teeth of the maxilla and the teeth of the mandible. The muscles of the cranium need to relax and become bilaterally equilibrated. This can be done by use of a Tanner appliance (made of hard acrylic) on which the maxillae may slide across the mandible without any fixed reference point.

If the temporomandibular joint is disturbed and the articular disc is clicking or locking, then a Stack appliance can be used to try and recapture the disc. A Stack appliance will bring the mandible forward, and increase the vertical by increasing the distance between the condylar head of the mandible and the glenoid fossa of the temporal bone.

Once a point of equilibration has been reached, a second and third stage of treatment may be looked at. Overlays may be used on some of the posterior teeth in order to increase the vertical while allowing the unencumbered teeth to erupt higher and maintain that vertical. In due course the overlays from the original teeth may be removed so that the original teeth may supererupt up to the new occlusal point.

Distorted patterns within the maxillae may mean that expansion of the maxillae is required. An orthopaedic appliance may need to be used in order to remove any torquing, side-bending, torsion or distorted pattern that has appeared as a result of long-standing malocclusion or anterior or posterior pivot involvement. Once the orthopaedic appliances have made the required changes, orthodontic appliances can be used to bring the teeth into a balanced position, thereby keystoning each arch in order to ensure that retention is maintained. Later, a retainer can be used to ensure that there is retention. Where there is lack of dentition, implants or bridgework can be applied in order to ensure that the upper and lower jaw have their full complement of teeth or at least that the surfaces come into contact equally on both sides without any interference at the incisal junction.

While this dental treatment is in progress it is imperative that the pelvis is balanced, and that the sacroiliac joints move in a normal cyclic motion without any interference or lesion at the auricular boot. There must be total freedom at the lumbar-sacral junction and the spine must be subluxation free. In order to enhance orthopaedic and orthodontic appliance treatment, it is important for the craniopath to ensure that the cranial sutures are at all times free, movable and uninhibited. Posturally the pelvis, diaphragm, shoulder girdle and cranial base need to be horizontal and level. If at any time these levels are not maintained, especially when a patient is in fixed upper appliances whereby the maxillae will be jammed together, distorted patterns can take place lower down in the spine.

It has been suggested by John Upledger, author of 'Craniosacral Therapy',[4] that fixed appliances across the mid-line of the maxillae can and will cause a scoliosis in pubescent children when one maxillae is fixed in internal rotation and the other fixed in external rotation. In other words the cranial base is disturbed and fixed at an abnormal level, creating a compensation and an adaptation through the shoulders into the diaphragm and into the pelvic girdle.

## Signs and symptoms of temporomandibular dysfunction

The aetiology of temporomandibular dysfunction can be either a pelvic problem, a cranial problem or a dental/cranial problem. They can produce a wide range of seemingly unrelated symptoms. For clarity, these symptoms will be discussed below, in relation to various anatomical sites.

### The eyes

Common symptoms are pain behind the eyes, bloodshot eyes, bulging eyes, sensitivity to light, photophobia and visual disturbances.

Pterygoid muscle spasms on the pterygoid plates of the sphenoid bone will disrupt and change the position of the lesser wing of the sphenoid affecting the superior orbital fissure. This may affect cranial nerves III, IV and the ophthalmic division of V and nerve VI. The optic nerve will also be affected through the optic canal.

Pterygoid muscle spasms may constrict the maxillary artery which passes between the superior and inferior heads of this muscle. Constriction of the maxillary artery results in a reduced blood supply to the orbit and subsequent visual disturbances. The visual aura preceding a migraine may be caused in this way.

**The jaw**

Jaw symptoms include clicking and popping of the jaw joint, pain in the cheek muscles, and uncontrollable jaw and tongue movement.

The mandible will become distorted in relation to the maxillae through premature contact, incisal interference or loss of vertical. This affects the relationship of the condyle within the glenoid fossa, the articular disc, the retrodiscal tissue area and the articular eminence.

The muscles controlling jaw movement will be under strain, leading to uncontrolled movement and/or spasm. Spasm will result in pain in the muscles and/or referred pain to areas such as the cheek.

**The head**

Headaches can take the form of frontal, temporal, parietal and occipital.

The temporalis muscle inserts into the periosteum of the cranium. This area of the skull will be affected by temporalis muscle spasm pulling on the periosteum and tightening the sutures. Sutural jamming affects the endosteal dura and will ultimately affect venous drainage which may create pockets of hydrostatic pressure change in the cerebrospinal fluid within the cranium.

**The face**

Symptoms include facial neuralgia, tic doloreaux and Bell's palsy.

Changes at the mandibular condyle/glenoid fossa of the temporal bone may change the internal acoustic meatus which carries the facial nerve (VII) and the vestibular cochlear nerve (VIII). This will affect facial muscles, facial function, closing and opening of the eyelids, hearing, balance and cause loss of function to the semicircular canals and ossicles of the ear.

**The throat**

Symptoms include swallowing difficulties, hoarseness, laryngitis, voice irregularities, constant clearing of throat, coughing, and the persistent feeling of a foreign object in throat.

The retruded mandible will change the tone of the digastric, geniohyoid, mylohyoid and sternomastoid muscles affecting the oesophagus, trachea, larynx and pharynx.

**The neck**

Symptoms includes stiffness, muscle spasms, shoulder girdle and upper trapezius pain and paraesthesia into the arm and fingers.

These signs and symptoms will arise as a result of the loss of lordosis in the cervical spine, particularly C3/C4/C5, creating irritability of the brachial nerve plexus and changes of the trapezius and sternocleidomastoid muscles (SCM). Changes at the occiput can affect the jugular foramen through which passes the vagus, the glossopharyngeal and spinal accessory nerves. The spinal accessory nerves innovate the upper trapezius and the SCM.

Changes in the SCM and trapezius affect latissimus dorsi which can stretch the brachial nerve distribution into the arm and finger, resulting in paraesthesia of this area.

### The teeth

Changes in the maxillae and mandibular create occlusal changes that will alter the lines of force through the teeth, producing damage to the cusps. Premature contact results in compounding pressure into the alveolus around one tooth and loosening, with possible loss of the tooth.

## An interdisciplinary approach to treatment

The interdisciplinary collaboration between a dentist/orthodonist and a chiropractic craniopath indicates that with a good working relationship between the two disciplines the required results can be achieved.

When looking at skeletal balance it is vital to ensure that the arches of both feet are supported properly and that there is no pronation or supination of the feet. If this is not corrected by stabilizing the pelvis, a third discipline, in the form of a podiatrist, will be required to assess the feet and prescribe the correct orthotics to support the arch which in turn will support the pelvis and consequently support the cranium.

Many patients who require cranial/dental treatment have, as a result of this condition, become exhausted and run down. Their energy level is low, their diet is sometimes harmful and, because of the pain and discomfort, their medication level has been high. Nutritional supervision is needed, particularly in the early stages, to allow the body to re-establish some stability.

Nutrition in the form of enzymes, minerals and vitamins are essential in order to support the body physiologically while the structural changes are being made. Reduction of analgesics and anti-inflammatory drugs must be stressed and guidance on good nutrition needs to be emphasized. These patients are usually frequent coffee drinkers, with high levels of chocolate and sugar intake, artificially stimulating the adrenals and overloading the pancreas.

## Conclusion

An attempt has been made to demonstrate a need for an integrated interdisciplinary relationship between chiropractor and dentist. The aetiology of a problem can then be defined and diagnosed early, so that the correct treatment can be applied.

While the cranium is influenced by pelvic distortions, dental malocclusions can also influence the pelvis. Pelvic and cranial distortions are commonplace among the patients of cranial chiropractors, but a dental malocclusion will not automatically be balanced by chiropractic treatment. However, stabilization of the cranium may produce muscular changes which affect the mandible in its relationship with the maxillae.

Conversely, correction of the malocclusion by a dentist will produce stabilization of the cranium but not necessarily have an effect on pelvic distortion. It is therefore important that a cohesive treatment plan be structured to incorporate a balance between the pelvis and cranium and the occlusion and cranium.

A descending major stress area is a primary dental problem requiring a chiropractic back-up to ensure a return to biomechanical stability. An ascending major stress area is a primary chiropractic problem requiring dental back-up to ensure that premature contacts of teeth, loss of dentition and incisal interference can be monitored while the sacroiliac lesion is stabilized.

The number of patients presenting with obscure, unusual and apparently unrelated symptoms not responsive to conventional medical tests is on the increase. A logical conclusion to this state of affairs, despite our sophisticated technology, is the iatrogenic effects of dental extractions. Their long-term effect is exhaustion of the body from a structural standpoint. This chronically lowers the immune system and culminates in pathophysiology and a breakdown in homeostasis. These problems cannot be resolved by a conventional medical or dental approach. An understanding of the effects that structural instabilities have on the nervous system and their mimicking symptomatic pictures is essential.

It is inherent in these new holistic, multidisciplinary treatments to address all the issues and challenge aesthetic irrationality for a rational functional protocol. These groups with the knowledge of dynamic structural change must persevere regardless of criticism, to influence orthodox thought for the benefit of all our patients in the twenty-first century.

# References

1  Strang V V. *Essential Principles of Chiropractic*. Davonport, Iowa: Palmer College, 1984.
2  Smith G. *Cranial Dental Sacral Complex*. Newton, Pennsylvania, Gerald Smith, 1983.
3  Retzlaff E W, Mitchell F L Jnr. *The Cranium and its Sutures*. New York: Springer-Verlag, 1987
4  Upledger J, Vredevoogd J D. *Craniosacral Therapy*. Seattle: Eastland Press, 1983.

# Bibliography

Bevelander G. *Essentials of Histology*, 5th edn. St Louis: C V Mosby Co, 1965.
Breig A. *Adverse Mechanical Tension in the Central Nervous System*. John Wiley & Sons, 1978.
Brookes D. *Lectures on Cranial Osteopathy*. Wellingborough: Thorsons Publishing, 1981.
Buddingh C C. *Sphenomaxillary Craniopathy*. Los Angeles, CA: Woodland Hill, 1988.
Clemente C D. *Regional Atlas of Human Body*, 3rd edn. Baltimore, MD: Urban & Schwarzenberg, 1987.
DeJarnette B. *Cranial Technique*. Nebraska: DeJarnette, 1979.
DeJarnette B. *Sacro Occipital Technique*. Nebraska: DeJarnette, 1979.
DeJarnette B. *Sacro Occipital Technique*, 3rd edn. Nebraska: DeJarnette, 1984.
Denton D G. *Craniopathy & Dentistry*. Los Angeles, CA: David Denton, 1979.
Enlow D H. *Facial Growth*, 3rd edn. Philadelphia: W B Saunders & Co, 1990.

Ferreri C, Wainwright R. *Breakthrough for Dyslexia Learning Disabilities*. Pompano Beach, FL: Exposition Press, 1984.

Fonder A C. *Dental Physician*. Rock Falls, Illinois: Medical-Dental Arts, 1985.

Fonder A C. *Dental Distress Syndrome*. Rock Falls, Illinois: Medical-Dental Arts, 1990.

Gelb H. *Clinical Management of Head, Neck and TMJ Pain and Dysfunction*. Philadelphia: W B Saunders & Co, 1985.

Gray H. *Gray's Anatomy*, 28th edn. Philadelphia, NJ: Lea & Febiger.

Guyton A C. *Neuroscience – Basic Anatomy and Physiology*, 2nd edn. Philadelphia: W B Saunders & Co. 1987.

Howat A P, Capp N J, Barrett N V J. *Colour Atlas of Occlusions & Malocclusions*, Aylesbury: Wolfe Publishing 1991.

Kraus S L. *TMJ Disorders: Management of the Craniomandibular Complex*. Edinburgh: Churchill Livingstone, 1988.

McCatty R R. *Essentials of Craniosacral Osteopathy*. Bath: Ashgrove Press, 1988.

Magoun H I. *Osteopathy in the Cranial Field*, 3rd edn. Kirksville, Missouri: The Journal Printing Co, 1976.

Netter F H. *The CIBA Collection of Medical Illustrations*, Vol. I; *Part 2: Neurological and Neuromuscular Disorders*. West Caldwell, NJ: CIBA, 1986.

Rees M L. *The Art and Practice of Chiropractic*. Newton, Pennsylvania: M L Rees, 1984.

Smith G. *Cranial Dental Sacral Complex*. Newton, Pennsylvania: Gerald Smith, 1983.

Snell R S. *Clinical Neuro Anatomy for Medical Students*. Boston, Massachusetts: Little, Brown & Co, 1978.

Strang V V, *Essential Principles of Chiropractic*. Davenport, Iowa: Palmer College, 1984.

Upledger J, Vredevoogd J D. *Craniosacral Therapy*. Seattle: Eastland Press, 1983.

Upledger J. *Craniosacral Therapy II. Beyond the Dura*. Seattle: Eastland Press, 1987.

Walther D S. *Applied Kinesiology*, Vol. II: *Head, Neck and Jaw Pain and Dysfunction – The Stomatognathic System*. Pueblo, Colorada: Systems DC, 1983.

Wilson-Pauwels L, Akesson E, Stewart P. *Cranial Nerves – Anatomy and Clinical Comments*. Philadelphia: B C. Decker Inc, 1988.

Witzig J W, Spahl T J. *The Clinical Management of Basic Maxillofacial Orthopedic*. St Louis: Mosby Year Book Inc, 1991.

# Associations

International Chiropractors' Association
Suite 1000
1110 Glebe Road
Arlington
Virginia 22201
USA
Tel: 001 703 528 5000
Fax: 001 703 528 5023

American Chiropractic Association
1701 Clarendon Boulevade
Arlington
Virginia 22209
USA
Tel: 001 703 276 8800
Fax: 001 703 243 2593

World Federation of Chiropractic
78 Glencairn Avenue
Toronto
Ontario M4R 1M8
Canada
Tel: 001 416 484 9601
Fax: 001 416 484 9665

European Chiropractic Union
9 Cross Deep Gardens
Twickenham
Middlesex TW1 4QZ
UK
Tel: 0181 891 2546
Fax: 0181 744 2902

British Chiropractic Association
Equity House
29 Whitely Street
Reading RG2 0E9
UK
Tel: 0118 975 7557
Fax: 0118 975 7257

Chiropractors' Association of Australia
PO Box 241
Springwood
NSW 2777
Australia
Tel: 00 614 751 5644
Fax: 00 614 751 585

# Courses

Information on general chiropractic courses can be obtained from the organizations listed above. For information on the courses and seminars on the sacro-occipital technique, contact one of the chiropractic organizations listed below which specialize in the that method.

SOTO Europe
3 Sittingbourne Road
Maidstone
Kent ME14 5ES
Tel: 01622 661883
Fax: 01622 671611

SORSI
Sacro-Occipital Research Society
  International
P.O. Box 8245
Prairie Village
Kansas 66208
USA
Tel: 001 913 649 3475
Fax: 001 913 649 2676

Pacific Asia Association of Chiropractic
  (PAAC)
6th Floor, Yamanote Bld
Higashi-kan 1-19-12
Minami Ikebukuro
Toshima-ku, Tokyo 171
Japan
Tel: 0081 339 88 0704
Fax: 0081 339 86 1297

SOTO Australasia
PO Box 5346
SCMC
Nambour
Queensland 4560
Australia
Tel: 0061 7 5476 1122
Fax: 0061 7 5476 1129

### *SOT Education – Module Series*

Modules 1 and 2. Basic Sacro-Occipital Technique
Module 3. Anatomy and Physiology of SOT
Module 4. Extremities
Module 5. Chiropractic Manipulative Reflex Technique – Visceral and Soft
          Tissue
Module 6. Introduction to TMJ Cranial Ranges of Motion Sutural Work
Module 7. Cranial Dental Sacral Complex
Module 8. Intraoral Specifics
Module 9. Cranial Specifics and Non-specifics

# Cranial osteopathy

**Richard Holding**

## Introduction

The temporomandibular joint (TMJ) has a surprising fascination for many different therapists, both orthodox and complementary. Dentists could be said to have first claim to the area, but osteopaths and chiropractors have shown interest in the TMJ for some time. This is because its function has such an enormous influence on the whole posture of the patient from the feet to the cranium.

There are many important acupuncture points in the area of the TMJ so its function is also of interest to acupuncturists. George Eversaul[1] noted that each tooth has a relationship to an acupuncture meridian and this in turn gives a relationship to both muscle and organ function throughout the whole body (see *Table 10.1*). The TMJ is also of interest to practitioners of biofeedback and psychotherapy, since the masseter muscle is well known for maintaining its level of tension following any emotional trauma long after ordinary muscles have relaxed.[2]

None of these disciplines can have quite the same interdependence and mutual interest than that of the two disciplines of cranial osteopathy and dentistry. The necessary but slight motion in the cranium means that the articulation of the temporal bone and the condyle of the mandible are in motion. The maxillae and the mandible and hence the maxillary teeth and the mandibular teeth are also in motion.

The idea that the mandible is articulating with a moving glenoid fossa may be an unnerving concept for dentists. This is not the static relationship that has usually been assumed and this has far reaching applied anatomical and clinical significance.

### Development of the cranial approach

#### DR A. T. STILL

Osteopathy was founded in 1892 when Andrew Turner Still, a doctor and travelling preacher from Kirksville, Missouri, founded the American School of Osteopathy. He had lost three children through meningitis and was deeply distressed at his inability to help them with conventional medical methods. Convinced that God had given mankind the capacity to heal themselves, he began to look for ways to enable this capacity to be utilized.

Through detailed observation and palpation, he learned to use his hands as therapeutic tools. He refused to teach specific techniques and used to say that he would not teach lazy students to 'push and pull at bones'. He believed that a detailed knowledge of anatomy, combined with finely tuned palpatory skills, would enable the doctor to develop the techniques necessary to allow the body to correct itself. According to Still, osteopathy was not just bone manipulation but the law of mind, matter and motion.[3] The osteopathy that he developed was a complete system of healing rather than a branch of minor orthopaedics as it later became.

### DR W. G. SUTHERLAND

Dr William Garner Sutherland, a former journalist, was one of Dr Still's students. He asked Still, who had a disarticulated skull in his office, why the sutures were bevelled in a manner that suggested motion, if as was generally believed the cranial bones were unable to move. Sutherland then spent the next 20 years trying to find the answer to this question. In order to do so, he had to acquire an understanding of the function of the anatomical structure and physiology of the whole body. This is as important as the applied anatomy and physiology of the cranial bones themselves.

By using techniques such as compression bandages to limit sutural movement, he became confident that the cranial bones were designed for motion. He then developed techniques to evaluate and correct any restrictions in cranial bone motion. As he came to understand what causes the motion in the cranial bones, he was able to develop his approach further to include dural and cerebrospinal fluid techniques.

Interestingly, there are only two accounts of the way that Still actually treated. One is in the 'History of Osteopathy' by Dr Booth and the other in 'Contributions of Thought' by Sutherland. The latter description is as follows:

*In technique we endeavour to follow Dr Still's methods. That is, getting the point of release with no jerking and then allowing the natural agencies to return the bones to their normal relations and positions. What are the natural agencies? The ligaments, not the muscles are the natural agencies for the purpose of correcting the relations and positions of joints. Dr Still's application of the technique is the gentle exaggeration of the lesion that allows the natural agencies to draw the bones into place. Dr Still has taken my hand in his and allowed me to feel the lesion as it was being exaggerated and then as the natural agencies pulled the bones back into place. There is reason for applying that technique in the cranial mechanism. The difference between spinal technique and cranial technique is like the difference between an automobile mechanic and a watch maker. We do not force anything into place in the reduction of the lesion. We have something more potent than our own forces working always in the patient towards the direction of the normal.*[4]

Since there are no muscular agencies between the bones of the skull, the question 'How did the cranium move?' took Sutherland into another area of study – the dura mater. The dura mater is described as a continuous sheet that covers the outside of the brain and spinal cord, blending with the outermost layer of the periosteum of the cranial bones. Internally there are three sickle-shaped invaginations of the dura that meet together in the area of the junction of the straight sinus. These sickles are the two tentorium cerebelli and the mid-line falx cerebri. Taking a look at the whole cranial-sacral inelastic dura as a totally interconnected mechanism where if one part moved, everthing moved, he was able to explain the changes in bevel in the sutural articulations in terms of applied anatomy. He was then able to describe the changes in the shape of the skull that could be expected from these changes in sutural bevel. This inelastic dural membrane that joined the cranial bones and the cranium to the sacrum he called the *reciprocal tension membrane* – 'a structure that moves the cranial articular mechanism *to* and *fro* between two distinct positions that result in two distinct shapes of the cranium'.[5]

These two shapes he called *flexion* and *extension* and he postulated that the whole movement took place around an automatic shifting suspended fulcrum in the area of the straight sinus – the junction of the falx and the tentorium. He still did not have an agency for the motion and as his palpatory skills developed and his capacity to 'see' what was happening under his fingers, what he would eventually call his 'feeling, seeing, knowing fingers',[6] he was able to discern a fluctuation type of motion in the cranium as distinct from the to and fro motion of the dura. This he called the *fluctuation of the cerebrospinal fluid*. This fluctuation is the direct result of the motility of the central nervous system.

So now Sutherland had the basis of a new anatomical physiological system of cranial motion. This included:

- a fluctuation movement of the cerebrospinal fluid;
- the to-and-fro movement of the reciprocal tension of the dural membranes;
- motility in the brain;
- minute movement of the 22 cranial bones and the sacrum between the ilea.

What was left was to find out how clinically relevant this movement was and how it could be utilized in the treatment of people's health problems.

After 20 years of research he was able to demonstrate that the craniosacral mechanism's motion was not just clinically important but vitally important to the proper functioning of the individual's physiology. The motion was shown to have the following characteristics:

- it is involuntary;
- it has a respiratory function;
- it has a lubricating function to the whole spinal cord;
- it controls venous return in the skull;
- it provides drainage and balance to the orbit eight bones;
- it is independent of thoracic respiratory motion;
- it is independent of arterial fluctuation.

**DR R. BECKER**

The next main influence on osteopathic development in the cranial field was Dr Rollin Becker. Becker was a pupil of Sutherland and specially trained by him. After Sutherland's death, Becker continued to teach and develop the approach. He was particularly interested in the therapeutic benefit of stillness and in the way that it enables the tissues to reorganize themselves in the most efficient pattern possible. I was privileged to have my first cranial course with Dr Becker and to teach with him on several subsequent courses.

**OTHER INFLUENCES**

A list of those instrumental in developing the craniosacral approach and influential on my own research and development must also include Dr Anne Wales, who helped me to understand the principles of reciprocal tension of the dural membranes; Dr Harold Magoun, who wrote the first textbook and taught us the power of observation; and Dr Robert Fulford, who introduced me to the 'energetics' of the system and from whom I first heard of Dr George Goodheart, the founder of applied kinesiology.

Gradually, their gentle approach began to attract others. Initially the therapists that studied under Sutherland were all osteopaths. Through the results that they got with the patients, dentists soon became interested and started to train with him. In fact, ever since, dentists have made up a significant percentage of the students of this approach. Today there is a keen nucleus of osteopaths in the USA and Europe who use only this approach, whereas others combine cranial and manipulative techniques, depending on the patient's problem. Since 1987 I have been teaching chiropractors in the USA and we now have a faculty of chiropractors there using and teaching this approach. Similarly in Sweden I have been teaching varied therapists (naturopaths and osteopaths) the cranial approach since 1991 and a faculty is developing there also.

**FURTHER DEVELOPMENT**

After 10 years with the cranial approach, I became interested in the effect of the dental occlusion on cranial motion and began to do dental courses to understand the biomechanics of the TMJ. One of these was a course in dental kinesiology given by Dr George Eversaul. This was the first time that I was exposed to muscle testing and to the chiropractic 'hard-handed' approach to the craniosacral system. Applied kinesiology made me realize that nutrition was important for the functioning of the craniosacral system. It was not until I was introduced to clinical kinesiology that I really began to further my understanding of the craniosacral system. Over the last few years I have developed treatment procedures in clinical kinesiology which have expanded our understanding of the craniosacral system, and these procedures within that system are as a result much more efficient. More recently, an evaluation of the fundamental principles of traditional Chinese medicine has enabled the treatment procedures within the craniosacral system to be refined still further.

### Skills required in cranial therapy

Sutherland emphasized that osteopathy, with its cranial approach, is a science, not a therapy. It 'is a science that deals with the natural forces of the body'.[7] The basic skills that we need to learn are not a collection of techniques but those in the following paragraphs.

#### RIGHT AND LEFT BRAIN AWARENESS

One of the skills needed by practitioners using the craniosacral approach is the integration of right and left brain awareness. Those people who are right brain dominant rely on their intuition to tell them what is happening under their hands. Those who are left brain dominant tend to learn this approach through the analytical and systematic application of anatomy and physiology. Unfortunately, the use of either of these approaches to the exclusion of the other will not allow the real beauty of this way of working to be appreciated. One needs to understand the inherent simplicity of its action and the complexity of its manifestation in the tissues of the body. The predominantly right-brained practitioner tends to fall into a pattern of 'windscreen wiping', treating every patient in the same way and missing important clues as to how the body is best able to unravel its stress patterns. The predominantly left-brained practitioner will usually find that his mind tends to interfere with his proprioceptive awareness, restricting his ability to read the sensory data from the tissues. The optimum way of learning this approach is to use both right and left brain to develop 'thinking, feeling, seeing, knowing fingers'[8] which, according to Sutherland, is the way to obtain knowledge, rather than information.[9]

#### GENTLE TOUCH

The usual osteopathic approach is to take a firm grasp on the body to 'work our way to the bone'. This is the exact opposite of what we need in this work. Our touch should be very light and gentle. In fact the more gentle the touch, the less invasive we are and the more the tissues under our hands are able to demonstrate what they wish to do. If we apply too great a pressure, then the system locks up and we feel nothing. So always place your hands *gently* on the patient's body, make contact with the tissue, then back off slightly to be sure that you are not interfering with the motion of the craniosacral mechanism. As Sutherland used to say, you should alight like a bird onto a branch: 'Finger contacts should be *firm* and *gentle*, applied like the bird's digits in contacting the bark of a twig on a tree – alighting gently and gradually increasing firmness without injury to the bark.'[10]

#### PROPRIOCEPTIVE AWARENESS

When we touch things we activate the touch fibres of the central nervous system. In order to work with the craniosacral system we need to use the nerve fibres associated with our sense of awareness of position in space, i.e. the proprioceptive nerve fibres. This means that we are able to experience not only the motion of the tissues under our hands, but also to differentiate distinct directional components within the craniosacral system, allowing us to analyse accurately what is happening within the body. An individual used to operating a mechanical digger can 'feel' the hardness of the ground through the metal bucket and up to his controls. Our hands should operate as listening posts so that we are able to read what is happening under them.

### ANATOMICAL VISUALIZATION AND AWARENESS OF NORMAL FUNCTION

The ability to visualize the anatomy is essential. Because of the continuity of the fascia and reciprocal tension of the dural membranes, it is possible to project our awareness to different parts of the body. The more one works with the craniosacral mechanism, the more tuned one becomes to the levels of kinetic dysfunction throughout the body. When normal anatomy is understood, we can detect conditions that are abnormal.[11]

### DEVELOPMENT OF SENSOR MOTOR SKILLS AND THE USE OF FULCRA

In practice, one of the most important skills is to be able to move automatically with the tissues, in direct response to their motion, rather than having to go through the agency of the conscious awareness. That is not to say that the motion should not be analysed by the conscious mind at the same time in order to decide where to provide a fulcrum for change in the tissues.[12] The creation of a fulcrum, e.g. with our hands or elbows, enables us to project our awareness more accurately. Dr Rollin Becker says it helps us to 'think our way in'. By adding light compression to the fulcrum, one's proprioceptive awareness will remain relatively superficial. The more compression that is added to the fulcrum, the deeper one's projected awareness will go.

### PATIENCE

It can take a long time to develop these skills.

# Motion

One of the first things that we were taught in biology was that motion characterizes life. However, it was soon forgotten in our anatomy classes, where we learned by examining the dead, rather than living bodies in motion.

It is important to recognize that there are two types of motion working independently but concurrently in the body – voluntary and involuntary motion.

## Voluntary motion

Voluntary motion is the motion with which we are most familiar. We often utilize it at a subconscious level in our corrections or at a conscious level when we do muscle work. There are several ways of utilizing voluntary motion and several structural therapies have been developed based on these:

- exercise: movement by the patient with no intervention by the therapist.
- muscle energy technique: movement by the patient with guidance by the therapist.
- long lever articulation: therapist moves the joint with no involvement from the patient.
- ligamentous articular release technique: therapist moves the joint with movement by and respiratory co-operation from the patient.

## Involuntary motion

Involuntary motion is not under our conscious control. It is a driving force for normalization in the tissues. The characteristic of this motion is that it has only one pattern of expression in which all structures move rhythmically and alternately into expansion then recession. In expansion, all mid-line structures flex and all bilateral structures rotate externally, whereas in recession all mid-line structures extend and all bilateral structures rotate internally. The overall motion is one of the rhythmic shortening and widening of the whole body in the expansion phase, followed by a rhythmic lengthening and narrowing of the whole body in the recession phase.

This involuntary motion, which is the motion of the primary respiratory mechanism, operates throughout life, starting in the early stages of fetal development until the death process. This phased motion occurs 10–12 times a minute and is called the cranial rhythmic impulse (CRI). The CRI is accelerated by fever and slowed down by infection, trauma and drugs. Dr Viola Frymann was able to show quite clearly that craniosacral motion is distinctly separate from respiratory motion and the arterial pulse and that it oscillates between 7 and 14 expansion and recession cycles per minute.[13]

Although the craniosacral motion is slight, Frymann was able to measure the movement to be between 0.0005 and 0.001 in (0.013 and 0.03 mm).[13] Sutherland had to develop new ways of working with this motion to evaluate and increase its function. Nearly a century later, we are still continuing to expand on Sutherland's work to develop our understanding of this fundamental respiratory motion and to understand how it affects all malfunctioning and pathological states in the body.

### PHYSIOLOGICAL EFFECTS OF INVOLUNTARY MOTION IN THE TISSUES

There are at least three different ways that this involuntary motion affects the tissues:

- it acts as a very powerful hydraulic system that initiates fluid-balanced interchange between all the tissues of the body;
- it has a lubricating function, which enables the tissue to protect itself against stress and trauma;
- the involuntary motion of the primary respiratory mechanism is the primary energetic system of the body – the level of activation of other energetic systems, e.g. subtle body energy and Qi energy, is dependent on it.

## The primary respiratory mechanism

The craniosacral system is the primary respiratory mechanism of the body. Physiologically it is *the highest known element* in that it carries 'the breath of Life' into the tissues.[14] Sutherland distinguished 'the breath of Life' from 'the breath of air', describing the former as 'the spark' and the latter as 'merely one of the material elements that the "breath of Life" utilizes in man's walkabout here on earth'.[15]

---

HEALTH : DISEASE

- WHAT IS HEALTH?
- maximum capacity to resist trauma and disease
- to be fully functioning in all planes of being
- to be fully open to all experiences
- to be fully open to change

- WHAT IS DISEASE?
- a reminder?
- a lack of motion in all or part of the person
- a lack of integration of HEAVEN–MAN–EARTH

---

OPTIMUM HEALTH

- The natural state is an integrated state of optimum health
- Optimum health can be read in terms of freedom of motion in all areas of being

---

Careful balancing of the primary respiratory mechanism will correct unwanted adaptation to stress, trauma and disease. Dr Rollin Becker[16] said of adaptation that 'we have a way of reading the microlevel of motion in the tissues and therefore we are able to assess the kinetic patterns of dysfunction that the tissue's adaptation has accepted'. The more efficiently the primary respiratory mechanism functions, the more the body is able to resist trauma and disease in the future.

Although Sutherland always stressed that the primary respiratory mechanism was a unit of function, he recognized that it is easier to understand if it is broken down into four constituent parts of CSF, dura, brain and bones. Since osteopathy meant 'starting with the bones', he always taught the bones first, then the dura, then the cerebrospinal fluid, then the central nervous system. Much later he admitted that the constituent parts have a hierarchy of function, which he listed in the following order:[17]

- the fluctuation of the cerebrospinal fluid;
- the reciprocal tension of the dural membranes;
- the motility of the brain and spinal cord;
- the mobility of the 22 cranial bones and the sacrum between the ilia.

**Fluctuation of the cerebrospinal fluid**

An understanding of the potency inherent within the fluctuation of the cerebrospinal fluid (CSF) is central to the cranial osteopathic approach. Sutherland found quite early on in his research that the CSF fluctuates in a rhythmic fashion. He considered that this fluctuation was extremely important to physiology in that it provided a driving force towards normal function. This fluctuation could be harnessed internally by the homeostatic mechanisms of the body and externally by the physician to achieve homeostasis.

It is possible to use the dural membranes to induce balance in tissues or even use the bones as levers to initiate change, but the effects on the physiology of the body as a whole are totally insignificant compared to the effect of utilizing the innate potency of the CSF. It is not clear how Sutherland came to understand how to utilize the potency of the CSF. The philosophical basis had already come from Still, who describes it in the following way:

*The cerebro-spinal fluid is the highest known element in the human body, and unless the brain furnishes this fluid in abundance a disabled condition of the body will remain';*[18] *and 'He who is able to reason must see that this great river of life must be tapped and the withering fields irrigated at once or the harvest of health will be forever lost.*[18]

Creating a state of stillness in the CSF is one of the keys to its management. We can only assume that Sutherland came to understand the biomechanics and healing potential of the CSF through observation and direct experience of the way that the body corrects itself. This was probably the same way that Still formulated the original philosophy of osteopathy. Sutherland observed that one way in which the body's physiological system initiates change is by inducing stillness in the tissue. Then he began to develop techniques to help the body to find stillness.

---

**CSF FLUCTUATION**

STILLNESS

⇩

FLUID BALANCED
INTERCHANGE

⇩

ACTIVATES INNATE POTENCY
TOWARDS NORMAL IN
STRUCTURE AND FUNCTION

---

By causing the CSF to cease fluctuating, the master fulcrum will then change, and the CSF will re-establish itself as a more potent and powerful balancing force. If the CSF fluctuation is abnormal, it will cause abnormal fluid balance between all the tissues.[19] The adaptation of the tissues to inadequate CSF fluctuation leads to subclinical malfunction. It is as though the CSF is not able to penetrate these tissues so that on palpation they feel starved or 'dead'. By balancing the CSF fluctuation, the tissue's innate potency for self-healing is activated so that it is able to reverse these changes.

This utilization of the body's natural search for stillness is a wonderful discovery and healing tool. Dr J. Upledger makes the point that the most effective forms of treatment are those that follow the pattern the body adopts to correct itself:

Nature makes the best designs. Every design in nature is for a purpose and is the most efficient way to accomplish a task. We should study the way nature does things and try to emulate it, rather than clumsily and egotistically try to invent our own. We cannot improve on natural design; we need only to understand it.[20]

### The reciprocal tension of the dural membranes

The dural membranes are a tough and inelastic sheath for the whole brain and spinal cord. The concept of reciprocal tension can be likened to the operation of a mobile; when one part moves, the remaining parts will shift to adapt to this change.

Reciprocal tension is made possible by the inner layer of the cranial dura forming three sickle-shaped membranes called the falx cerebri (the mid-line membrane) and the two tentorium cerebelli (the lateral membranes). Because the sickle-shaped membranes are formed by a reduplication of the dura, they are of double thickness and carry the valveless venous sinuses. The outer layer of the dura is continuous with the outer layer of the periosteum covering the cranial bones. Embryologically they develop as different layers, but for practical purposes they appear to be the same layer. The significance of this is that if there is a shift in the functional position of the dura, then the cranial bones *en masse* have to move also. This is why Becker says that the bones 'go for the ride'.

These three sickles are united in the area of the straight sinus, a common junction or fulcrum point for the operation of the reciprocal tension. This fulcrum is called the 'master fulcrum'. From a functional point of view, this master fulcrum attempts to resolve all the adaptation to stress induced by any pathological fulcra in the body. Therefore when the master fulcrum is no longer able to adapt to the demands made on it, the efficiency of the primary respiratory mechanism is seriously impaired and dysfunction and disease develop.

#### ARTICULAR POLES OF ATTACHMENT

There are six articular poles where the dura of falx cerebri and the tentorium cerebelli attach to various points inside the skull. There are two anterior articular poles: a superior and an inferior. These attach to the ethmoid bone and the clinoid processes of the sphenoid. There is a posterior inferior pole attaching to the occipital bone, two lateral poles attaching to the temporal bones and an inferior pole which attaches the spinal dural sleeve to the second sacral segment and then descends to blend with the coccygeal fascia.

It is important to be able to visualize the way that the articular poles of attachment of the reciprocal tension membrane move in different directions during the flexion and extension phases of motion.

### Flexion phase of motion

The anterior articular poles move in a posterior and inferior direction. The posterior articular pole moves in an anterior and superior direction. The lateral articular poles move medially, tipping all bilateral structures into external rotation. The skull therefore shortens in the anterior posterior plane and widens in the lateral plane.

### Extension phase of motion

The anterior articular poles move in an anterior and superior direction. The posterior articular pole moves in a posterior and slightly inferior direction. The lateral articular poles move laterally, tipping bilateral structures into internal rotation. The skull therefore lengthens in the anterior posterior plane and narrows in the lateral plane.

---

## PATTERNS VERSUS LESIONS

- PATTERN
  - ARRANGEMENT OF FORCES THAT CAN ADAPT TO AN ADDED FORCE

  - a dynamic answer

- LESION
  - ARRANGEMENT OF FORCES THAT CANNOT ADAPT TO AN ADDED FORCE

  - a static answer

---

CRANIAL PATTERNS OF MOVEMENT

In optimum health, the capacity of the craniosacral mechanism for flexion and external rotation, and extension and internal rotation, is evenly balanced. If, however, the craniosacral system has had to adapt to trauma or disease, the master fulcrum is likely to be limited in function and the reciprocal tension of the dural membranes will express itself in one or more of the following patterns (1–6).

*1. Exaggerated flexion*

All quadrants are held in external rotation.

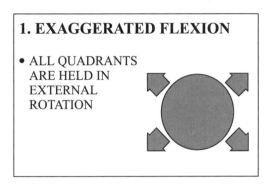

*2. Exaggerated extension*

All quadrants are held in internal rotation.

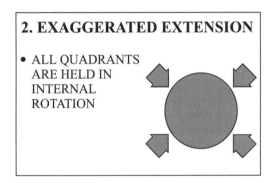

*3. Side-bending rotation or 'cranial bulge'*

Both quadrants on one side are held in external rotation, whereas the opposite quadrants are held in internal rotation.

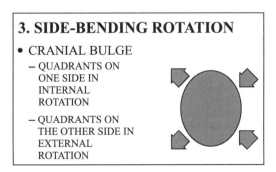

The preceeding three movements are what we call physiological constricted movements. The next three movements are pathological.

### 4. Torsion or 'cranial twist'

The anterior quadrant on one side is in internal rotation, whereas the posterior quadrant on the same side is in external rotation; on the opposite side, the anterior quadrant is in external rotation and the posterior quadrant is in internal rotation.

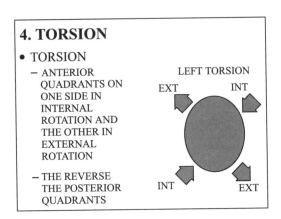

### 5. Lateral strain or 'cranial shear'

Both anterior quadrants are shifted laterally in one direction, whereas both posterior quadrants are shifted laterally in the opposite direction.

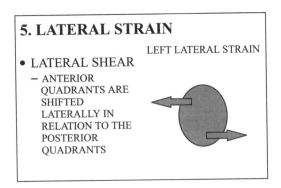

### 6. Vertical strain or 'cranial shear'

Both anterior quadrants are shifted in a superior direction, whereas both posterior quadrants are shifted in an inferior direction or vice versa.

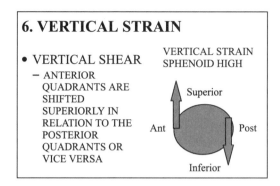

## 6. VERTICAL STRAIN

- • VERTICAL SHEAR
  - – ANTERIOR QUADRANTS ARE SHIFTED SUPERIORLY IN RELATION TO THE POSTERIOR QUADRANTS OR VICE VERSA

VERTICAL STRAIN
SPHENOID HIGH

Superior

Ant          Post

Inferior

### The motility of the brain and spinal cord

In order to understand the motility of the brain and spinal cord, it is useful to look at the brain from a mechanical view. During fetal development, the different areas of the brain grow at different rates, resulting in a coiled structure around the laminar terminalis, the embryological anterior portion of the neural tube. This coiled appearance in the adult brain can best be seen in the 'ram's horns' appearance of the lateral ventricles.

Because of this pattern of development, the brain is able to coil and uncoil in response to the fluctuation of the CSF. The coiling and uncoiling of the central nervous system is further facilitated by the fact that the brain 'sits' on a series of cisterna filled with CSF. Sutherland likened these cisterna to a series of waterbeds which cushion the brain as it expands and contracts rhythmically within the cranial vault.[21] The main cisterna are:

- • the interpenduncular cisterna under the pons and laminar terminalis;
- • the pontine cisterna under the pons and spinal cord;
- • the cisterna magna under the medulla oblongata and cerebellum;
- • the cisterna ambiens under the corpus callosum and superior cerebellum.

### The mobility of the 22 cranial bones and the sacrum

The cranial bones are divided functionally and embryologically into two types, those comprising the cranial base and those comprising the cranial vault.

#### THE CRANIAL BASE

This ossifies from a cartilaginous base. It consists of the following bones:

- • sphenoid;
- • occipital bone;
- • the cribriform plate of the ethmoid bone;
- • the petrous portion of the temporal bones.

It should be noted that all the articular poles of attachment of the dural membranes are to the cranial base. The sacrum functions as part of the cranial base, being formed in cartilage like the rest of the cranial base, and is functionally part of the cranial base through the dural attachment of the inferior pole at the second sacral segment.

### THE CRANIAL VAULT

The vault is formed in membrane, which eventually ossifies. The bones of the vault are adaptive in function and controlled by the motion in the cranial base and, because of their attachment to the dural membranes via the periosteum, they also move with the changes in the reciprocal tension membrane.

It is the movement of the cranial bones that the practitioner uses to assess and treat the various lesions, as described earlier, of exaggerated flexion, extension, vertical strain, lateral strain, etc.

In order to be able to visualize the patterns and restrictions present in the primary respiratory mechanism of your patient, it is essential to understand the anatomical interrelationship of the individual cranial bones and the sacrum. More specifically, it is necessary to look for the reasons for each change in bevel of the various bones, not just in relationship to each other but also in relation to the dural attachments, venous sinuses and cranial nerves. For this, a disarticulated skull is essential. Bassett slides (3-D dissection slides) are also very useful.

## Patterns of motion in the primary respiratory mechanism

- All the cells of the central nervous system expand simultaneously, taking in CSF. The brain therefore swells.
- Because of its spiral shape the brain coils bilaterally.
- This coiling exerts a compressive force on the inelastic dural membrane.
- The compressive force initiates an automatic shift in the master fulcrum at the straight sinus. The whole primary respiratory mechanism and the fascia move into flexion and external rotation as a result.
- The automatic shifting of the master fulcrum causes the cranial bones and sacrum to move and therefore the skull to change shape.
- As the brain expands into its inelastic dural bag, the incompressible CSF will fill the central ventricular spaces from the cisterna and the subarachnoid space.
- All the cells of the central nervous system contract simultaneously, expelling the CSF. The whole brain therefore reduces in volume.
- The brain uncoils.
- The master fulcrum shifts again causing the membranes and fascia to move into extension and internal rotation.
- Once again the cranial bones and the sacrum move causing the skull to change shape.
- The CSF moves outwards from the central ventricular system to the surrounding cisterna and subarachnoid spaces.

This rhythmic expansion and contraction of the neural tube means that the brain stem shortens and thickens towards the laminar terminalis; then it lengthens and narrows. Thus the spinal cord is raised and lowered; the cerebral hemispheres coil and uncoil; the cerebellum folds and unfolds like a pair of bellows.

## Cranial motion and the dentist

The initial fascination of cranial motion to the dentist was the complex applied anatomy of the temporal bone. Because of its intricate sutural articulations, Sutherland was able to demonstrate that it moved not just in external and internal rotation, but also medially and laterally on the petrous ridge of the occipital bone. This means that it has a sort of 'wobbly wheel' motion. The condyle of the mandible, as it moves on jaw opening, is not therefore moving in a fixed articular space. If the temporal bone is held in an asymmetrical position relative to other bones of the skull, especially the mandible, then the functional length of the muscles between these two bones will be altered and this will alter the muscle's tone.

Because of the complex interrelationship of inhibition and excitation of muscle tone between the different muscles of the stomatognathic system, this has an effect on not just the TMJ but the whole posture of the body. It is not just the muscle tone that is affected. We know that the firing sequence of the muscles in mastication is complex. If there is a change in balance between the sphenoid, temporal or parietal bones and the mandible, then the sensory engram of muscular action is impaired. This impairment occurs through changes in the proprioceptive information between the co-ordination centres in the brain and the muscles themselves and further stresses the craniosacral mechanism so a vicious circle is set up. Any appliance that bridges the maxillae will limit cranial motion and tooth extraction, especially the last molars, could possibly disrupt the functioning of the craniosacral mechanism. This meant that a lot of dentists felt the need to learn the cranial approach.

In the flexion phase of the craniosacral mechanism, the overall motion of the temporal bones will be in external rotation with the squama spreading laterally. The shift in the junction of the falx and tentorium (the fulcrum of the reciprocal tension membrane) is in an anterior and inferior direction. So the tentorium cerebelli will flatten and move in an anterior direction. The occipital bone circumducts and 'ploughs' the temporal bones apart. The basiocciput wedges the temporal bones apart, with the petrous portions being rolled in an anterior and lateral direction. The anterior portion of the temporal bone at the zygomatic process moves in an anterior and inferior direction, while the posterior portion at the mastoid tip moves in a posterior and superior direction. As the superior squamous areas move apart and broaden, the mastoid tips move medially because of the gliding action of the petrous ridge. Sutherland likened the combined effect of this tipping motion and medial lateral gliding to the action of a wobbly wheel.

In terms of the TMJ, the dentist needs to know that the condylar fossa of the temporal bone is moving both posteriorly with the overall external rotation movement and medially in the lateral expansion movement of the skull. In the internal rotation movement the reverse occurs; that is, the condylar fossa moves anteriorly as the superior margin of the squama moves posteriorly and laterally as the superior margin of the squama moves medially.

The result of this is that:

- if the functional resting position of one of the temporal bones is in internal rotation, then the mandibular condyle on that side will be held relatively anterior;
- if the opposite temporal is also in a relative rotation, then the mandible will be protruded;
- if the opposite temporal is held in relative external rotation, then the mandible on that side will be relatively posterior so it will be twisted.
- the reverse occurs in external rotation.

There is now a pattern in the cranial base that can explain the retruded and protruded mandible.

## Cranial techniques useful in dentistry

Cranial techniques can be useful to dentists before and after adjusting occlusal splints and orthodontic appliances, and also after the extraction of teeth or any other potentially traumatic application to the maxilla, mandible or surrounding bones.

### CSF techniques[22]

#### The still point technique

Sutherland described the still point as the point where the craniosacral mechanism is motionless, like a balance between two scales. 'This is the point where the mechanism is idling, neither ebbing out or flowing in, but right on the neutral point'.[23] That is why we say 'rhythmic balance interchange', for it is the period where all the fluids of the body have an interchange. Furthermore, he stressed that the still point change is not an outflow down the nerve but a transmutation in the CSF that flows into the lymphatics.[24]

In fact, all the fluid techniques use the still point as an initiation for a change towards normal. Sutherland described this as 'an unerring intracranial and intraspinal force, with the tendency towards normal as the motive power for the reduction of lesions'.

To initiate a still point through the occipital bone, **Occipital Hold 1** is used (see Appendix). The following procedure then applies:

Add slight compression to the occipital bone as it goes into its flexion phase, i.e. limit the flexion phase and exaggerate the extension phase. Continue to limit the flexion and exaggerate the extension phases until you feel that the body's physiological system has itself taken over the process. It will feel as though the extension continues to be exaggerated until all motion ceases briefly. It then starts up again with a new potency in the CSF and a new functional position in the reciprocal tension of the dural membranes, i.e. there is a new adaptability in the functional position of the master fulcrum. This is a still point. Physical signs in the patient include deeper breathing, perspiration on the forehead and heat in the occipital area.

LATERAL FLUCTUATION TECHNIQUE

This procedure is designed to exaggerate the fluctuation of the CSF, then induce a still point. This increases the potency of the CSF in situations of low energy, toxicity or trauma.

To initiate a lateral fluctuation through the temporal bones, **Occipital Hold 3** is used (see Appendix). The following procedure then applies:

With the little fingers crossed at inion and the thumbs resting on the anterior mastoid process, gently initiate one of the temporal bones into external rotation as the opposite temporal bone goes into internal rotation, and then vice versa. Repeat this procedure until, as with the still point technique, the body takes over the fluctuation of the CSF. When this occurs, gently reduce the alternating external and internal rotation, until all motion ceases and the craniosacral system goes through a still point. When the motion starts back up again, there will be a feeling of increased energy and movement in the tissues.

LONGITUDINAL FLUCTUATION TECHNIQUE

When neurological control over a particular area has been lost, this technique can be used to bring that area back into phase coherence with the rest of the body.

To induce a longitudinal fluctuation through the temporal bones, **Occipital Hold 3** is used. The following procedure then applies:

Induce a synchronous motion in the tentorium cerebelli by compressing the mastoid processes in a medial and posterior direction and then allowing the craniosacral mechanism to move into its extension phase. Repeat this procedure until, as with the still point technique, the body takes over the fluctuation of the CSF. When this occurs, gently reduce the alternating flexion and extension motion as in the still point technique, until all motion ceases and the craniosacral system goes through a still point. When the motion starts back up again, there will be a feeling of increased energy and movement in the tissues, and the tissue to which the longitudinal fluctuation was targeted will now feel more integrated with the rest of the body.

FLUID DRIVE TECHNIQUE

This is an indirect action technique developed by Sutherland to release impacted sutures by utilizing the potency of the CSF fluctuation. This technique can also be used to free or direct energy to other parts of the body. It is extremely useful to check that the occipitomastoid sutures are free after a dental extraction. This can be done by going to the opposite diagonal on the frontal bone, while placing the testing fingers either side of the occipitomastoid suture.

To release a cranial suture using a fluid drive, the following procedure is applied. Identify the suture that is locking up the craniosacral system and which, in your opinion, will allow the mechanism to unwind. Place the index and the middle finger of one hand on either side of the suture to be freed. Initiate a fluid drive across to the opposite side of the skull, i.e. find the opposite diagonal. Place the middle finger of the other hand on the opposite diagonal and send a fluid drive in the direction of the locked suture. At the same time, as you feel the fluid drive hit the suture, gently assist the release by spreading the fingers on either side of the suture. Continue the fluid drive until the suture has released.

After completion of this technique, it is always best to check that the whole craniosacral system has integrated the change by using the still point technique and then checking that the atlas has allowed the change.

## Dural techniques

### Membranous articular release technique

EVALUATION PROCEDURE

A cranial lesion is where the cranial dura have moved a little beyond their normal range of movement and become fixed in that position. If the dura are held in the direction of flexion, there would be lack of mobility that would prevent movement in the direction of extension. In order to assess the strain pattern of the dural membranes at any one time, it is necessary to know how to initiate cranial motion in all its possible ranges of motion. It is necessary therefore to evaluate each of the movements.

*Flexion*
The procedure here is to exaggerate the flexion phase by approximating the index and little fingers, i.e. approximating the greater wings of the sphenoid and the occipital bone. The mechanism will glide into flexion.

*Extension*
The procedure here is to exaggerate the extension phase by separating the index and little fingers, i.e. separating the greater wings of the sphenoid and the occipital bone. The mechanism will glide into extension.

*Side-bending rotation*
The axes for this pattern are:

- an axis of rotation from opisthion to nasion, as in torsion, except that the anterior and posterior portions of the head rotate ipsilaterally;
- side-bending axes which are parallel and vertical, one through the body of the sphenoid and the other through the foramen magnum.

On the divergent side, i.e. the side that bulges, the sphenoid and occipital bone are raised. The pattern is called right or left side-bending rotation, depending on which side bulges the most. Sutherland describes the side-bending lesion as follows:[25]

If the side-bending is convex to the left then the petrous portions of the temporal bones are included in the lesion, the right in internal rotation, the left in external. The basilar process is tipped upwards on the right and downwards on the left; while the greater wing of the sphenoid is upward on the right and downward on the left. The cranium, from front to back, is shorter on the right and longer on the left. If one were to observe this type of lesion from the front, one would see the right orbital cavity wider while the left would be narrower. The right zygomatic bone would be turned outwards and the left inward. The right eyeball would be forward while the left would be backward. Such observation would indicate the type of lesion at a glance and it would easily be verified by palpation.

The procedure is to exaggerate left side-bending rotation, add compression to the right side of the head to expand the left side, by approximating the index and little finger on the right side and separating the index and little finger on the left side. Reverse the procedure for right side-bending rotation. The mechanism will glide into side-bending rotation.

*Torsion*

The axis of rotation for torsion is from opisthion to nasion, so that the anterior portion of the head (controlled by the sphenoid) rotates in a contralateral direction to the posterior portion of the head (controlled by the occipital bone). The pattern is called right or left torsion, depending on which side the sphenoid is uppermost.

The procedure here is to exaggerate right torsion by inducing a lift or external rotation on the right greater wing of the sphenoid and the left side of the occipital bone. Lift with the right index finger and the left little finger. Reverse the procedure for left torsion, i.e. lift with the left index finger and the right little finger. The mechanism will glide into torsion.

*Lateral strain*

The axes for this pattern are variable, although the sphenoid will always be lateral to the occipital bone, relative to their mid-line axes.

The procedure is to exaggerate a right lateral strain and initiate movement of the sphenoid to the right while the occipital bone shears to the left; in other words, move both index fingers to the right and both ring and little fingers to the left. Reverse the procedure for a left lateral strain pattern. The mechanism will glide into lateral strain.

*Vertical strain*

The axes for this pattern are variable, although the sphenoid will always be superior or inferior to the occipital bone in relation to their axis from nasion to opisthion.

To exaggerate a vertical strain sphenoid high, the procedure is to lift the index fingers, simultaneously pulling down with the ring and little fingers so that the sphenoid shears in a superior direction and the occipital bone shears in an inferior direction. The mechanism will glide into vertical strain.

CORRECTION PROCEDURE

Having evaluated which of the above patterns is locking the craniosacral mechanism, the practitioner can then develop a strategy to assist the mechanism to correct that pattern or patterns.

*Stacking*
The most efficient way to help the body release these locked patterns is to hold in turn, or 'stack', each pattern that the mechanism likes, until sufficient patterns are stacked for the mechanism to go through a still point, or in this case a membranous articular release leading to a still point. When the mechanism restarts, the reciprocal tension of the dural membranes will operate from a more efficient point of balance.

The procedure for stacking is as follows:

- exaggerate flexion and then extension; assess which of the two feels freer, i.e. feels less blocked, with the greatest range of movement and more apparent energy; hold the mechanism in this pattern;
- still holding the mechanism in this pattern, exaggerate right and left torsion; assess which of the two feels freer and hold the mechanism in this pattern;
- still holding the mechanism in this pattern, exaggerate right and left side-bending rotation; assess which of the two feels freer and hold the mechanism in this pattern;
- still holding the mechanism in this pattern, exaggerate right and left lateral strain; assess which of the two feels freer and hold the mechanism in this pattern;
- still holding the mechanism in this pattern, exaggerate vertical strain patterns sphenoid high and low; assess which of the two feels freer and hold the mechanism in this pattern.

During this procedure, as soon as you feel that the involuntary motion of the body has taken over this stacking process, follow the unwinding of the membranes through to a still point. The process can be repeated until the mechanism feels free in all its patterns.

COMPRESSION PROCEDURE

If one analyses the restricted patterns of motion within the reciprocal tension of the dural membranes, there is a common element that they will exhibit and that is the element of compression. This element of compression can manifest itself evenly and unilaterally, as in side-bending rotation, or unevenly between the anterior and posterior portions of the skull, as in torsion.

If compression is initiated through the sphenobasilar symphysis, it is possible to disengage the individual compressive elements so that the mechanism can slowly unwind from its strain pattern.

# The temporomandibular joint

## Functional aspects of muscles affecting the TMJ

### TRIGGER POINTS

Trigger points have been extensively researched by Dr Janet Travell.[26] The main characteristic of trigger points is that there will be referred pain from individual muscles to the same side of the body as that muscle. The other characteristic is that these trigger points are painful on digital pressure. The stress level that initiates the pain is also very variable. On palpation, these muscles feel hypertonic, over-contracted and immobile, with specific areas of extreme discomfort. These trigger points can produce autonomic and proprioceptive disturbances that are quite worrying to the patient.

### TEMPORALIS

In cases of emotional stress or loss of the vertical dimension of the bite, the temporalis muscle becomes hypertonic and after compressing the TMJ, it causes a stress in the temporoparietal suture. If the temporal bone is locked, then the temporalis muscle will pull the parietal attachment in an inferior direction and exert a strain on the temporoparietal suture.[27] The three divisions of temporalis are innervated separately by the anterior and posterior temporal nerves and branches of the mandibular division of the trigeminal nerve.

Any trigger points in the three divisions of temporalis muscle should be examined with the jaw slightly open. They are all palpated on the skin except any trigger points on the inner surface of the coronoid process, which should be palpated inside the mouth. Referred pain from the trigger points in the different sections of the temporalis muscle occurs as follows:

- anterior portion: to the supraorbital ridge and down to the upper incisor teeth;
- middle portion: into the mid-temporal area and down to the upper front teeth;
- posterior portion: into the posterior temporal fossa.

Successful correction of temporalis imbalance often requires cranial treatment, applied kinesiology (AK) procedures and a dental splint to alleviate the effects of malocclusion before permanent reconstructive dentistry is undertaken.

### MASSETER

Travell[28] has found the mean incisal opening in patients with no history of temporomandibular joint dysfunction nor any palpable trigger points in masseter to be 50 mm in men and 45 mm in women. The simple test is whether the second, third and fourth knuckles of the non-dominant hand fit between the upper and lower incisor teeth. If only two knuckles can be inserted into the incisal opening, there will usually be a trigger point in the masseter muscle. However, it is not just the masseter that restricts incisal opening. Other mandibular muscles can also restrict incisal opening, so can sternocleidomastoid, trapezius, scalene and pectoral trigger points and these should be examined. The masseter muscle has the greatest number of trigger points, after the lateral pterygoid muscle.

Referred pain from the trigger points in the different sections of the masseter muscle occurs as follows:

- from the upper portion of the superficial layer: to the upper molar teeth and adjacent gums, and the maxilla;
- from just below the middle belly of the muscle: to the mandible and lower molar teeth;
- from the area of the angle of the mandible: to the lower jaw and across the greater wing of the sphenoid and over the eyebrows;
- from the deep layer of the muscle (palpated from within the mouth), into the TMJ itself.

There is also a trigger point just adjacent to the posterior zygomatic attachment of the deep layer of the masseter, from which pain is referred deep into the ear, which sometimes produces a 'low roaring' tinnitus. The trigger point near the attachment of the masseter to the mandible can restrict the emptying of the maxillary vein where it emerges between the masseter and the mandible. This will cause back-pressure in the pterygoid plexus and hence the orbital and deep temporal veins. The back-pressure in the orbital vein will cause puffiness behind the eyes and narrowing of the palpebral fissure. Stress to the masseter caused by reduced vertical dimension, e.g. due to wearing down of the teeth, ill-fitting dentures, loss of alveolar bone or loss of posterior teeth, will normally require both cranial and dental work. Stress due to emotional factors may require AK and/or clinical kinesiology (CK) clearing techniques.

### BUCCINATOR

The buccinator muscle functions in conjunction with the tongue in mastication and suckling; it also affects the ability to purse the lips and blow air. The relationship between the buccinator muscle, the orbicularis oris muscle and the tongue also affects the position of the teeth. Its innervation is the buccal nerve, which is a branch of the facial nerve.

The muscle is challenged for weakness by having the patient purse their lips and hold in the maximum amount of air whilst the therapist presses the cheeks for strength and at the same time palpates for trigger points or contracture in the muscle. It is sometimes necessary to look for reactive muscle weakness with the masseter, i.e. one muscle must be activated just prior to the testing of the other to show weakness in the latter.

### MEDIAL PTERYGOID

Trigger points in the medial pterygoid muscle refer pain to the general area of the TMJ, deep in the ear and into the oropharynx, rather than to specific areas. In the resting state, pressure from the medial pterygoid muscle helps to keep the Eustachian tube closed. Also, when the tensor veli palatini opens the Eustachian tube, it has to push the medial pterygoid to one side. If this is not possible due to contracture or trigger points, the Eustachian tube is unable to open, causing the ear to be blocked.

When there is a trigger point in the medial pterygoid, the incisal opening is often reduced to the width of two knuckles, or even one. Trigger points in the medial pterygoid can be primary and interfere with the rhythm of mastication and hence cause occlusal problems, or secondary to an occlusal imbalance. They may also be secondary to trigger points in the lateral pterygoid muscle. The trigger points should be palpated with the mouth open wide enough to stretch the muscle. The muscle should be palpated as close to its attachment on the ramus of the mandible as possible, to prevent gagging. With the patient alternately clenching and unclenching the teeth against a tongue spatula, in order to identify the muscle with accuracy, palpate up towards the pterygoid plate.

The fact that the medial pterygoid muscle is attached to the pterygoid plate of the sphenoid means that any imbalance has an effect on the mobility of the sphenoid and hence the rest of the craniosacral system. After correction of the trigger points, to prevent their recurrence, it may be necessary to use a mandibular repositioning appliance as part of the therapy.

LATERAL PTERYGOID

From the resting position the superior head closes the jaw and the inferior head opens the jaw. It is generally accepted that the superior and inferior heads function as two separate muscles. The superior head of the muscle pulls the articular disc of the TMJ in an anterior direction as the jaw closes. The inferior head of the muscle pulls the head of the condyle in an anterior direction as the jaw opens. Both the superior and inferior heads guide the mandible during chewing. Its innervation is from the lateral pterygoid nerve, which is a branch of the anterior mandibular division of the trigeminal nerve. The inferior head should be palpated intraorally. The mouth should be slightly open and to one side. Place the examining finger between the maxilla and the coronoid process, posterior to the molars and medially towards the lateral pterygoid plate. The superior head should be examined extraorally, with the mouth slightly open (when the mouth is closed, the superior head is behind the zygomatic arch).

Differential diagnosis between trigger points in the masseter muscle and trigger points in the superior head of the lateral pterygoid is necessary. Referred pain is to the area of the maxilla and the area of the TMJ. Any trigger points in the lateral pterygoid muscle alter the position of the jaw and can also cause deviation to the jaw on opening and closing. Trigger points in either head of the muscle can produce premature contacts of the teeth. These prematurities cause trauma to the teeth and gums, muscle spasm, trigger points and disorganization in the sequence of muscle activity of the TMJ. Contracture of the inferior head of the lateral pterygoid causes an anterior displacement of its mandibular condyle. A tongue spatula placed between the molars not only relieves pain in the muscle on clenching the teeth, but also facilitates release of the pterygoid plate of the sphenoid. Chronic tension in lateral pterygoid will cause stress to the sphenoid, causing a bulge or twist in the skull if there is unilateral tension and flexion if the tension is bilateral.

DIGASTRIC

The anterior digastric opens the jaw when the hyoid bone has been immobilized by the infrahyoid muscles. The lateral pterygoid initiates the movement and the anterior digastric completes it. Its pull is posterior and inferior, i.e. it is a mandibular retractor. When the anterior and posterior bellies of the digastric contract together and the mandible is immobilized by the jaw elevators in centric occlusion, e.g. as in swallowing, then the digastric elevates the hyoid.

Stimulation of the periodontal ligaments during chewing activates the jaw opening reflex whereby the posterior belly of the digastric is active and the mandibular elevators are inhibited so as to protect the teeth.

The anterior belly is supplied by the myelohyoid nerve, which comes from the alveolar branch of the mandibular part of the trigeminal nerve. The posterior belly is supplied by a branch of the facial nerve.

The trigger points of the anterior belly are just behind the chin and refer pain to the lower four incisor teeth and the adjacent alveolar bone. Trigger points are commonly found in the posterior belly, just behind the angle of the jaw. Pain is referred into the upper belly of the sternocleidomastoid, up into the occipital area and across the throat and under the chin. However, trigger points in either belly can cause difficulty in swallowing. Trigger points in masseter should be treated first, as any trigger points in digastric are often secondary to trigger points in masseter.

## Functions of the TMJ

MANDIBULAR POSITION

### Resting position

This is the position of the mandible when the muscles of the TMJ are inactive. The tongue is on the roof of the mouth, the lips are lightly touching, there is nasal breathing and the teeth are slightly apart. The distance between the teeth of the upper and lower jaw in the resting position is known as the freeway space. The resting position adopted depends on the individual's whole postural balance. The mandible may be held too open if the person habitually breathes through the mouth (creating habitual tension in the jaw openers); or the mandible may be held too closed if the person is under emotional stress or is a pipe smoker (creating habitual tension in the jaw closers).

### Centric occlusion

The relationship of the mandible to the maxilla with the teeth in maximum intercuspation is known as centric occlusion. In this position, the teeth of the upper and lower jaw are fully articulated. It is the habitual position when clenching the teeth and controlled by the teeth themselves.

*Centric relation*

This is the relationship of the mandible to the maxilla and cranial base when both condyles are properly related to their articular discs and in their most superior position in the glenoid fossae and stabilized against the posterior surface of the articular eminence. This position is recorded with the teeth slightly apart.

In practice, however, it is not always possible to know the correct position of the condyle. There is considerable controversy among dentists as to where the ideal position actually is. The position of the condyle takes into account the complex relationship between the cranial bones; it depends on the position of the temporal bone, the ligaments and muscles affecting the TMJ and the overall balance and posture of the body.

CONDYLAR POSITION[29]

*Anterior displacement*

In this position, the patient postures his jaw forward to use the incisors. Long-term chronic forward posturing causes strain on the muscles and an unstable joint.

*Distal displacement*

Here, the condyle is driven too far posteriorly in the glenoid fossa, due either to loss of the first molar and a subsequent shifting of the remaining teeth or to premature contact of the incisors or any tooth, which drives the mandible posteriorly.

*Contralateral interference*

The condyle shows degenerative changes following long-standing malocclusion.

*Loss of posterior support*

The condyle moves superiorly in the glenoid fossa, due to loss of posterior teeth or to retrusion of the teeth, so that chewing has to be done with the anterior teeth. This causes hypertonicity of the lateral pterygoid and masseter muscles, which exacerbates the anterior and superior position of the condyle.

MANDIBULAR MOVEMENT

There are three main forces in operation during opening of the mandible:

- gravity;
- contraction of the suprahyoid muscles, in particular the digastric;
- contraction of the inferior head of the lateral pterygoid muscle, pulling the disc and condyle anteriorly.

For the first 21 mm the mandible opens as a hinge joint in the inferior compartment of the TMJ. Then, the inferior head of the lateral pterygoid muscle pulls the condyle anteriorly, causing the mandible to glide anteriorly and inferiorly. This is called translation. The elastic retrodiscal laminar is stretched posteriorly keeping the disc, condyle and the glenoid fossa in contact with one another throughout the whole range of motion.

The mandible closes through contraction of the temporalis, masseter and medial pterygoid muscles. The slope of the glenoid eminence guides the condyle posteriorly and superiorly. The disc rotates anteriorly at the head of the condyle due to the removal of tension on the superior retrodiscal laminar, as the condyle translates posteriorly.

### NORMAL DISC–CONDYLE RELATIONSHIP

The disc is considered to be a friction reducer between the condyle of the mandible and the glenoid fossa of the temporal bone. It caps the head of the condyle, being attached both medially and laterally. During opening of the jaw, the disc rotates posteriorly on the head of the condyle at the same time as the condyle and the disc move anteriorly and inferiorly against the posterior slope of the eminence in the glenoid fossa. In this way, the disc always maintains its position between the mandible and the temporal bone.

### ABNORMAL DISC–CONDYLE RELATIONSHIP

The weak point in the TMJ mechanism is the articular disc and its posterior elastic ligament. This ligament is easily damaged and loses its ability to resist the pull of the lateral pterygoid muscle when in spasm. Internal derangement occurs when there is damage to the disc and posterior ligament. It produces an abnormal relationship between the glenoid fossa, articular disc and the condyle of the mandible. These abnormalities or internal derangements can be classified as follows:

- Reciprocal clicking (i.e. dislocation of the disc with reduction) is classified according to the stage in the opening of the jaw at which it occurs.
- Intermittent locking (i.e. dislocation of the disc with intermittent reduction):
  (i)    unilateral;
  (ii)   bilateral.
- Closed lock (i.e. dislocation of the disc without reduction):
  (i)    unilateral – acute or chronic;
  (ii)   bilateral – acute or chronic.

### Reciprocal clicking

The click indicates that the disc is dislocated anteromedially when the mandible is in the resting position. The click is in fact the disc reducing the dislocation, i.e. 'popping' into its correct position at some point during the opening of the jaw.

*(i) Early phase clicking*
The disc is dislocated anteriorly. The condyle is behind the disc and reduces to its normal position in the centre of the disc as the jaw begins to open. It then dislocates again at the late stage of closing the jaw.

*(ii) Middle phase clicking*
The disc is again dislocated anteriorly, but in this case the condyle articulates against the retrodiscal laminar. The condyle reduces to its normal position in the centre of the disc when the jaw is open about 1 inch (25 mm). When closing from a wide-open position, it then dislocates again in the middle stage of closing the jaw.

*(iii) Late phase clicking*
The disc is again dislocated anteriorly and does not find its normal position until late in the opening of the jaw. From a wide-open position it will dislocate early in the closing movement. Since the reduction of the disc can be painful, the patient will tend not to open the jaw wide enough to reduce the dislocation. To challenge this situation clinically, ask the patient to yawn.

*Unilateral reciprocal clicking*
- occurs after trauma such as dental, cranial or whiplash;
- produces unilateral clicking, with no limitation of interincisal opening but a semilunar opening pattern of the chin to the right where the left disc is dislocated;
- the clicking then stops but the semilunar opening pattern continues;
- this will in time stress the disc on the other side and produce bilateral clicking.

*Bilateral reciprocal clicking*
This is the most common pattern and is caused by:

- trauma such as dental, cranial, whiplash, etc.;
- this produces bilateral clicking with no limitation in interincisal opening, but a sigmoidal opening pattern as one disc articulates before the other;
- the clicking then stops as both sides become locked (i.e. a closed lock situation – see below) and the interincisal opening is reduced to 21–24 mm;
- the interincisal opening gradually increases to 38–44 mm, but the movement remains silent, even though there may be bone-to-bone contact;
- crepitus eventually develops.

**Intermittent locking**

The patient will complain of intermittent clicking and intermittent locking of the jaw. This will inevitably progress to the closed-lock situation just described above and expanded on below. This means that reduction of the dislocation of the disc is becoming more difficult.

- periodic locking occurs, e.g. on awakening or with yawning;
- the patient is able to free the jaw by manipulating the TMJ;

- the jaw remains locked for longer periods and the patient finds it increasingly difficult to free it himself by manipulation;
- one side becomes permanently locked (acute unilateral closed lock);
- this will stress the other side so that eventually this will also lock, producing a bilateral closed lock (see Bilateral reciprocal clicking, above).

### Closed lock

The disc is dislocated both in the resting position and throughout opening and closing of the TMJ. The head of the condyle articulates against the retrodiscal laminar. The laminar was not designed to be a load-bearing structure, so the patient will complain of pain. During opening the jaw, the mandible will be deflected away from the mid-line. In the chronic stage after the clicking has stopped, there is destruction of the retrodiscal laminar, with eventual perforation by the condyle. This can lead to osteoarthrosis with bone-on-bone contact between the condyle and the base of the skull. In time this may produce crepitus on movement of the jaw. The osteoarthrosis begins in the lateral pole of the condyle due to the pull of the superior head of the lateral pterygoid muscle, and it may eventually destroy the whole head of the condyle.

In time, osteoarthrosis may become bilateral. It may take the following path:

- One or both discs become dislocated without reduction (i.e. closed lock). First one disc and then the other may dislocate, or both may dislocate at the same time.
- Dislocation may be acute or chronic. In the acute stage, the interincisal opening will be reduced to 21–24 mm and there will be premature occlusal contact on the side of the dislocation. During the chronic stage, the interincisal opening gradually increases to 38–44 mm and the teeth occlude again on both sides. The contracture or trigger points in the muscles of mastication generate considerable force on the TMJ. The dentist will notice fractures of the cusps of the posterior teeth or excessive wear to any splint that has been fitted.
- Crepitus develops, possibly followed by osteoarthrosis.

## The interrelationship between cranial osteopathy and dentistry

The relationship between the mandible and the temporal bones is reciprocal, in that the position of the temporal bones can alter the occlusion just as the occlusion can affect the position of the temporal bones.

On some of the early cranial courses, we used to ask students to feel their own craniosacral mechanism while chewing, in order to demonstrate the concept of reciprocal tension. It was noticed that some of the beginners found it easier to feel the craniosacral mechanism after this. The reason was that, provided there was no gross abnormality in the occlusion, chewing would allow a locked cranial mechanism to free temporarily.

'If the cranium is the pump for the cerebrospinal fluid, then the mandible is the pump handle.' (W. B. May, personal communication)

**Diagnostic procedures**

When assessing the occlusion and the TMJ it is important to consider the effects of the cranial mechanism. The following simple but effective diagnostic procedures should be useful.

- During assessment of cranial rhythmic impulse (CRI), if the CRI decreases when the jaw is closed, then it is reasonable to suspect the jaw as a limiting factor in cranial motion. If the CRI increases with the jaw closed, this indicates that the occlusion is helping to correct a cranial fault.
- Palpate the muscles of the TMJ for hypotonicity, hypertonicity and trigger points (see Trigger points, above, with descriptions of techniques for individual muscles).
- Place the little fingers in the external auditory meatus and ask the patient to close his jaw. If this produces excess pressure on the fingers and/or pain in the joint, the mandible is being pushed too far posterior on closure and may need to be corrected with an anterior mandibular repositioning appliance.

Dr Harold Magoun[30] lists four categories of overlapping interest between the dental and the osteopathic professions in the area of the TMJ:

- developmental problems;
- the effects of dental trauma on the cranium;
- movement and position of the mandibular fossae;
- positional shifts in the maxillae.


**Developmental problems**

Another way of looking at the overlapping interests of the two professions is by defining the relationship between the cranial bones and how during development they affect the whole stomatognathic system.

We know that sometimes the normal overriding of the neonate cranial bones within the birth process fails to be cleared by the suckling at the breast or crying. This allows the development of intraosseous lesions within the cranial bones (intraosseous lesions are spatial distortions between different areas of ossification in the same bone). These occur during the first 7 years of growth while the bones are still ossifying.

We also know that possible warping or crowding of the fetal skull *in utero* can occur secondary to maternal stress. Major trauma to the neonate skull can occur in the birth process from factors such as disproportion, abnormal presentations, forceps, induced births or maternal fatigue. Whatever the cause, facial asymmetry is often seen in the newborn without any history of trauma. Fortunately, the condylar squama and the condylar parts of the occipital bone fuse in the fifth year; the condylar parts of the occipital bone and the basiocciput fuse in the seventh year; and no sutures form before the age of 7 years. This gives time for the body to correct these problems.

In dental terms the eruption of the deciduous dentition starts at 6–8 months of age and finishes with the second deciduous molars at 30 months. The permanent teeth erupt at about 6 years of age, with the lower central incisors and the first molar, the first molar's position being in direct response to the position of the second deciduous molar. All further growth in the dentition will come from this first molar point of reference and continue through to the eruption of the third molar between 18 and 21 years of age.

THE EFFECT OF CRANIAL DEVELOPMENT ON THE OCCLUSION

The relative balance of the infant's posture, not just of the spine but of the TMJ, is intimately connected to the relationships of the two temporal bones to each other – the sphenoid to the occipital bone and the maxillae to the mandible. When assessing the occlusion and the TMJ in relationship to developmental problems in these cranial bones, it can be evaluated in at least three ways:

- When there is a change in the spatial relationship of the two temporal bones. In cranial terms one of the temporal bones will be held in internal rotation and the other in relative external rotation. The end result will be a twist in the craniosacral mechanism, but from a dental point of view a potential crossbite. Although the degree of motion in the cranium is only slight, with the combination of leverage and/or locking over many years during development of the skull significant changes can result in the position of the bones.
- When there is a change in relationship between the sphenoid bone and the occipital bone without any major twist between them. In cranial terms this implies a flexed or extended head. In dental terms this means a protruded jaw with the extended head, as the temporal fossa moves anterolaterally in internal rotation, or a retruded jaw with the flexed head, as the temporal fossa will be displaced posteromedially in external rotation.
- When there is a change in the relationship between the mandible and the maxillae in their transverse planes. In cranial terms this implies intraosseous strains of either the mandible or the maxillae or both. The mandible and maxillae are bilateral structures; they either externally rotate or internally rotate, so if the two maxillae are relatively internally rotated on an externally rotated mandible, there will be a tendency towards a crossbite and a change from the optimum freeway space and vertical dimension.

Early co-operation between dentists and osteopaths would therefore seem to be fundamental to these young children. Everything flows from here: if the infant is corrected after birth by either a dentist or an osteopath with craniosacral skills, the only problems that should occur with the development of the bite and the rest of the posture will be from postnatal trauma, malnutrition or genetic factors.

DEVELOPMENTAL RETARDATION PATTERNS

When assessing the function of the cranium we are looking at craniosacral mobility, but also the various developmental retardation patterns in the

cranial bones. This is another area of mutual interest to the cranial osteopath and the dentist.

The commonest abnormalities are:

- Intraosseous strains of the premaxilla on the maxilla with either over or
  underdevelopment.
- Compression of the maxillae into internal rotation, causing a high arched
  palate and restricted lateral space for the tongue.
- Restricted growth of the lateral masses of the ethmoid and/or the lateral
  turbinates so that breathing through the nose is difficult.
- Trauma or restricted growth of the nasal septum, resulting in a deviated
  septum, which can also affect the ethmoid or the vomer. A rupture of the
  vomer through the hard palate is called a taurus palatinus and is particularly common during birth with face presentations and as a result of
  severe perinatal trauma.
- Restricted development of the frontal ossification centres, which can
  produce asymmetry of the face.
- Compression of the condylar part of the occipital bone, which will limit
  the motion of the temporal bone and hence the mandible. Although the
  mandible is suspended from the sphenoid by two main ligaments, and the
  main muscles that move the mandible originate from the sphenoid, it is
  more common to find functional imbalance of the mandible caused by
  compression of the condylar part of the occipital bone than by developmental abnormalities of the sphenoid.

This brings us to the three main points that the dentist must consider
cranially.

- if the temporal bone is held in internal rotation, the mandible will be held
  in an anterior direction;
- if the temporal bone is held in external rotation, the mandible will be held
  in posterior direction (i.e. in a retruded position);
- if the temporal bones are held in torsion, one side of the mandible will be
  held in an anterior direction and the other side in a posterior direction.

**The effects of dental trauma on the cranium**

It is not only that cranial distortions affect the occlusion but that occlusal
problems may have an effect on the cranium. It is not a one-way street.
Some common occlusal problems are outlined below.

LACK OF VERTICAL DIMENSION

Lack of vertical dimension will limit cervical mobility, especially in the area
of C3. A good check is to increase the vertical dimension of the bite and
observe if there is an increase in cervical rotation. Lack of vertical dimension
will also cause hypotonicity in the muscles of mastication, which in turn
limits motion in the sphenoid and temporal bones and hence the face.

PREMATURITIES

Premature contacts of the teeth cause hypertonicity in the TMJ muscles which in turn limit cranial and cervical motion. The position of the prematurity in the mouth will affect the degree of hypertonicity in the muscle. The more distal the tooth with the prematurity, the greater the stress on the muscle. As in a nutcracker, the closer to the hinge, the greater the force on the nut.

The size and angle of the prematurity will also have an effect, as will the patient's adaptive capacity to cope with the interference. This last factor is related to the patient's stress levels.

LACK OF POSTERIOR SUPPORT FOR THE BITE

Lack of posterior support to the bite (i.e. posterior molars missing) will cause weakness of the psoas, lumbar and abdominal muscles during lifting. This is because the usual reflex during lifting is to clench the teeth to stabilize the craniomandibular complex. If, however, there is no posterior support to the bite, this reflex is inhibited, which in turn inhibits the psoas, lumbar and abdominal muscles (see Effort closure, in Chapter 9).

## Movement of the mandibular fossae

THE EFFECT OF CRANIAL PATTERNS ON THE OCCLUSION

### Flexion pattern

This is typified by the short wide head. The maxillae, frontal bones and zygomas are all in relative external rotation. On examination, one finds a low wide palate. The glenoid fossa will be in relative external rotation, causing the head of the mandible to be held posteromedially. This is similar to the Calcarea carbonica type of person, as discussed in Chapter 1.

### Extension pattern

This is typified by the long thin head. The maxillae, frontal and zygomatic bones are all in relative internal rotation. On examination, one finds a very high palate but narrowed in its transverse plane. There is insufficient room for the tongue, nasal breathing will be difficult and there will be a deviant swallow. The glenoid fossa will be in relative internal rotation, causing the head of the mandible to be held anterolaterally. However, the mandible may be underdeveloped if the narrow intercanine and bicuspid width has not allowed the mandible to come forward enough to achieve its full growth potential. Normally the arches are long and thin. This is the Calcarea phosphorica type of person.

### Side-bending pattern

This is typified by the head with a bulge. One side of the head is held in internal rotation and the other is in external rotation. The roof of the mouth will therefore show a buckling of the palate, high and narrowed on the compressed (internally rotated) side and wide and low on the expanded (externally rotated) side. The head of the mandible will be anterior on the compressed side and posterior on the expanded side. This is the Calcarea fluorica type of person.

### Torsion pattern

This is typified by the head with a twist. Since the mandible has no choice but to follow the temporal bone's position, the mandible will have the same patterns as in the 'bulging' head. The added complication is that the temporal bone will be in internal rotation as the sphenoid tries to take the frontal and hence the rest of the face into external rotation in the expansion phase of cranial motion. This will stress the TMJ because the main influence on the TMJ is from muscles and ligaments derived from the sphenoid.

### Occlusal pattern

The bite has an effect on the cranium. It is not a one-way street.

## Positional shifts in the maxillae

MAXILLARY EXPANSION APPLIANCES

Although these appliances are very efficient at initiating remodelling at the frontozygomatic, frontomaxillary and intermaxillary sutures, they will lock the craniosacral mechanism into relative flexion as they widen the maxillae into external rotation.

MAXILLARY SAGITTAL APPLIANCES

These appliances are necessary to move the mandible from its retruded position, but they tend to lock the craniosacral mechanism into relative extension, the maxillae into internal rotation and restrict cranial movement in general. One will find that the problems associated with weakness in masseter, temporalis, sternocleidomastoid and sacrospinalis muscles may be induced by the craniosacral extension. Using a mandibular appliance instead of a maxillary one will help to avoid this problem.

## Developing a treatment procedure

Dr Rollin Becker used to say that it takes patience with a 'C' and patients with a 'T' to practise cranial osteopathy. One has to admit that this is true and constant practice is necessary, as in the development of any skill. In your practice rooms, consciously set out to train yourselves in the palpation skills that you need.

Regardless of how you practise, be it pure cranial, dental, clinical or applied kinesiology, or any other system, add palpation to your routine.

When you make a correction to the bite, release any of the TMJ muscles, correct a subluxation or fixation in the neck, then feel the involuntary motion in that tissue before and after the correction. Go and palpate the potency of the primary respiratory mechanism before and after any correction.

Ask yourselves these questions:

- Has the correction been successful at the microlevel of motion in the body?
- Has the correction been integrated by the rest of the body via a shift in the efficiency at the master fulcrum in the dural membranes?
- Can you feel that should you introduce a still point in the fourth ventricle, while you projected your awareness to that lesioned area, that the correction would be better integrated and less likely to recur?

Eventually, try correcting subluxations and fixations only by treating through the primary respiratory mechanism and feel the depth of change that can be achieved. This would be an ideal framework for a treatment programme. Diagnose the overall pattern of function in the primary respiratory mechanism and the occlusion. Is the rate too fast or too slow? Is the overall impression one of a positive direction and purpose? Is the overall impression of a cranial compression or a dragging down from the sacrum? Does restriction of the TMJ or clenching the teeth limit the primary respiratory mechanism? Does the motion of the sacrum appear synchronous with the cranium?

Initiate the stacking procedure in the dural membranes. Stack in flexion, in extension, in torsion, in side-bending rotation, in vertical strain, in lateral strain and hold the mechanism in the pattern that has the greatest range of motion. Still holding that pattern, keep adding those patterns that have the greatest ranges of motion until a still point is achieved.

Following the still point, check the freedom of the atlas, the second and third cervical vertebrae and the sacrum because of the dural attachments. Release any areas of restriction.

Re-evaluate the motion in the dural membranes. If the membranes do not feel that they have the energy for continued correction, then proceed to a fluid balance therapy procedure. You can initiate a still point through a direct still point technique if there is an overall compression, or through a lateral fluctuation if there is not enough energy to initiate a change.

The aim is to provide an environment for change, both in the potency of the CSF fluctuation and in the adaptation available at the master fulcrum.

With an increased potency in the CSF fluctuation and increased mobility in the reciprocal tension of the dural membranes, one can then decide to free any local areas of restriction that require correction. These are often fascial areas like the masseter, diaphragm and the pelvic floor. Correct these in the same way that you corrected patterns in the reciprocal tension membranes.

Now you can re-evaluate the TMJ and the occlusion and make any adjustments that are necessary from this new balanced position.

# Conclusion

As the biomechanics of the craniosacral mechanism become more widely appreciated, certain dental procedures such as extractions, orthodontics and splint work can be developed utilizing the palpatory skills that are taught within the postgraduate osteopathic teaching programme for the craniosacral system. This will have major repercussions in our patients' health and greatly facilitate our working with the more difficult or problem patient.

# References

1 Eversaul G. *Dental Kinesiology*. Las Vegas: privately published, 1977.
2 Yemm R. Variations in the electrical activity in the human masseter muscle in association with emotional stress. *Arch Oral Biol* 1969; **14**: 873–878.
3 Still A T. *Autobiography*, p 282. Kirksville, Mo: Still, 1908.
4 Sutherland A S, Wales A L (eds). *Contributions of Thought: Collected Writings of William G Sutherland*, p 112. Fort Worth, Texas: The Sutherland Cranial Teaching Foundation, 1967.
5 Wales A. The work of Willam Garner Sutherland, DO, DSC (Hon). *J AM Osteo Assoc* 1972; **71**: 789.
6 Sutherland A S, Wales A L (eds). *Contributions of Thought: Collected Writings of William G Sutherland*. Fort Worth, Texas: The Sutherland Cranial Teaching Foundation, 1967.
7 Sutherland A S, Wales A L (eds). *Contributions of Thought: Collected Writings of William G Sutherland*, p 147. Fort Worth, Texas: The Sutherland Cranial Teaching Foundation, 1967.
8 Sutherland A S, Wales A L (eds). *Contributions of Thought: Collected Writings of William G Sutherland*, p 243. Fort Worth, Texas: The Sutherland Cranial Teaching Foundation, 1967.
9 Sutherland A S, Wales A L (eds). *Contributions of Thought: Collected Writings of William G Sutherland*, p 157. Fort Worth, Texas: The Sutherland Cranial Teaching Foundation, 1967.
10 Sutherland A S, Wales A L (eds). *Contributions of Thought: Collected Writings of William G Sutherland*, p 178. Fort Worth, Texas: The Sutherland Cranial Teaching Foundation, 1967.
11 Still A T. *Philosophy of Osteopathy*, p 33. Kirksville, Mo: Still, 1899.
12 Sutherland A S, Wales A L (eds). *Contributions of Thought: Collected Writings of William G Sutherland*, p 166. Fort Worth, Texas: The Sutherland Cranial Teaching Foundation, 1967.
13 Frymann V. A study of the rhythmic motions of the living cranium. *J Am Osteo Assoc* 1971; **70**: 9.
14 Still A T. *Philosophy of Osteopathy*, p 38. Kirksville, Mo: Still, 1899.
15 Sutherland A S, Wales A L (eds). *Contributions of Thought: Collected Writings of William G Sutherland*, p 97. Fort Worth, Texas: The Sutherland Cranial Teaching Foundation, 1967.
16 Becker R. *Motion* (unpublished).
17 Sutherland A S, Wales A L (eds). *Contributions of Thought: Collected Writings of William G Sutherland*, pp 206–210. Fort Worth, Texas: The Sutherland Cranial Teaching Foundation, 1967.
18 Still A T. *Philosophy of Osteopathy*, p 39. Kirksville, Mo: Still, 1899.
19 Sutherland A S, Wales A L (eds). *Contributions of Thought: Collected Writings of William G Sutherland*, p 142. Fort Worth, Texas: The Sutherland Cranial Teaching Foundation, 1967.
20 Upledger J E, Vrendevoogd J. *Craniosacral Therapy*, p 3. Seattle: Eastland Press, 1983.
21 Sutherland A S, Wales A L (eds). *Contributions of Thought: Collected Writings of William G Sutherland*, p 242. Fort Worth, Texas: The Sutherland Cranial Teaching Foundation, 1967.
22 Holding R A, DO MRO. *The Craniosacral System. Part 1*. London: Ark International Training Seminars, 1994.
23 Sutherland A S, Wales A L (eds). *Contributions of Thought: Collected Writings of William G Sutherland*, p 142. Fort Worth, Texas: The Sutherland Cranial Teaching Foundation, 1967.

24 Sutherland A S, Wales A L (eds). *Contributions of Thought: Collected Writings of William G Sutherland*, p 140. Fort Worth, Texas: The Sutherland Cranial Teaching Foundation, 1967.

25 Sutherland A S, Wales A L (eds). *Contributions of Thought: Collected Writings of William G Sutherland*, pp 123–124. Fort Worth, Texas: The Sutherland Cranial Teaching Foundation, 1967.

26 Travell J, Simons D. *Myofascial Pain and Dysfunction: The Trigger Point Manual*, Vol. 1. Baltimore/London: Williams and Wilkins, 1983.

27 Upledger J. *Craniosacral Therapy II. Beyond the Dura*, p. 173. Seattle: Eastland Press, 1987.

28 Travell J. Temporo-mandibular joint pain referred from muscles of the head and neck. *J. Prosth Dent* 1960; **10:** 745–763.

29 Walthur D S. *Applied Kinesiology*, Vol. II, pp 300–301. Pueblo, Co: Systems DC, 1983.

30 Magoun H I. Osteopathic approach to dental enigmas. In: *Academy of Applied Osteopathy Year Book*, p 131. Colorado: American Academy of Osteopathy, 1967.

# Bibliography

Gehin A. *Atlas of Manipulative Techniques for the Cranium and Face*. Seattle: Eastland Press, 1985.

Magoun H I. *Osteopathy in the Cranial Field*, 3rd edn. Kirksville, Missouri: The Journal Printing Co, 1976.

Retzlaff E W, Mitchell F L Jnr. *The Cranium and its Sutures*. New York: Springer-Verlag, 1987.

Ricard F. *Osteopathic Treatment of Pain Originating in the Craniocervical Area*. France: Editions de Verlaque Aix en Provence, 1990.

Still A T. *Philosophy of Osteopathy*. Colorado: American Academy of Osteopathy, 1889.

Still A T. *The Philosophy and Mechanical Principles of Osteopathy*. Kirksville, Mo: Osteopathy Enterprise, 1902.

Still A T. *Autobiography*. Colorado: American Academy of Osteopathy, 1905.

Still A T. *Osteopathy: Research and Practice*. Colorado: American Academy of Osteopathy, 1910.

Sutherland A S. *With Thinking Fingers. The Story of William Garner Sutherland DO*. Fort Worth, Texas: The Cranial Academy, 1962.

Sutherland A S, Wales A L (eds). *Contributions of Thought: Collected Writings of William G Sutherland*. Fort Worth, Texas: The Sutherland Cranial Teaching Foundation, 1967.

Sutherland W G. *The Cranial Bowl*. Mankato, MN: The Free Press, 1939.

Sutherland W G. *Teachings in the Science of Osteopathy*. Wales A L (ed). USA: Rudra Press, 1990.

Upledger J. *Craniosacral Therapy II. Beyond the Dura*. Seattle: Eastland Press, 1987.

Upledger J. *Craniosacral Therapy III. Somato Emotional Release and Beyond*. Florida: UI Publishing.

Upledger J, Vrendevoogd J. *Craniosacral Therapy*. Seattle: Eastland Press, 1983.

Walther D. *Applied Kinesiology*, Vol. II. *Head, Neck and Jaw. Pain and Dysfunction – The Stomatognathic System*. Pueblo, Co: Systems DC, 1983.

# Appendix

## Hand hold positions

OCCIPITAL HOLD 1

| | |
|---|---|
| Purpose | This hold is ued to evaluate craniosacral motion through the master fulcrum or to still the cerebrospinal fluid fluctuation. |
| Patient position: | Supine with the legs uncrossed. Remove spectacles and dental splints. |
| Therapist position: | Seated at the head of the table, forearms on the table providing a fulcrum. |

Contact points

| | |
|---|---|
| Thumbs: | Touching the mastoid process. |
| Index and middle fingers: | Either side of the occipitomastoid suture. |
| Ring fingers: | On the occipital squama. |
| Little fingers: | Crossed at the external occipital protuberance in order to provide a fulcrum. |

OCCIPITAL HOLD 3

| | |
|---|---|
| Purpose: | To assess the motion of the occipital bone and the tentorium cerebelli, or to induce a still point through control of the motion of the tentorium cerebelli. |
| Patient position: | Supine with the legs uncrossed. Remove spectacles and dental splints. |
| Therapist position: | Seated at the head of the table, forearms on the table providing a fulcrum. |

Contact points

| | |
|---|---|
| Fingers: | Overlapping or intertwined under the occipital bone. |
| Thumbs: | Parallel to the anterior border of the mastoid with the thenar eminences on the mastoid processes. |

VAULT HOLD

| | |
|---|---|
| Purpose: | This hold is useful in assessing cranial motion as a whole and membranous motion in particular. |
| Patient position: | Supine with the legs uncrossed. Remove spectacles and dental splints. |
| Therapist position: | Seated at the head of the table, forearms on the table providing a fulcrum, fingers spread out but relaxed, holding the patient's vault. |

Contact points

| | |
|---|---|
| Thumbs: | Touching above the cranium to provide another fulcrum. |

| Index fingers: | On the greater wings of the sphenoid behind the external occipital ridge of the frontal bone to provide a slight lift. |
| Middle fingers: | Slightly anterior to the external auditory meatus. |
| Ring fingers: | Posterior to the ear at asterion to feel the parietal notch and the mastoid processes. |
| Little fingers: | Onto the lateral angle of the occipital bone. |

## Associations

General Council and Register of Osteopaths
56 London Street
Reading
Berkshire RG1 4SQ
UK
Tel: 0118 957 6585
Fax: 0118 956 6246

Cranial Osteopathic Association
478 Baker Street
Enfield
Middlesex EN1 3QS
UK
Tel: 0181 367 5561
Fax: 0181 202 6686

Craniosacral Therapy Association
8 Warren Road
London SW19 2HX
UK
Tel: 0181 543 4969
Fax: 0181 543 4969

## Courses

Ark International Training Seminars
144 Cloudesly Road
London N1 0EA
UK
Tel: 0171 833 3454
Fax: 0171 833 3454

British School of Osteopathy
1–4 Suffolk Street
London SW1Y 4HG
UK
Tel: 0171 930 9254
Fax: 0171 839 1098

European School of Osteopathy
104 Tonbridge Road
Maidstone
Kent ME16 8SL
UK
Tel: 01622 671558
Fax: 01622 662165

The Upledger Institute UK
52 Main Street
Perth
Scotland PH2 7HB
UK
Tel: 01738 444404
Fax: 01738 442275

Upledger Institute Inc USA
11211 Prosperity Farm Road
Palm Beach Gardens
Florida 33410
USA
Tel: 001 561 622 4334
Fax: 001 561 622 4771

Sutherland Cranial Teaching Foundation (USA)
4116 Hartwood Drive
Fort Worth
Texas 76109
USA
Tel: 001 817 656 1700

Sutherland Cranial Teaching Foundation (Australia)
687 White Horse Road
Mont Albert
Victoria 3127
Australia

# Applied kinesiology

**Joseph Shafer**

## Introduction

Pain is a word found in all languages. It is a feeling common to all peoples. Some seek pain for its hedonistic gratification and some religions embrace suffering for its spiritual rewards, but most try to avoid it. Like night is to day, pain is our indispensable partner, often met with forms of analgesia which tend to lull the nervous system into complacency. The doctor hopes that the body will take care of the cause before the false sense of well-being wears off and the pain returns. More effective drugs and the availability of modern medicines, together with our demand to be free from pain, have made it easier for us to treat the pain in a reflex fashion rather than attempting to understand the reason behind its onset.

Our desire to be free from pain is probably the most important catalyst for the evolution of witch doctors, acupuncturists, modern-day medicine, dentistry, psychiatry, homoeopathy, osteopathy and even applied kinesiology. No healing profession can be more thankful for its existence than for the pain and suffering of mankind.

We now have a better understanding of the mechanisms causing the sensation of pain. We know how it is perceived, we know how it is transmitted, and we know how it is registered in the brain. For those who continue to experience intractable pain this is of little consolation. Far too often diagnostic conclusions are made and therapy begins, but the pain persists unabated. Each new idea as to how to alleviate pain brings with it another professional specialty. Billions are spent each year by people who are searching for an answer to their question of pain, but must resign themselves to combing the health-care jungle in what sometimes becomes a futile search for a cure.

Pain is frequently a reflex symptom far removed from the origin of the problem. When obvious pathology cannot be demonstrated the doctor must rely upon functional testing in order to arrive at a probable diagnosis. Too often, in the absence of clear diagnostic indicators, an educated guess is offered as to the cause of the pain. A therapeutic trial is begun, hoping that despite the lack of diagnostic markers the therapy will be helpful to the patient. Sometimes the therapy works and sometimes it does not.

The continued suffering of the patient is not the intent of the doctor. Medical schools have had more of a love affair with pathology than with normal functional analysis, and the young doctor has been led to believe that a measure of health is the absence of disease. It is a wide gap which greatly limits the doctor's capacity to help the patient. To do so the doctor must become skilled in methods that allow a holistic and functional evaluation of the patient. Applied kinesiology (AK) provides a basis from which this functional understanding can be found.

The word 'holistic' does not mean that one has to accept Eastern philosophy. It does mean, however, that we should try to look at the body in a multi-dimensional way, bearing in mind that each individual part is inextricably linked to all the others. Any method of diagnosis allowing this kind of flexible approach becomes a powerful tool in the hands of the clinician skilled in its use. In AK, examination procedures based on simple muscle tests provide valuable information as to local biomechanical function and central nervous system regulation. The doctor willing to devote the time necessary to learn simple muscle testing procedures will open a whole new world of therapeutic possibilities for his own benefit and that of the patient.

## Dentistry and AK

Applied kinesiology is unique in its ability to help the doctor 'break free' from the limitations of a medical specialty while not giving up their specialist identity. One can think of AK as a 'diagnostic bridge' enabling the doctor to follow almost any path leading to patient recovery. Once the muscle testing skill is learned, AK techniques are readily adaptable to almost any health profession. There is no need to give up the specialty which took years to learn only to become a 'jack of all trades and a master of none' in order to fulfil a new trend in medical thinking. On the contrary, the doctor using AK maintains the security found in practising the specialty and gains the ability to test the efficacy of a wide range of therapeutic inputs.

One of the best examples of this is found in dentistry. The dentist, in most countries, is supposed to treat problems originating from the mouth and jaw. Anything below the shoulders is considered taboo and only a few rogue dentists dare to extend their borders beyond these limits. Dental specialists in the temporomandibular joint (TMJ) know that it can negatively influence posture from the neck all the way down to the feet. The reverse is also true.

The TMJ is exquisitely sensitive to imbalances in the body far removed from the head and neck. Yet dental training really does not provide the tools necessary to understand, let alone evaluate, parts of the body below the neck as they relate to the TMJ. What then does the dentist do: return to four or more years of schooling to learn biomechanics and orthopaedics? Unless dental schools incorporate this new knowledge into their programmes, it is the only way for the dentist to understand how the jaw relates to the rest of the body.

In response to this need, an increasing number of dentists are following postgraduate courses in AK. Using simple AK muscle tests they are not only better able to evaluate patient response to therapy, but to determine when and where other disturbances in the body are influencing the jaw joint. Iatrogenic reactions to bridges, crowns, splints, fillings and other dental procedures, can make the dentist and patient very frustrated. Problems arise when the patient is unable to tolerate the change created in the mouth by the dental therapy. These occur most often when the dentist has been unable to monitor the whole body reaction to what is being done. Instead, local responses and functional tests of the jaw alone frequently provide the only basis for a conclusion.

Applied kinesiology improves the dentist's ability to uncover hidden imbalances in the patient that can cause unwanted side-effects to therapy. Muscle testing a patient before and after the therapeutic input allows the doctor to evaluate immediately the effectiveness of the therapy and the potential side-effects. Applied kinesiology does not require any special tools. It is simple and effective. Few diagnostic techniques can boast this capability. The specialist skilled in this technique is able to isolate quickly areas of dysfunction and cross-reference these to the area being examined. In the long run, everyone benefits and that means less pain for the patient.

## The historical perspective

Applied kinesiology originated in the USA in the late 1950s through astute clinical observations of George Goodheart DC. Because he was a chiropractor, his education prepared him to look primarily at problems related to the spine and the way it affected the nervous system to bring about pain and disease. An insatiable reader, he was especially interested in books with new concepts of health maintenance and the prevention of disease. A colleague gave him a book on manual muscle testing written by the physiotherapists, Kendall and Kendall. This husband and wife team had spent many years observing and treating patients who suffered from nerve trauma and other pathologies. Muscle weakness related to the involved nerve roots was a consistent finding and they were able to develop manual tests to evaluate precisely the muscles inhibited by improper nerve function.

Goodheart thought that these testing procedures might provide him with an instrument through which to help some of his more difficult patients. This proved to be correct. He was surprised at first to realize that weak muscles were a far more common cause of structural imbalance than hypertonic and contracted ones. The current belief was that muscles became taut and contracted rather than weak in response to structural imbalances. After further investigation he found that the contracted muscle was, more often than not, due to a weak opposing muscle. By correcting the weakness, the tight muscle returned to normal on its own.

This was a revelation, because at the time almost everyone believed that tense, overworked contracted muscles, not weak ones, were more common. For this reason, most conventional therapies had been designed to relax and elongate the tense fibres, rather than to reinforce weakened muscles. Until Goodheart began testing otherwise normal patients and finding weaknesses, no one appreciated the significance of the weak muscle as a primary factor for structural instability leading to pain. The work done by Kendall and Kendall was performed mostly on patients with frank nerve pathology. One would have expected muscle weakness to ensue in pathology. The observations of Goodheart are that the muscle weakness patterns are also present in patients who have no nerve pathology, but have functional or structural imbalances as the cause of pain and disability.

**Early observations related to muscle weakness**

As with most new developments, muscle testing in the beginning seemed to pose more questions than answers. Goodheart was puzzled to observe that patients showed muscle weakness not related to any obvious nerve or structural problem. The muscles remained weak despite there being no apparent problem in the spine or nerve to that muscle. Soon, one of many undeniable new patterns emerged. He found that when he had patients with a disease in a specific organ like the liver, kidney or gallbladder, certain muscles would always test weak. Although he had no answer for his observations, these findings remained consistent in all patients.

### THE MUSCLE ORGAN REFLEX

Goodheart hypothesized that skeletal muscles must have some sort of reflex relationship to the internal organs and vice versa. When an organ was diagnosed as having a pathology, the corresponding muscle would usually test weak. Furthermore, the muscle would remain weak until the organ recovered from the pathology. As research in the human body continues to improve, it is hoped that a more precise definition of what occurs can be made with respect to this phenomenon. The fact that it does happen is noted every day by applied kinesiologists throughout the world. Although some minor changes have been necessary with time, these reflexes continue to be valid today, almost 40 years later.

Armed with this knowledge, Goodheart discovered that not only organ problems, but many other imbalances such as nutritional deficiencies, blocks in lymphatic drainage and emotional conditions could adversely change the resistive strength in muscles both locally and diffusely. His finding that aberrant changes in normal, co-ordinated muscle function could be caused by imbalances anywhere in the body, gave us a new dimension to what we knew and believed about the integration of the body. As AK continued to develop and Goodheart began to understand many more of these inter-relationships, he would often describe the situation with the phrase, 'The body is simply complex and complexly simple'.

**End-organ response**

More recent research in neurology is beginning to support the basic concepts of Goodheart and AK. Some theories have been revised and others will continue to be revised as our understanding of AK improves. Even so, the fundamental basis of AK remains unchanged. Nothing happens in the body without being registered by the nervous system. Based on the type and strength of the stimulus, an appropriate response is then made. When the nervous response is to an abnormal situation, changes in muscle resistance patterns will and do occur. In fact, any sensory or mechanical stimulus in the human body that is registered by the nervous system has the potential to create changes in the 'end-organ'. The end-organ in this context is understood to be that organ or tissue which is the final receptor of the nervous impulse. In muscle it would be the neuromuscular spindle cell that contains the motor unit for muscle contraction. Failure of the nervous system to co-ordinate contraction against a dynamic resistance is called in AK the 'weak muscle'.

## Failed neuromuscular co-ordination

For some time, in AK, it was believed that the muscle weakness noted in the manual muscle test was reflected in a lack of strength in the muscle, but this idea has since been cast aside. New research indicates that the weak muscle phenomenon is most likely a failure of the neuromuscular complex to co-ordinate and maintain contractile force against dynamic resistance. Disturbances can be found locally in muscle and can change the ability of a single muscle to maintain contraction. These disturbances could be things like strains, contusions and old injuries. When more than one muscle has changed its resistance pattern, the cause becomes more diffuse. A joint problem might cause several muscles to respond with weakness, whereas a metabolic problem like hypothyroidism or dehydration will show a more diffuse muscle reaction.

The nerve factors responsible for adverse muscle reactions can be centrally located in the brain, or they can be spinal or peripheral in nature. Aberrant signals from the nervous system will cause changes in muscle resistance that are not necessarily measured as a loss of strength. We understand this to be a failure of the nervous system to control and co-ordinate muscle contraction.

Just how the body responds at the level of the skeletal muscle depends upon what area of the nervous system is adversely stimulated. During manual muscle testing, the nervous system must be involved from the brain down to the terminal endings of the motor nerves and then back up again. The continual changes in test pressure demand constant compensation from the nervous system. When there is no disturbance causing nervous system irregularity, the patient has the capacity to keep the extremity from moving by what is called 'locking' the muscle in contraction.

## Central v. peripheral disturbance

Usually, the more peripheral the disturbance, the more local is the reaction and the fewer the adverse muscle reactions involved. In general, the greater the number of muscles involved, the more likely that the disturbances influence central nervous control. The body then responds with a more global reaction.

The AK muscle test can be combined with other external stimuli. This requires the patient to respond neurologically to at least two sets of incoming information. When the nervous system is in some way compromised by an adverse stimulus, the patient may have a reduced ability to register and respond correctly if the muscle is tested immediately thereafter. This is understood to be a form of 'neurological disorganization'. The level and severity of the disorganization will determine the type of muscle response that is made. How the muscle responds, before and after the stimulus, forms the basis for diagnostic input.

## Body language

The weakness patterns proved to be consistent and Goodheart has called this a non-verbal 'body language'. Any reaction in the body, regardless as to whether it be normal or abnormal in character, is registered, monitored and modified by the nervous system. Muscles reflect these changes in nervous output through changes in resistive capacity. These changes are consistent and reproducible. But Goodheart knew he had discovered a new language for which there was no dictionary and no written rules. Because these neuro-muscular reactions were so varied and had never been observed before, early AK practitioners were often left confused and questioned the validity of the testing procedures. As time passed, thanks to the insight of Goodheart and the persistence of the first AK doctors, most of the early problems have now been resolved and the muscle test can be performed with knowledgeable confidence by any practitioner.

This does not mean that the manual muscle test is a foolproof method of diagnosis. On the contrary, like most things, it is only as good as the person performing the task. Manual muscle testing, although becoming more scientifically accepted, is still very much a learned art and skill. Since diagnostic input is based on the muscle responses, the skill with which a doctor performs the test is paramount to making proper diagnostic conclusions. Those lacking sufficient training in precise manual muscle testing will often unconsciously change a testing parameter and a muscle will appear to weaken when in fact it did not. False conclusions may ensue and the diagnosis becomes founded on intuition rather than on reality.

Age, sex and the state of health play significant roles in every individual's response and each patient will test a little bit differently from another. This is why the 'art' of manual muscle testing is so important. Experience enables the doctor to distinguish between abnormal and normal patterns in patients who, due to age or other factors, do not have the resistive capacity, for example, of an athlete in his or her twenties. In reality, anything less than normal must be considered as some degree of abnormal. Therefore, if the practitioner must test a patient more slowly and carefully, it is an indication of nervous ability. In a child younger than 5 years, this might be an indicator of the stage of nervous development and be normal. In an older person, it is an indicator of the degree of nervous degeneration and, although a normal consequence of ageing, the quality of the test gives the doctor much information as to the vigour and vitality of the individual.

## Over-zealous testing

Sometimes, practitioners have been misled by over-zealous, unskilled proponents of manual muscle testing who, as in the days of the travelling medicine man, tended to brandish AK as a prophetic cure-all for mankind. Applied kinesiology helps the practitioner arrive at a more precise diagnosis through the pre- and post-muscle test. Any information gathered by the doctor is ultimately dependent upon the quality of the muscle test. If the test is not performed correctly, it becomes the weakest link in the chain and transforms AK into a New Age phenomenon equal to pyramid power, the pendulum and the Ouija board, rather than a useful tool for the serious practitioner.

## Weak *v.* over-facilitation

Today, we have a much better understanding of the muscle weakness patterns, what kind of problems create the reactions and how to test for them. We also know that muscles seem to respond by becoming over-facilitated rather than weak. At first, this made it difficult for AK practitioners as the muscles tended to remain abnormally resistant to muscle testing. They had more convoluted methods of testing for this type of response than we do today. Under normal testing procedures, these muscles tested as if they were truly normal, when, in fact, they were not.

We are still not exactly sure just how to define this reaction. It has been called 'hypertonic', 'frozen', and 'over-reactive' among others. We know the muscle is not hypertonic because it is not contracted and shortened. The other two terms do not seem to identify the reaction adequately. Over-facilitation appears to be the result of increased neural tonus in response to some stressor. More often than not, this stress is of a metabolic (chemical/ nutritional) nature, but it can be psychological as well. True mechanical problems do not seem to create increased neural tonus. The over-facilitation phenomenon provides us with more insight into human compensatory mechanisms and the way the body tries to compensate for perceived imbalances.

## Development of AK

Applied kinesiology developed slowly, due to a natural tendency in doctors for scepticism of anything new, especially something so seemingly iconoclastic as AK. Still small in number compared to other major health professions, applied kinesiologists can now be found in almost every major country in the world. In the beginning, a severe lack of qualified teachers created a knowledge vacuum and interested doctors were often left to their own trial and error methods to learn the skill of manual muscle testing. To the untrained eye, manual muscle testing seems very simple, but it does require hours of training in order to perform it with the precision necessary for accurate diagnosis.

Most health professionals tend to resist change if it seems somewhat radical in nature. Patients do not; especially those who are seeking relief from pain. Word about how people were helped by doctors using AK spread much more quickly than did the number of qualified doctors skilled in its use. In response to this, a world-wide group of non-professionals grew who were using muscle testing to diagnose and treat anyone who would sit still for the testing procedure. Some were seriously trying to help people, some were just curious fad-followers and others turned it into a side-show, selling AK as the master key to understanding the deepest secrets of the body.

Although the number of people exposed to manual muscle testing grew quickly, due to this grass-roots phenomenon, it was a double-edged sword. On the one hand, they rapidly spread the word about the potential of AK. On the other hand, AK was frequently dismissed as lacking any scientific foundation or clinical worth because it appeared to be a system of diagnosis comparable to palm reading or the divining rod.

This trend initially upset many doctors and AK suffered for years under the stigma of being considered as just another cult fad. The change came slowly, due to the persistence of a dedicated group of doctors who continued to use AK and refused to be intimidated by presumptuous professional bias. Today, AK is making great strides among health-care professionals throughout the world and our understanding of the mechanisms responsible for this phenomenon are being supported by new and innovative scientific research able to document responses within the central nervous system.

## Basic principles of AK – 'Body language never lies'

Attributed to Dr Goodheart, the idea that body language never lies is the essence of the philosophy behind AK. It is this ability to interpret body language that is the key to success in functional diagnosis. Specific muscle tests are used by the doctor to determine where the problem originates and how to treat it. Once muscle weaknesses are found, the doctor tries to find what will return them to normal by different forms of stimuli that are registered and interpreted by the nervous system.

### The challenge mechanism

A specific sensory stimulation is called a 'challenge' and is combined with the muscle test to aid in both diagnosis and treatment. The ways in which a doctor can perform a challenge are many and only depend on what area or condition he is trying to examine. In general, however, the challenge can be broken down into a few main categories that cover most of the conditions for which it is used.

#### MECHANICAL CHALLENGE

A mechanical challenge can be made to a joint, muscle, ligament and tendon receptors and can be osseous or soft tissue in nature.

#### Osseous-articular challenge

A directional pressure is applied to a bone on the skull, spine or any joint complex of the body. This is used mostly in manual medicine in order to aid in locating the lesion and the precise correctional vector needed for the therapy.

#### Soft-tissue challenge

This is used for diagnosis of muscle, tendon, ligamentous and visceral problems. For example, temporary ischaemic pressure might be applied to an area of a muscle thought to contain an active trigger point. This is an attempt to correct a weak muscle when the problem lies within the muscle itself. Changes in muscle strength response indicate the type of problem and what therapy choices can be made.

Many other mechanical challenges exist, but they do not need to be discussed in detail here. All are designed to aid in diagnosing the problem and finding the best method of treatment.

## SENSORY CHALLENGE

A sensory challenge is made by the stimulation of the sense of smell, hearing, taste, vision and touch. Diagnostic conclusions can be made by varying the type of sensory stimulation to match the requirement of the doctor and the type of problem the patient may be experiencing. Most often used in applied kinesiology is the sense of taste in order to evaluate nutritional responses.

### Nutritional

The lingual receptors are challenged with various substances, usually nutritional in character; and muscle response is observed. If a muscle weakens or becomes over-facilitated while the lingual receptors are 'challenged', it indicates the patient has difficulty in coping with the substance which has been placed on the tongue. If the substance helps a muscle return to normal strength, it is an indication that the patient needs the substance in question in order to aid healing.

### Medicinal

This same procedure can be used for medicinal drugs. If a pharmacological agent causes abnormal muscle responses, the doctor can expect side-effects to its use. Ideally, the doctor should choose the medicine causing the fewest changes in muscle strength, indicating the least harmful drug of choice. Very simply, the procedure can be taken one step further. If a patient is suffering from a throat infection and needs an antibiotic drug, the agent of choice should do two things:

- it should strengthen the muscles reacting to the throat infection;
- it should not weaken any other muscles.

In this way the doctor is sure that the drug of choice has been determined and that it will have few, if any, negative side-effects.

The other primary senses are stimulated in the same fashion. The doctor changes the type of stimulation to fit the area being tested. For example, the patient may sniff a substance for the olfactory challenge, listen to tones and vibrations for the auditory sense and react to changes in light, accommodation and position for the visual sense. Certainly, the depth to which each of the senses can be tested is dependent upon the doctor's need and knowledge of the sensory area being examined. All that is required is that the doctor make a stimulation which is specifically designed to activate the central neuronal pools in question. Corresponding changes in pre-tested muscle response help the doctor in making a more precise diagnosis.

EMOTIONAL CHALLENGE

A patient is asked to visualize or recall a psychologically demanding situation and muscle strength is evaluated. When an emotional component is suspected, the doctor may try to determine the type of emotional stress experienced by the patient through specific positive and negative suggestions which the patient is asked to repeat. A patient may be asked to repeat phrases like, 'I am loved', 'I can love' or 'I don't have anger'. There are innumerable combinations and suggestions that can be made; the only restriction being the doctor's depth of knowledge in psychology. Muscle strength is re-evaluated after each suggestion and the doctor has a valuable input which will aid in making a more specific conclusion into the emotions and behaviour.

PSYCHOLOGICAL REVERSAL

A technique developed in AK is used for the evaluation and treatment of a problem called 'psychological reversal'. The technique has proved to be beneficial in many cases where the patient's problem tends to persist despite what seems to be proper treatment. When this is suspected, the patient is asked to repeat a positive phrase like, 'I can see myself in the future without pain', or 'I can see myself as a non-smoker in the future'. For example, the dentist has a patient suffering from TMJ pain that gets better, but always seems to return after a period of time. If the doctor suspects an emotional involvement, he might ask the patient to repeat the phrase, 'I can see myself in the future without pain in my jaw'. Other phrases may be substituted that are more specific or change the suggestion somewhat. The main idea is to be as precise as possible and that the patient understands the suggestion. One should not use the word 'want'. Many people want something, but that does not necessarily indicate that they have the capacity to accomplish that want. In that respect it is also wise to ask the patient to repeat the phrase in his/her own language to avoid any misunderstanding in translation.

If a previously normo-facilitated muscle changes its strength pattern after the suggestion, it indicates that the patient might be consciously or unconsciously resisting any change in the situation. Hence the term psychological reversal. Obviously, it is important to have the patient working together with the doctor to aid in a return to better health and this technique helps to break any emotional patterns which might inhibit this process. The treatment for this condition is a combination of nutrition, homoeopathy and acupuncture, together with having the patient repeat the positive phrase. It has been very effective in many difficult cases.

ELECTROMAGNETIC CHALLENGE

In AK, electromagnetic challenge is a specific stimulation to the meridian receptors, often known as acupuncture points. Research has shown them to be electromagnetic in character. One or several of these acupuncture points is challenged by tapping, needling, laser activation or electrical current. The method of stimulation most often used is manual tapping of the point in question. Other methods of stimulating the points exist, but are not as often used for diagnostic input or therapy in AK.

After the specific stimulus, the muscles are tested for changes in pre-challenge strength. Meridian challenge is used both diagnostically and to locate specific points affecting therapy. By assimilating the many different challenges, the doctor has the ability to examine a problem from many points of reference. AK practitioners never try to use the muscle test as the sole indicator for or against a diagnosis or therapy. Combining the positive muscle responses with clinical experience and other medical tests the doctor can arrive at a conclusion which is more specific to the patient and their needs.

# Using applied kinesiology in dentistry

### The temporomandibular joint

Applied kinesiology has been given great support by many in the dental profession because of its ability to help the dentist locate and correct the many causes of TMJ pain and dysfunction. Most dentists are aware of the influence of the jaw joints and dental occlusion on the whole body. When the jaw and occlusion function within normal limits patients will usually present with good posture, balanced emotions and a digestive system without many problems. Should the teeth and the jaw be out of balance, any one of the above can be part of the symptom complex in the suffering patient.

Dentists specializing in the TMJ know that successful results can be obtained by balancing the jaw. There are stories of hypothyroidism, pituitary dysfunction, scoliosis and digestive disorders being restored to normal by balancing the mechanical function of this area. Problems began to arise, however, when backed by enthusiasm from early successes, dentists started recommending splints and appliances for a majority of patients who appeared to have measurable jaw joint asymmetry. Believing the occlusal problems to be the cause of the other symptoms, it became all too simple to attempt equilibration. Soon it was found that not all patients presenting with imbalance of the jaw responded with the awaited success to corrective therapy. In fact, some became worse which confused matters even more. What is understood today, partly due to the efforts of dentists who use AK, is that not only can the jaw joint create havoc all over the body, but that the rest of the body can also create havoc in the jaw joint.

### Inter-professional communication

Treating the jaw has become more demanding. The dentist must be able to evaluate the relationship of the whole body to the jaw and vice versa. Most dentists, like most specialists, have a love affair with their area of expertise and to go out of that zone is like sending them on a mission to uncharted territory. To compensate for their inability, it is sometimes necessary to employ the help of a diverse group of professionals, ranging from physiotherapists to chiropractors, speech therapists and even podiatrists. Each with their own specialty, they would attempt to evaluate and eliminate other problems, often far removed from the jaw, but possibly reflected in the jaw area. The job of the dentist became less frustrating, but the extra care is passed on as an extra expense to the patient.

Yet even the cooperation of all these specialists did not remove the difficulties involved in TMJ treatment. Too often the dentist wrongly assumed that the new specialist was able to make a comprehensive evaluation and relate the rest of the body to the jaw. In many instances, the other practitioner suffered from the very same problem as the dentist, only in reverse. As with many relationships based on this premise, it frequently ended up with each doing their own thing; neither understanding the work of the other, but both crossing their fingers in the hope that the dual effort would come to fruition for them and the patient.

Based strictly on statistics, the final result should be better than any one of the two alone. Adding one or another of the various specialists would again increase the positive response to therapy. Yet this, too, has problems of cost-effectiveness to the patient. The real problem in this kind of inter-professional relationship is that one specialty usually does not have the capacity to understand the other specialties fully, let alone to communicate with them using the same language or set of diagnostic tools.

Applied kinesiology helps inter-professional understanding by bridging the gap between practitioners and allowing them to use a common denominator – the muscle test – through which to evaluate both the local and the global effect of each therapeutic input. More importantly, the use of AK techniques indicates to the specialist in one area when the patient is in need of care from another area of expertise. This might be thought of as a form of 'rapid deployment' and sends the patient more quickly to the professional who is able to remove the imbalance.

### TMJ examination

In applied kinesiology the TMJ examination is a combination of many procedures; some of them dental, others osteopathic/chiropractic, but all combined with the manual muscle test. Where the practitioner decides to begin the evaluation may vary according to professional specialty and patient history. Usually, however, visual and palpatory evaluation is begun both statically and dynamically. Very important to the applied kinesiologist is the sense of palpatory pain experienced by the patient over the muscles of mastication and the TMJ joint. Normally, two indicators of correct therapeutic input are used:

- the muscles must return to normal tested function;
- palpatory pain should be significantly reduced almost immediately after the therapy has been applied.

In conjunction with this, muscles of the shoulders and neck are tested and their responses recorded. These muscles may or may not be used later for final and more precise confirmation of the diagnosis.

The sternocleidomastoid (SCM) and upper trapezius (UT) muscles are especially useful as they have a dual innervation: one from cranial nerve XI and the other from the upper cervical area. Frequently, when the TMJ is disturbed, it influences the temporal bone which in turn compromises the area of the jugular foramen. Because the cranial portion of the innervation for these muscles must pass through this foramen, it is not uncommon to find TMJ problems coupled with weakness of one or both these muscles. Compounding the effect is the fact that the SCM attaches primarily to the mastoid process of the temporal bone and the UT to the occiput. Failure of proper muscle co-ordination between the two can increase the effect of any imbalance. Realizing this, it becomes easy to understand that anything causing an aberrant muscle reaction in these muscles must be regarded as a potential factor in TMJ dysfunction.

### Correlating the TMJ with other areas of the body

At this point, the AK practitioner might decide to remain in the area above the shoulders or proceed to eliminate possibilities arising from other areas of the body. Several methods are employed in which to do this, the most simple being to begin testing each of the major muscles associated with the area being examined. Once a discrepancy is located, the practitioner has the possibility of correlating the problem with that of the jaw or eliminating it as a local problem having little or no influence.

The method is quite simple. If the imbalance was found in the pelvis or the foot, one might ask the patient to assume different body positions which are designed either to increase or decrease the mechanical stress in the area. For the pelvis the patient might be asked to stand in a gait stance which would increase stress on the sacroiliac joints by mimicking walking. As for the feet, the patient could be asked to invert or evert the feet in order to stress the ankle mortise. After each change, the practitioner tests the SCM and/or UT muscles for changes and palpates the previously noted painful areas for changes. Any change noted in muscle patterns and pain response is a good indication that the problem is related to the TMJ symptomology. This procedure may be done with any part of the body as long as the doctor tries to isolate the part being tested and then checks it against the response at the head and neck.

When these extraneous factors have been found and eliminated the practitioner may return to the TMJ area and evaluate the jaw joint in greater depth. The SCM and UT muscles are still very important in this examination as they will help to confirm any diagnosis reached by other means. The TMJ complex is very often referred to as the craniomandibular complex, which probably is a much better description. A skilled practitioner is quite capable of evaluating all components of this complex. Harmonious occlusion must be correlated with the mandible, the maxillae, the muscles of mastication and deglutition, the cervical spine, head and neck lymphatic drainage and cranial bone motion. This becomes no small task when one realizes that they are all intricately interrelated and an incremental change in one will often cause a change in the others. Therefore, it would seem most appropriate to be able to simply and effectively evaluate each of the parts individually without losing sight of the others. Without using AK muscle testing as an adjunct to other methods, this task becomes impractical.

**Cranial imbalances**

The patient should be tested for cranial imbalances using manual muscle testing and other methods that have already been described in this text. Respiratory phasing, along with specific mechanical challenges, are used in AK to locate and treat cranial lesions. Although some of the procedures might differ, the corrective intent is the same. After each treatment the SCM/UT muscles are re-evaluated along with patient response to palpatory pain. Any changes are noted. (For more detailed discussions see Chapter 4.)

**Therapy localization**

There are many different tools at the disposal of the practitioner which help to make a diagnosis more precise. One of these is called 'therapy localization'. Goodheart observed that patient muscle resistance could change if they were allowed to place their hands on certain parts of their bodies. There was no real consistency from one patient to the next and for a while this reaction caused him concern.

Experimenting with this phenomenon, Goodheart realized that when the fingers were placed over a problem area, pre-tested muscle strength would often change. Sometimes the dorsal aspect of the hand could give the same result, but overall, the palmar aspect of the fingers gave the most consistent response. He then found that by opposing the thumb and the little finger and touching the skin over problem areas of the body, a much greater result was forthcoming. He likened it to turning up the 'squelch' on a walkie-talkie for a better signal. Neurologically, we know that only humans can oppose the thumb and little finger, the action requiring higher centres of cerebral function. Goodheart hypothesized that the opposition of the digits somehow activates more of the neuronal pool which, in turn, couples more of the central reflexes into the test.

THE UNCONSCIOUS REACTION

We are still not quite sure what causes the phenomenon of the unconscious reaction, but it does change muscle strength responses and it is used extensively. The nerve endings in the fingers measure differences in pressure (touch), heat, vibration and pain. There is also evidence that changes in electromagnetic balance can be detected at the fingertips and hands. Subtle changes in heat, vibration and frequency may not be immediately apparent to us. They end up as an unconscious reaction because we have not trained ourselves consciously to recognize them. However, we can train ourselves consciously to respond to very minute stimuli. Blind people offer a very good example of this. Their sense of touch, smell and hearing becomes much more heightened. Many of them have been taught to 'feel' the frequency given off by a colour. By learning the different frequencies, the blind can learn to distinguish between each colour.

Therapy localization in AK probably utilizes these 'unconscious' nervous reactions that are coupled with the sense of being touched. Each of the specialized nerve endings may be stimulated singly or in combination with one another. Every input is processed in the thalamus, which in turn creates an appropriate response depending upon the signals received. If the brain registers that something is amiss, it can respond accordingly. If nothing seems to be out of order, no response is necessary.

Perhaps this is why it is quite impossible to tickle yourself under normal circumstances. All sensory impulses from the fingers to the central nervous system (CNS) must pass through the thalamus. At the same time the fingers are sending signals to the brain that they are doing the touching, and the part being touched is sending signals that it is being touched. The brain quickly assesses the situation and realizes that no neurological response is necessary. Hence we do not feel the tickle. When 'other' hands are doing the touching, no such correlation is made by the brain and we often end up in spasms of laughter.

The phenomenon of therapy localization may be related to these same CNS responses. Very often, problems in the body are reflected on the skin by changes in temperature and electrical conductivity. Touching a part with the fingers allows the brain to register the difference between the fingers and the area being touched. When this is put together with the manual muscle test, the CNS appears to be temporarily disorganized and previously strong muscles will change their capacity to resist the testing pressure. For now, this is at least a plausible beginning of a neurological explanation of therapy localization.

In dentistry, therapy localization may be used to help locate teeth with caries or pathological disturbance in the jaw. The patient is asked to touch the tooth and its gingiva with a finger. A strong muscle is tested against the therapy localization. When pathology exists in the tissue underlying the touching finger, the strong muscle will change its resistance pattern and become either weak or over-facilitated. Toxic amalgams, granulomas, hidden infections and other problems can be located in this fashion. Once the area is located, the dentist can choose the appropriate procedure to identify the problem further.

TMJ EVALUATION

Therapy localization for TMJ problems begins over the joint itself and the patient is asked to open, close, bite down, chew, swallow, phonate and perform many other movements. After each change, muscle response is re-evaluated. When a positive reaction is noted, the practitioner tries to confirm the result by testing different muscles related to the TMJ area. If no positive test is forthcoming the practitioner has no evidence of mechanical disturbance in the joint. They may, unless diagnostic tests indicate otherwise, proceed to evaluate other non-mechanical causes of the patient's symptoms.

For example, let us assume that a therapy localization screening test for a patient is positive when the patient bites down with a cotton roll between the molars on the right side, but not on the left. The vertical dimension (VD) of the TMJ on the right will be kept open by the cotton roll, while the condyle and meniscus on the left will be pushed higher into the glenoid fossa by the force of mastication. Should therapy localization be positive on the side of the cotton roll, it indicates a possible myofascial problem. Positive therapy localization over the joint opposite the cotton roll usually means a decreased vertical dimension problem on that side. Excess and uneven wear of dentures or a bridge or crown that is too high on the non-involved side can also cause the same positive test results.

Once the screening procedure is positive, the skilled applied kinesiologist will attempt to confirm this by using other muscle tests that are more specific to the TMJ. The most important muscles for this area are the SCM and the UT.

### Craniosacral influences

The TMJ is intricately related to the craniosacral mechanism through the temporal bone and the attachments of the muscles of mastication to the bones of the skull. When the jaw joint is adversely influenced, the craniosacral mechanism will reflect these changes. If the jaw is unbalanced, it creates abnormal tension in the muscles of mastication and the cranium becomes restricted in one way or another.

Many of the muscles attached to the skull have a pumping effect and aid in normal cranial movement. The body will try to compensate for cranial restriction by contracting some of these muscles in an almost futile attempt at liberating cranial motion. Some of these muscles can be easily tested.

The SCM is one of these important muscles. It is a muscle not unfamiliar to most dentists because it is used as an indicator for occlusal disturbances. Frequently this muscle is taut and tender in patients exhibiting some TMJ problem. The reason for this is logical. The SCM attaches to the mastoid process of the temporal bone. Restriction of the temporal bone will reflexively inhibit the SCM as the body tries to remove anything that might hinder a return to normal motion. In the example above, with the patient biting down on the cotton roll on the right side and the therapy localization screening positive on the left, we should be able to confirm this with the SCM.

The left SCM of the patient should test strong when there is no cotton roll on the right or when there is no masticator pressure on the roll. The muscle must only test weak when the patient occludes on the cotton roll. If true, the initial screening procedure has been confirmed and the doctor now has two methods for evaluating the effect of proper therapy. If the SCM does not weaken, the doctor must re-evaluate to find the cause for positive screening test. By carefully combining different mechanical variables with the muscle tests, it is possible to confirm or eliminate the many different causes of jaw joint dysfunction.

Once the applied kinesiologist has examined all of the many influencing factors for TMJ evaluation, they are ready to form a diagnosis and to recommend or perform appropriate therapy. Ideally, upon completion of a therapeutic input, muscle strength should be normalized and palpatory pain preferably reduced by at least 50%. This does not mean that the patient will be spontaneously pain-free upon leaving the office, but it does mean the patient should begin returning to more optimum health as quickly and efficiently as possible.

# Possible toxic effects in dentistry

Dentistry has more to concern itself about than just the TMJ. Dentists routinely use substances that may or may not cause harm to themselves as well as their patients. The most publicized in recent years is mercury. Hal Huggins, a dentist in Colorado, has probably done more to make us aware of the health hazards linked to mercury than any other person. Although still very controversial within the dental profession, more scientific evidence is being accumulated every year that supports the belief that we should find an alternative to the mercury-based amalgam.

## The battery effect

To complicate matters, not every amalgam has the same metals mixed together in the same ratios. For example, research in Sweden has shown that amalgams with a higher level of copper would, when new, have residues of pure mercury on the exposed surfaces. When several amalgams of differing composition are put in the mouth together with gold crowns, bridges and other metal-based objects, it is not uncommon to find that the patient has the equivalent of a small battery in their mouth. When combined with the chemical make-up of the saliva and different food substances, it is possible to create a continual micro-current in the mouth.

Micro-currents in the mouth are linked to muscle tension, headaches, loss of taste and various other symptoms caused by a simple reaction called bimetallism. Remember the experiment almost every child does in school where a small piece of steel and copper are connected to small wires they place opposite each other in a halved lemon? The current created is strong enough to light a small flashlight bulb. The same reaction can occur in the mouth when different metals are combined with a more acid saliva.

## Mercury

Galvanic current from the bimetallism is important because it alone can be responsible for many unresolved problems in our patients. However, the presence of a current with mercury amalgams is even more important. When an abnormal current is measured between fillings or a filling and another material, it creates a 'streaming potential' and tends to liberate metal ions into the saliva where they are absorbed by the body.

This does not mean that everyone should immediately get their mercury amalgams removed. First, the improper removal of amalgam may create a health crisis in some individuals. Second, not everyone has mercury amalgam intolerance as the primary cause of their symptoms. Third, the dentist cannot guarantee that new filling materials will not have any negative effects. Yet those individuals who have long-term suffering will very often cling to any glimmer of hope in an explanation for their condition and ask their dentist for advice or even demand that all their amalgams be removed.

This puts the dentist in a difficult position. Having been taught in school that mercury amalgams are totally safe, many are not prepared to accept, let alone evaluate and treat patients who may have true amalgam intolerance.

Yet if the right answers are not given, the patient may choose to seek the advice of another colleague who is perhaps more prone to do what the patient asks. The problem here is not so much that the patient chooses another colleague, but that the patient is left with the responsibility of making the correct diagnosis rather than the person who should be trained to do it – the dentist.

The dentist's problem is that no one has given him the tools with which to make this type of diagnosis. Most allergies and intolerances can be put in the category of functional disturbances whereby the patient has not developed a true pathology and diagnosis is often a hit-or-miss affair. With few metabolic markers as stepping stones to correct conclusions, the dentist may end up on a merry-go-round from which there is no beginning and no end.

### Other toxins

What is important to remember here is that even though mercury amalgams can be quite harmful to the patient, the true answer to the problem may be that the patient is suffering from the plethora of different toxins which have accumulated in the body over time. Many toxins may be responsible for the accumulated negative effect in man. Other toxins like heavy metals, radiation, chemicals and hydrocarbons are placing noxious reactions in our bodies. We live with them every day, swallowing them and inhaling them. We need to protect ourselves as best we can from each of these harmful factors.

Mercury toxicity has a list of symptoms not unlike a host of other chemical and heavy metal toxins, not to mention those of a fungal, viral and parasitic nature. One must eliminate one from the other in order to make a more precise diagnosis. If left only to blood and urine analysis and a few other specific tests, the process becomes expensive for the patient. Applied kinesiology may help the dentist to specify precisely what is the cause of the problem. Armed with this knowledge the dentist can then order specific tests to confirm the initial diagnosis. This saves time for the dentist and money for the patient.

### Testing for toxins

The applied kinesiologist uses the same procedure for testing any substance that might cause patient intolerance. The classic method used is to introduce the substance into the mouth, stimulating the lingual receptors. These send impulses directly to the brain, again via the thalamic control centres. When the brain registers a substance that initiates an abnormal response, previously tested muscles will dramatically change their strength reaction. The doctor is immediately alerted to look more closely at the offending substance.

Dentists can use this simple technique quite effectively in their surgeries. Prior to using a foreign substance in the mouth, a minute portion of the material can be put on the tongue and the patient asked to taste it. A muscle strong prior to the oral challenge, is tested again. If the patient changes muscle strength, the dentist may wish to use another type of material, preferably one that does not change the pre-tested muscle strength. This technique is especially useful when confronted with patients who are highly sensitive or suffer from multiple allergies.


## Conclusion

Many useful techniques are found in AK. When combined with the knowledge of the individual doctor or specialist, AK provides a welcome bridge from which we can understand the complexities of the human body. Institutions such as Tufts in the USA have programmes incorporating research into applied kinesiology and showing its effectiveness in the dental field. Applied kinesiology is standing the test of time and withstanding the onslaught of scientific scrutiny because it is based on sound neurological principles. Dentistry has much to gain from AK principles and dentists have much to give back in return as AK continues to develop and grow for the benefit of all.


## Bibliography

Esposito V., Leisman O. Neuromuscular effects of temporomandibular joint dysfunction. *International Journal of Neuroscience*; **68**: 3–4.

Goodheart G. *Applied Kinesiology Annual Research Manuals (1964–1996)*. 200567 Mack Ave, Grosse Point Woods, Michigan 48236: Privately published.

Goodheart G. Applied kinesiology in dysfunction of the temporomandibular joint. *In* Gelb H (ed). *Dent Clin N Am*; **27(3)**: 1983.

Lawson A., Calderon L. Interexaminer reliability of applied kinesiology manual muscle testing. *Perceptual and Motor skills*, 1997 (in press).

Lee T N. Thalamic neuron theory: theoretical basis for the role played by the central nervous system (CNS) in the causes and cures of all diseases. *Med Hypoth* 1994; **43**: 285–302.

Leisman G., Shambaugh P., Ferentz A., Somatosensory evoked potential changes during muscle testing, *International Journal of Neuroscience*, 1989, Vol. 45, pp. 143–151.

Leisman G. *et al*. Electromyographic effects of fatigue and task repetition on the validity of estimates of strong and weak muscles in applied kinesiology muscle-testing procedures, *Perceptual and Motor Skills* 1995; **80**: 963.

Magoun H I. *Osteopathy in the Cranial Field*. Kirksville, Missouri: Magoun, 1976.

Perot C., Meldener R., Gouble F. Objective measurement of proprioceptive technique consequences on muscular maximal voluntary contraction during manual muscle testing, *Agressologie* (French journal) 1991; **32(10)**: 471–474.

Saw I, Lewis R J. *Dangerous Properties of Industrial Materials*, 7th edn. Reinhold, NY: Van Nostrand, 1989.

Sigel A, Sigel H. 'Mercury and its effects on environment and biology' from the series *Metal Ions in Biological systems*. New York: Dekker, 1980.

Sigel H. *Metal Ions in Biological Systems*. New York: Dekker, 1980.

Walther D. *Applied Kinesiology*, Vol. II. *Head, Neck and Jaw Pain and Dysfunction: The Stomatognathic System*. Pueblo, Colorado: SDC Systems DC, 1983.

Walther D. *Applied Kinesiology: Synopsis*. Pueblo, Colorado: SDC Systems DC, 1988.

## Associations

Applied kinesiology is developing all over the world and inter-professional organizations for the International College of Applied Kinesiology (ICAK) are found in Russia, Japan, Europe, Australia, Canada and the USA. For information as to whom to contact in your area, it is best to write or call the International Secretary for the organization at the following address:

ICAK
6405 Metcalf Ave
Suite 503
Shawnee Mission
KS 66202
USA
Tel: 001 913 384 5336
Fax: 001 913 384 5112

ICAK UK
Downsview
New Hall Lane
Small Dole
West Sussex BN5 9YJ
Tel: 01273 493492
Fax: 01273 493694

## Courses

For details of courses in your area contact ICAK at the above address.

# Acupuncture

Simon Hayhoe

## Introduction

Acupuncture is used to some extent in the majority of hospital pain clinics[1] and many general medical practitioners include it in their armamentarium. For most people, however, there still seems to be a psychological chasm between Western medical logic and mediaeval Chinese theory. This is an unnecessary and artificial division. Acupuncture is in fact a simple technique that can be readily practised by doctors and dentists with a minimum of theoretical and practical training. It requires no knowledge of Daoist philosophy, but does need the expertise in anatomy and physiology that should have been acquired at medical or dental school.

### Historical background

There is good evidence that stone needles, 'Bian Shi', were used during the Stone Age to treat illness by pricking parts of the body.[2] Quantities of these Bian stones were found in the foothills of Eastern China, so it is thought that the practice of acupuncture originated in that area. Later, iron and bronze needles were used in other parts of China; and some fine examples of gold and silver needles were recently excavated from the tomb of a Han dynasty Prince in Northern China. There followed a long succession of Chinese physician acupuncturists, often handing their skills down through families that lasted many generations: the Xu family were noted acupuncturists for over 300 years.

There is some controversy over when the earliest known medical textbook, the 'Huang Di Nei Jing' (Yellow Emperor's Classic of Internal Medicine)[3] was completed. It is ascribed to the legendary Emperor Huang Di, the Father of the Chinese people, but it was probably started in the 5th century BC and added to by eminent physicians over the following several centuries. It contains an account of acupuncture theory, and it is clear that acupuncture was fully integrated into what was the conventional medicine of the day. Most of the masters of acupuncture used it in conjunction with drugs (herbs), something that receives little attention nowadays, despite knowledge that drugs can modify the acupuncture response. For instance, the tricyclic antidepressants, which are useful not only in depression but also in the relief of chronic pain through the enhancement of serotonin, can improve the analgesic action of acupuncture.

The acupuncture masters became the court physicians. Many books were written recording clinical observation and historical theory, when in the mid-17th century, Western influences began to deprive acupuncture of its status. By 1822 acupuncture had fallen from grace and the Emperor Dao Guang banned it from the Imperial Medical Institute. It remained a popular treatment with the people, but it was no longer practised by the court physicians. There was no research, no recording of observations and no new literature. This at a time when Western medicine had been making unprecedented advances that should have been incorporated into the theory and practice of acupuncture by leading lights of the Chinese medical profession.

It was not until the Great Leap Forward in the 1950s that acupuncture re-emerged and was enthusiastically promoted by the government. Unfortunately, the two centuries of stagnation had prevented acupuncture from advancing medically in step with modern physiological research. It was brought back undeveloped, in the same state that it had been in before its decline. This effectively prevented its assimilation into modern medical use. It was an alien subject, mediaeval in theory and outlandish in practice. Nevertheless, in recent years the Chinese have worked hard to bring their traditional medicine, including acupuncture, up to date medically, with some fine research into its basic physiology.[4] Surprisingly, there has been pressure from the West, notably from the non-medical practitioners, to retain acupuncture in its mediaeval state. The Chinese appear quite happy to provide courses in the old-fashioned theories; after all they bring in many much needed dollars. This has meant that acupuncture has three distinct types of practice in the West:

- A small number of fully trained Chinese doctors practise traditional Chinese medicine (TCM) in Western cities. They utilize the traditional Chinese teaching in the light of modern medicine, and are very often highly effective practitioners.
- A huge number of non-medical Westerners who have had some training in traditional acupuncture use it to treat medical problems with varying degrees of success. Some give great benefit to their clients, but their lack of basic medical knowledge means that care must be taken to dissuade patients from using their services without initial recourse to a general medical or dental practitioner.
- Medical, dental and veterinary practitioners tend to practise a Westernized, 'scientific' form of acupuncture in which little account is paid to the traditional laws and theories, but points are selected according to neurological and muscular patterns, with reference to the relevant neuropharmacology and physiology. The success is excellent in the relief of pain and for a few other medical problems, but less so for the majority of non-painful disease. So those practitioners who intend to use acupuncture for problems other than pain, should seek training in TCM and use this to augment their Western medical expertise.

## Relief of pain

The main use for acupuncture in dentistry is in the relief of pain,[5] for which it falls into the category of 'stimulation induced analgesia' that includes acupressure,[6] electrical point stimulators (electropuncture) and transcutaneous electrical nerve stimulation (TENS).[7]

Facial neuralgia, now being seen more often by dentists, is one of the most distressing and debilitating afflictions. This is particularly so as its conventional treatment can be poorly effective or even destructive. However, acupuncture is a highly effective (over 70% success), cheap, simple and non-intrusive treatment, sadly distinguished by its lack of use.[8] Indeed, it is of surprising benefit for most types of facial pain, which makes it all the more frustrating that the technique is so little known to dentists.

# Mechanism of action

Acupuncture itself can be used in a number of ways, related to the specific mechanism of action:

- segmental;
- distant;
- trigger point;
- traditional;
- microsystem.

In general, a combination of methods should be used for maximum benefit, but for ease of understanding each will be described separately.

### Segmental acupuncture

Pain is carried from the periphery to the spinal cord by two types of nerve fibre. Unmyelinated C fibres carry chronic, or what the anatomists call 'real' pain, while acute withdrawal or 'pinprick' pain is transmitted by small myelinated A-delta fibres.[9] The C fibres synapse at the substantia gelatinosa of the dorsal horn of the spinal cord for onward transmission to the brain, while the A-delta fibre impulses are transmitted along the spinothalamic tract, at the same time stimulating an inhibitory interneuron via a collateral within the dorsal horn. This inhibitory cell releases methionine enkephalin at the substantia gelatinosa, blocking release of the neurotransmitter substance P and thus inhibiting the transmission of pain impulses (Figure 6.1).[10]

The result of this is that pinprick (acupuncture) stimulation can block the perception of pain by neurotransmitter inhibition at a spinal level. This mechanism relies on the pinprick impulse arriving at the same segment of the spinal cord as the chronic pain impulses, hence the name 'segmental acupuncture', although it is in fact an application of Melzac and Wall's gate theory of pain.[11]

Segmental acupuncture is particularly effective for localized pain and neurological pain. At its simplest, needles inserted subcutaneously, parallel to the skin, along the line of a wound can induce a sensation akin to local

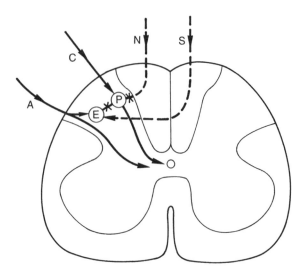

**Figure 6.1** Cross-section of spinal cord to show inhibitory pathways activated by acupuncture (A, myelinated A-delta nerve carrying 'pinprick' pain; C, unmyelinated C fibre carrying chronic pain; E, inhibitory cell releasing met-enkephalin; N, inhibitory noradrenergic fibres from brain stem; P, substantia gelatinosa cell releasing substance P; S, serotonergic fibres from higher centres; X, inhibitory neurotransmitter release)

anaesthesia for an inch or so around the wound. The needles need either manual or electrical stimulation to release sufficient enkephalin for a good spinal inhibitory effect. This is a reproducible phenomenon, quite sufficient to give good postoperative analgesia for skin wounds.

TENS, where conduction pads are applied to the skin and electrically stimulated, can induce the same local analgesic phenomenon, and electronic dental analgesia (EDA) is based on the same principle, only varying in the form of electrical stimulation. Low-frequency (2–5 Hz) gives a pricking sensation that activates the A-delta fibres in the same way as needling. This is sometimes termed 'acupuncture like electrical stimulation', as the frequency is similar to that of manual stimulation of a needle. Higher frequencies (100 + Hz) give a buzzing sensation that activate A-beta fibres which are sensitive to vibration. The spinal blockade induced by A-beta fibre stimulation is similar to that with A-delta fibres, but the inhibitory neurotransmitter involved is gamma amino butyric acid (GABA).

As might be expected, the inhibitory effect is not confined purely to a single segment. The enkephalin or GABA diffuses up and down the spinal cord to act on the segments above and below that which was stimulated. This is particularly important in the treatment of facial neuralgia, where there is small myelinated nerve degeneration, as in any long-standing neuralgia, allowing the normal sensations of touch, vibration and temperature change to be interpreted as pain. In some patients, needling into the neuralgic area thus exacerbates their pain rather than helping it. Fortunately it is possible to stimulate the segments above and below that affected, together with the same segment contralaterally. This gives good diffusion of inhibitory transmitter into the appropriate area with useful interruption of the pain pathway.

In practice, gentle low-frequency electrical stimulation is often needed and regular weekly treatments may be required over 2 or 3 months to give long term relief. Adequate, if not total, success is to be expected for most sufferers. Recurrence is likely if the patient has major physical or mental trauma, which are the usual triggers that cause instability of any neuralgia no matter what suppressant treatment is being used, even if there had been an effective response. A couple of acupuncture treatments will usually suffice to restore benefit.

Where then, should the needles actually go? Theoretically, any safe point within the distribution of the appropriate nerve root will do, superficially to stimulate within a dermatome and deeper to reach a myotome or sclerotome, bearing in mind that the nerve root supply to a muscle or bone may be very different from that of the overlying skin. However, the traditional Chinese acupoints provide a good basis for point selection as they have proved safe and effective over the centuries, and are now known often to be points at which A-delta nerves come to the surface, giving a good chance of entry into the spinal inhibitory pathways.

## Distant acupuncture

The folk remedy of dropping a brick on your big toe to relieve a toothache not only works, but can be physiologically explained. It is really using the well-respected principle of distraction, now graced with the name 'diffuse noxious inhibitory control' (DNIC), in which a strong stimulus of any sort can distract attention from chronic pain.[12] Neurologically, a strong peripheral stimulus feeds into the spinal pathway in the usual way, but this can have no segmental inhibitory effect as it is not close enough to the chronically painful area. However, arrival of the strong stimulus in the brain sets off a descending inhibitory system that has a whole-body effect. This has been well researched in experimental animals and is known to involve beta-endorphin and serotonin as inhibitory neurochemicals.[13] This acts not only along nerve pathways which have a generalized spinal feedback into the inhibitory segmental system with release of methionine enkephalin at the substantia gelatinosa, but also by humoral release of beta-endorphin from the pituitary.

The discovery of acupuncture's modulation of these neurohormones and transmitters is worthy of a detective story. Chinese experimenters joined the carotid arteries of two rabbits, thus providing a crossed circulation, and after giving acupuncture to one rabbit, found that both developed generalized analgesia, suggesting that some analgesic substance had been released into the blood by the first rabbit following acupuncture. Their second experiment was to take a sample of cerebrospinal fluid (CSF) from an acupunctured rabbit which had developed generalized analgesia and inject it into the 4th ventricle of a second rabbit, so that it entered the CSF circulation. The second rabbit was then found to have a generalized analgesia, effectively demonstrating that an analgesic substance had been released after acupuncture into the CSF as well as into the blood stream.

Some of the morphine receptors had been discovered by this time, so there was speculation that the analgesic substance released by acupuncture could be an endogenous opioid acting at these receptors. Naloxone is a specific opiate antagonist,[14] so Pomeranz in Canada gave this to rats to find out if it would inhibit the normal development of generalized analgesia. It did, but only if manual or low-frequency (4 HZ) electrical stimulation was used. Naloxone did not block the effect of 200 Hz stimulation, but further experiments showed that blockade did occur if the rats were pretreated with a serotonin inhibitor. Thus there appeared to be two mechanisms for acupuncture analgesia: opioid and serotonin.[15]

For the next stage in the story, Wen, a neurosurgeon at the Kwong Wah Hospital in Hong Kong, took CSF and blood samples from patients half an hour after electroacupuncture; these were flown to a team at St Bartholemew's Hospital in London, where they were analysed using newly developed, specific, radioimmunoassay techniques. It was found that low-frequency electroacupuncture was followed by a substantial rise in both CSF and blood beta-endorphin levels,[16] while higher frequency (125 Hz) induced release of methionine enkephalin.[17] Anatomists later took up the investigation to delineate the neurological pathways involved and used micro-techniques to demonstrate their relationship with the neurotransmitters.

The most dramatic application of distant acupuncture is the so-called 'acupuncture anaesthesia', in which the patient has sufficiently generalized analgesia to tolerate surgery.[18–20] When this works it is very effective, but unfortunately it is often inadequate, requiring additional analgesia and sedation; indeed it is normal practice in China to add a low dose of neurolept anaesthetic (tranquillizer and opiate analgesic) together with appropriate local anaesthesia. Despite this it seems worth while, as it improves the degree and speed of recovery and is reported as reducing postoperative complications such as infection and oedema. Surprisingly, although acupuncture has been known as an effective analgesic for so long, its use as an adjunct to surgery is very recent, with the first intentional use for surgical analgesia being in 1958 for a dental extraction. This was rapidly followed by use in tonsillectomy and now it is common practice in many Chinese hospitals and a few in the West for a variety of operations, particularly head and neck procedures for which it seems more reliable.

Bonica investigated the general Chinese claim of a 94% success rate for acupuncture anaesthesia and found that patients were graded into three levels of success and one of failure. Grade 1 (30%) was good analgesia, grade 2 (37%) was inadequate analgesia, grade 3 (27%) was pain that did not prevent the operation continuing and grade 4 (6%) was severe pain that disrupted the operation. From the Chinese point of view, the first three grades were successful since the operation was completed. From a Western point of view, grades 2, 3 and 4 would all be considered failures of the technique since the patients were in pain. Further, only those patients (about 10%) who were psychologically suitable and who had already demonstrated an analgesic response to acupuncture were selected for acupuncture anaesthesia. Thus the Westernized success rate was about 3% rather than the 94% quoted. This is reflected in the initial use that was made of the technique in China.

Despite a serious shortage of anaesthetists and anaesthetic equipment during the years of the political Great Leap Forward, acupuncture anaesthesia was little used except in a few centres in China. It was not until Mao Tse Tung's notorious Cultural Revolution that it was declared a suitably Chinese invention, and promoted with zeal. Unfortunately, this entailed substantial, politically motivated misuse. Surgeons and anaesthetists had been dismissed and were subject to political re-education, while the hospital porters and cleaners had to perform the operations. Acupuncture anaesthesia had to be seen to work, so patients were held down while their screams were drowned by the chanting of Mao's famous 'Little Red Book'; thus 100% success was obtained.

After Mao, when life had returned to normal in China, the ruling Gang of Four declared that acupuncture anaesthesia existed only in the imagination and that it had no clinical use. This was clearly untrue as thousands of operations continue to be performed annually with its benefit. The selection of patients has been refined, so that success is now the norm in those who receive it. Specifically, patients must be psychologically suitable and also develop the 'acupuncture state' on testing preoperatively: following needling there should be a one degree rise in skin temperature, a rise in pain threshold and a rise in pain tolerance.[21]

The foregoing highlights the problem of interpreting Chinese research papers, which often claim a success rate of over 90%, with many trials achieving 100%. It is not that there is any intention to mislead, as the true figures are usually given, but that the interpretation is of a culturally Oriental, over enthusiastic variety rather than the typically Western, phlegmatic reporting that we have come to expect from our research papers. Each Chinese report, therefore, needs to be re-evaluated with this in mind, rather than being dismissed as simply unbelievable.

So what points are most suitable to activate descending inhibitory pathways and induce DNIC? In theory, any distant point at which manual or electrical stimulation can be felt reasonably strongly should have the desired effect, but in practice a small number of points have become standard to use in most cases, in particular one on the hand (LI.4) for procedures in the upper half of the body and one in the foot (LR.3) for the lower half (see **'Point description'** section later in the chapter).

### Trigger point acupuncture

Trigger points are acutely tender spots in muscle, associated with a pattern of referred pain usually including or related to the involved muscle, but surprisingly often actually felt at some distance from it. The distinction between pain and tenderness needs to be clear. Pain is what the patient reports at rest or on particular movements. Tenderness is felt only on pressure. In the case of trigger points, tenderness is elicited by firm, rolling pressure with the tip of a finger on specific points in muscle. A hard muscle band can usually be felt. Often the patient is quite unaware of any muscle tender spots despite the sometimes severe, chronic pain associated with them.

Locating trigger points is a matter of experience and with careful musculoskeletal examination it is very straightforward, aided nowadays by some excellent manuals describing and illustrating the positions of trigger points associated with particular pain patterns.[22–24] These trigger point/pain patterns are remarkably constant, so you can surprise a patient by going straight to a previously unnoticed tender spot – tremendous for your diagnostic reputation! The anatomical positioning of trigger points corresponds closely with that of traditional acupuncture points,[25,26] suggesting that the development of traditional acupuncture was based substantially on the needling of tender points, known as 'Ah Shi' points. In chronic problems, abnormal use of the muscle containing the primary trigger point can activate secondary points in muscles further and further away, so that after a few months there may be multiple trigger sites to be treated.

The so-called 'myofascial pain syndrome', in which trigger points have become activated and tender, can mimic various facial problems: headache, facial pain, ear pain, temporomandibular joint (TMJ) pain or dental pain. In particular, those frustrating patients who complain of severe pain in an apparently normal tooth, and often insist on its extraction, may have trigger points in the masseter or temporalis muscles, needling of which can effectively eliminate the pain (Figures 6.2 and *6.3*).

### Traditional acupuncture

Acupuncture is only one part of TCM, which also involves herbal treatment, massage and moxibustion. TCM as a whole is based on the holistic concept that disease is due to an imbalance within the body, the family or the environment, and this is expressed by the relationship of Yin and Yang: negative/positive, black/white, female/male, in which, within a closed system, a deficiency of one inevitably produces an excess of the other.[27–29]

Traditional theory says that the body is kept in balance by a flow of vitality along 12 paired meridians, each of which is intimately related to an internal organ, e.g. the heart or the bladder, and maximally potent at a specific time of day when the flow of vitality is maximal within it. This is expressed in the Midday–Midnight Law which gives the time that the energy surge takes place for each meridian (Table 6.1).

In addition to the 12 main meridians described here, there are the Conception Vessel, Governing Vessel and Extra Points. These are covered under 'point description' later in the chapter.

The Mother–Son Law describes the flow of energy along the meridians from one to another (the order of flow can be seen from the time of energy surge). It states that in disease there is a blockage within a meridian, so that vitality is excessive in the meridian before the block and deficient after it. This blockage is said to be caused by one or more of the traditional Chinese 'pathogens': weather, emotion, wounds, infestation, food, drink and poison.

A traditional history and physical examination is undertaken. These are not so very different from their Western equivalents, but the examination concentrates on the pulse and tongue. Both of these formed the mainstay of Western examination in the old days before more mechanized methods became available, and many a good, old-fashioned GP will still use them in preference. The Chinese had integrated the information obtained into their traditional system. Thus, the pulse was taken at three points and two depths along the radial artery of both wrists, giving 12 readings, one

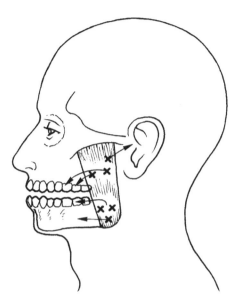

**Figure 6.2** Areas of referred pain from trigger points in the masseter muscle

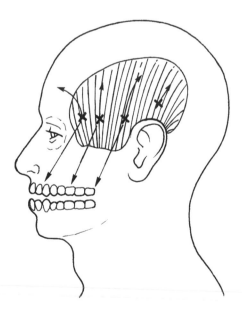

**Figure 6.3** Areas of referred pain from trigger points in the temporalis muscle

**Table 6.1 The 12 meridians showing the Midday–Midnight Law**

|  | Yin meridians (Interior, Zang Organs) |  | Yang meridians (Exterior, Fu Organs) |
|---|---|---|---|
| 4 a.m. | Lung (Hand Taiyin) | 6 a.m. | Large intestine (Hand Yangming) |
| 10 a.m. | Spleen (Foot Taiyin) | 8 a.m. | Stomach (Foot Yangming) |
| 12 m.d. | Heart (Hand Shaoyin) | 2 p.m. | Small intestine (Hand Taiyang) |
| 6 p.m. | Kidney (Foot Shaoyin) | 4 p.m. | Bladder (Foot Taiyang) |
| 8 p.m. | Pericardium (Hand Jueyin) | 10 p.m. | Triple energizer (Hand Shaoyang) |
| 2 a.m. | Liver (Foot Jueyin) | 12 m.n. | Gall bladder (Foot Shaoyang) |

relating to each meridian. This theory is expressed as the Husband–Wife Law, which describes the relationship between pulses on the left (dominant, husband) side of the body and those on the right. The trouble is, that despite this law there is dispute as to which position relates to which meridian.

A TCM diagnosis is then arrived at. Application of traditional laws, such as the Law of the Five Elements, helps to select acupuncture points that will relieve the blockage and allow a normal flow of vitality again. The five elements law arranges the organs in Yin–Yang pairs (as in the list above) around a five-pointed star, each corner of which relates to an element: earth, metal, water, wood and fire. Lines within the star show how the elements (and their organs) are creative or destructive to each other and thus how stimulation or sedation of a particular meridian should affect a diseased organ. It is intriguing to note that the Greek system, upon which Western medicine is based, had four elements: earth, air, water and fire.

The TCM theoretical explanation of the clinical observations may seem bizarre in the light of current anatomical and physiological knowledge that was not available at the time they were made, but the points selected by TCM theory are usually very similar to those suggested by the application of modern neurophysiology. This is certainly true when using acupuncture for pain relief but, effective as it is, there is often little logical explanation for the use of acupuncture in non-painful disease. So, perforce, traditional theory must be used until such time as Western research can come up with a more realistic approach.

The theory of acupuncture was initially based on observation of the clinical relationship between organs, diurnal variation and disease patterns. The Chinese cultural love of symmetry and order caused these practical observations to be adapted to fit a beautifully constructed, but artificial, pattern. It is now difficult to determine, from the laws and theories that have been handed down, where logic ends and fantasy begins.

Through the centuries the Chinese Masters have generally interpreted the tradition of acupuncture in a thoroughly pragmatic manner; the theory is there to be used only in so far as it helps in the selection of an effective point prescription. Our modern use of acupuncture must likewise avoid a slavish adherence to tradition; but it would be an enormous loss to reject it entirely.

The position of TCM in China today is as a true parallel system to Western medicine, with patients being able to choose an initial consultation in either and doctors being expected to treat within their own competence or refer into the alternative system. Thus physicians will have had a full medical training in TCM with a good grounding in Western medicine, or vice versa depending on their preference, both types of course being of equal length. So it is clear that traditional theory is not to be picked up after a few lectures or even after months of study, particularly for Westerners in whom a major shift in attitude towards health and disease is necessary. As a result, Western acupuncturists often opt for a 'cookbook' approach to treatment, selecting points that have been traditionally recommended for a particular problem, without fully understanding the rationale behind their use. The results may not be as good as with a full TCM diagnosis and prescription, although due to the lack of comparative controlled trials this must remain speculative, but for many problems they are quite acceptable.

## Microsystem acupuncture

In recent years, a multiplicity of 'microsystems' have been described: ear acupuncture,[30] hand acupuncture,[31] foot acupuncture (similar to reflexology), oral acupuncture,[32] scalp acupuncture,[33] 1st metacarpal acupuncture[34] and a host of others. Some are based on a homuncular representation of the whole body on the physical area of the microsystem, and some on a meridian system like that of traditional body acupuncture. None can offer much in the way of controlled clinical trials. Although their proponents are fiercely enthusiastic about the benefits of specific points within their preferred microsystem for specific problems, there is a feeling that this is merely an alternative route to inducing DNIC.

### ORAL ACUPUNCTURE

This is a system in which the meridians are represented by points in the buccal sulcus, beside specific teeth in each quadrant.[32] Thus: kidney and bladder are beside the incisors; liver and gall bladder are beside the canines; spleen and stomach beside the premolars in the lower jaw and the first two molars in the upper, while lung and large intestine are beside the upper premolars and lower first two molars; heart and small intestine are beside the third molars (see Table 10.1). Note that the meridians are in the same Yin–Yang pairs as in the five elements law (see the TCM section above). These have been termed the five functional circuits. Additionally there is a series of points in the retromolar space. Gleditsch[35] describes treatment by injecting a small amount of normal saline into the appropriate points with a fine dental hypodermic needle, since the use of acupuncture needles in the mouth is hazardous due to the risk of inhalation or swallowing.

### EAR ACUPUNCTURE

Probably the best known of the microsystems is auricular acupuncture,[36] which the Chinese claim to have been the first to use.[37] However, there is no doubt that its popularity is due to a Frenchman, Paul Nogier, who in the 1950s noted the French folk remedy of cautery to a point on the ear to relieve sciatic pain. Following this discovery, he mapped ear points that corresponded with painful areas throughout the body and constructed an

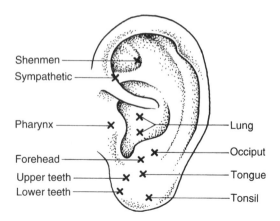

Shenmen
Sympathetic
Pharynx
Forehead
Upper teeth
Lower teeth
Lung
Occiput
Tongue
Tonsil

**Figure 6.4** Nogier acupuncture points on the ear, useful in dentistry

inverted homunculus planned out over the surface of the ear. Some of the Nogier acupuncture points useful in dentistry can be seen in *Figure 6.4*.

The standard method of treatment is to press over the ear with a blunt probe until a tender spot is found that should relate on the map to the painful body area, and then needle this briefly and superficially.

The concept of this technique, treating the whole body by needling specific points on the ear, seemed inherently unlikely until a research team at the UCLA School of Medicine tested the hypothesis by probing the ears of 40 patients with assorted, prediagnosed pain problems to find tender spots.[38] Patients were hidden under a sheet with only the ears visible while the experimenters attempted to predict their area of pain using Nogier's auricular map. They achieved a 75% success rate, well beyond the bounds of intelligent guesswork.

Following on from Nogier's original ear acupuncture, a number of variants of auriculotherapy are now popular. Taping a seed (*semen vaccara*) over the selected ear point and then using finger pressure to stimulate this is widely practised in China and is a popular and apparently effective way of expelling gallstones.[39]

The ear provides a very suitable site for the insertion of semi-permanent, indwelling needles which can be left for a period to give prolonged, continuous, gentle stimulation at specific auriculo-acupuncture points. The most common use for this technique is in the treatment of addictions,[40–42] particularly tobacco, when a tiny press-needle is placed over the lung point in the cavum conchae, so that it penetrates the skin surface but not into the cartilage, and is taped on to the skin. Stimulation can be provided if necessary by pressing with the tip of a finger whenever the addictive urge is felt. This gives a little endorphin boost that overcomes withdrawal symptoms and enhances relaxation. It is surprisingly effective, but must be looked upon as a useful adjunct to aid withdrawal rather than a magic replacement for will power.

Needles left penetrating the skin for more than brief periods can act as a nidus for infection. In the ear this is seen as a painful, red, swollen area around the indwelling needle. The needle should be removed at once and antibiotics commenced; despite this, auricular chondritis can leave the ear permanently disfigured.[43,44] Worse, if the patient has a cardiac defect, particularly valvular, the consequent bacteraemia can cause bacterial endocarditis;[45,46] there have been deaths from this. It is vital, therefore, that indwelling needles are left *in situ* for no longer than 1 week, that patients are warned to remove their needle if the site becomes red or painful and that a cardiac history is an absolute contraindication to the use of indwelling needles.

## Practising acupuncture

### Needles

Needles come in a range of types, lengths and thicknesses, but the most suitable for beginners is the pre-sterilized, disposable variety, ready packed in plastic guide tubes. They are extremely easy to put in with a minimum of practice and are virtually pain free. The method of insertion is to press the guide tube on to the acupuncture point and tap the needle into the skin. For the face, half-inch, gauge 34 needles are the most popular; elsewhere on the body 1 inch are usually better. Hypodermic needles have a cutting edge; acupuncture needles do not. So bleeding after needling is rarely a problem, since acupuncture needles tend to push blood vessels aside rather than slice through them. Despite this, bruising can be a problem in some places, such as around the eye.[47]

Although very fine, the needles are strong. None the less breakage can occur, leaving a piece of needle buried in the patient. In the majority of cases no harm comes from this; indeed there is a technique popular with a large group of licensed, non-medical acupuncturists in Japan, called Okibari, in which needle tips are intentionally broken off and left under the skin to provide continuous stimulation at the acupuncture point.[48,49] Unfortunately, needle tips can migrate elsewhere in the body. If they get into a blood vessel, they may be washed along to the heart;[50] and in Japan cardiac surgery has been needed to remove needle tips that were causing myocardial irritation.[51] Also, needle tips in the muscle of the back have been known to migrate to the spinal cord, where they have induced neurological symptoms.[52–54] So broken needles should be surgically removed without delay.

### Needle stimulation

The amount of stimulation required after insertion of a needle is still a source of controversy. Traditionally needles are pushed through into muscle and rotated to induce 'needling sensation', which is variously described as a 'deep-seated hurt' or an 'electric tingle', depending on the site stimulated. More commonly now, brief, superficial needling is considered sufficient, even for trigger point deactivation, as induced activity of the A-delta nerves overlying the trigger point often seems to be as effective as needling into the point itself.

When I first started acupuncture, I was upset to find that many of my patients went through a severe worsening of their condition before gaining benefit from my ministrations.[55] At that time I was an enthusiastic needler, giving all my patients either strong manual or electrical stimulation. It was not till I heeded the advice of my mentors to be gentle always, that I saw a change in pattern. My routine is now to use brief, superficial acupuncture on the first visit and to increase the amount of stimulation on subsequent visits until the maximum benefit is seen without upset; as a result I need electrical stimulation only rarely. This may mean that I sometimes have to treat for one or two more sessions, but worsening after treatment is unusual. It is particularly important to be very gentle in needling pregnant patients; indeed some authorities suggest that acupuncture should be avoided altogether, preferring acupressure or TENS, since it is possible that over-stimulation at some points could induce abortion.

Electrical stimulation of the needles should normally be left to later stages of treatment, but there are several occasions, such as chronic back pain, neuralgia and baldness, when electro-acupuncture is the most likely treatment to help, right from the start. There are a variety of complicated and expensive machines that offer types of electrical stimulation, but the simplest are perfectly adequate for needle stimulation. It is important to use a machine specifically made for electroacupuncture, as TENS machines intended for use with pads rather than needles may have a wide pulse width that allows excessive heating, with a consequent skin burn, when connected to a needle.[56] The method is to attach the positive and negative electrodes to a pair of needles inserted at acupuncture or trigger points, or within the muscle to be stimulated. Neural accommodation tends to occur if single-frequency stimulation is used, so commonly two frequencies alternating at brief intervals, or a modulated frequency in which stimulation is given in bursts, is fed through the needles.

As explained in the Mechanism of action section above, high-intensity, low-frequency acupuncture (2–5 Hz) generates a release of beta-endorphin, while low-intensity, high frequency (100+ Hz) stimulation releases met-enkephalin, both of which act as inhibitory neurochemicals blocking pain sensation. Low frequency should thus be given as strongly as possible without causing pain, with good muscular twitching visible. High frequency should be a pleasant, gentle vibration with little or no muscular movement. The maximum release of neurochemicals occurs after about 20 min, so it is rare to prolong treatment for more than this period. Sensitive patients who have had a good release of endogenous opioids become very relaxed and may be sleepy enough to make driving home after treatment dangerous.[57] Electrical stimulation on the neck can affect the baroreceptors situated around the carotid, causing a fall in blood pressure; and low-frequency electrical impulses can inhibit the normal activity of a demand pacemaker.[58]

## MOXIBUSTION

Another variant of stimulation popular in China is moxibustion. This is essentially the stimulation of an acupuncture point by heat. The dried leaves of Artemesia plants are teased into a wool-like state and burned, either on slices of ginger laid directly on the skin, or wrapped around the handle of an acupuncture needle, thus giving a very point-specific heating effect. Traditionally, this is used for diseases of the cold and damp, such as arthritis. The problem is that burns are common, and the smell is unacceptable in a Western surgery, so electrical heaters have been developed to attach to the needles that provide the same heating effect without the dangers. None the less, this is not a popular form of therapy medically.

## Treatment frequency

In China, treatment may often be given daily, but in the West it is rare to treat more than once a week. Apart from the obvious practical aspect of providing sufficient clinic time, weekly treatment seems logical since needling causes a small amount of injury, with consequent release of tissue injury factors, that last for about a week until the tiny wound has healed. As a rule, acute problems settle rapidly if they are going to respond, while chronic disease requires multiple sessions. Again, as a rule, if no response is seen within three sessions, it is unlikely that benefit will be obtained and there is little point in persevering with acupuncture treatment. The generalized success rate found in several large studies is around 70%, with about 20% of people seeming to be non-responders.[29]

## Side-effects

Not only is acupuncture sufficiently powerful that over-treatment can cause worsening but, like any other effective therapy, it can have side-effects, some dangerous. Indeed in the 1st and 2nd centuries the Chinese regarded acupuncture as far too dangerous for normal use, since the cult of ancestor worship had made anatomical dissection unacceptable and even physicians were therefore profoundly ignorant of internal anatomy. As a result, the practice of acupuncture at that time was all but forbidden. Most complications, like the puncture of internal organs, are due to inadequate anatomical knowledge or faulty technique, but some may be quite unexpected unless forewarned.

### FAINTING

One such side-effect is fainting, sometimes accompanied by an epileptiform fit, which occurs as an autonomic over-response to needling, particularly in young men at their first treatment session.[59-61] In general, therefore, a first acupuncture treatment should be given lying rather than sitting.

### PNEUMOTHORAX

The most common major complication of acupuncture that has many reports in a wide variety of journals is pneumothorax.[62-73] One would naturally take care when needling the chest not to insert a needle deeply, but patients with thoracic deformity may have a surprisingly thin chest wall. A British death occurred in a scoleotic patient when needling punctured a large emphysematous bullus that was less than an inch from the skin surface; it is therefore safest never to insert the needle more than half an inch (12 mm) into the chest wall.

A point on the ridge of the shoulder near the nape of the neck, GB.21, which is a very commonly used tender spot associated with neck pain and headache, has been the source of many pneumothoraces, as the apex of the lung comes close to the skin surface there; to avoid danger needles should be inserted superficially, parallel to the skin. However, unless there is major chest pathology, a small lung puncture may give minimal symptoms, so there is a consequent under-reporting of the problem. An American patient had 5 acupuncture treatments, 3 of which produced mild chest pain and shortness of breath, but all settled within a few days except the last. When she consulted her doctor about this, the pneumothorax was discovered. Typically, pneumothorax following acupuncture does not present for a few hours and may not be diagnosed for a few days, as X-ray changes are not always readily visible in the early stages.

INTERNAL ORGAN DAMAGE

There are reports of puncture of most other major organs, notably the liver, spleen and gall bladder in malarial areas when these organs are enlarged or abnormally positioned. Death from puncture of the heart has occurred, one recently due to needling at CV.17, in the centre of the sternum,[74] where a congenital sternal foramen is to be found in almost 10% of men and 5% of women. This does not show on a plain chest X-ray, so needling must be done with care. Acupuncture may give rapid pain relief. Occasionally someone discovers this for themselves and is tempted to try self-administered treatment with a darning needle. A woman developed cardiac tamponade and died after pushing a needle into her heart, apparently to relieve chest pain.[75]

EAR DAMAGE

There was at one time a vogue for attempting to treat deafness with acupuncture. Needles inserted behind the ear lobe have penetrated the ear drum and disrupted the middle ear. A major Chinese trial involving 1000 patients demonstrated no overall benefit in the treatment of deafness: a similar number worsened as improved, and one had cerebellar damage from deep needling at the base of the skull.[76]

EYE DAMAGE

The eye is at risk from inappropriate needling. There are several points that traditionally require a needle to be placed between the eyeball and the orbital fossa,[28] so occasional penetration of the eyeball and subconjunctival haematoma can be anticipated if traditional teaching is followed. Sensible medical usage avoids this risk.

Similarly, tradition recommends needle insertion into a number of other sites at which deep penetration or misdirection can cause serious damage. Treatment for respiratory problems may require a needle to be inserted at the suprasternal notch and to penetrate for one and a half inches (38 mm) directly behind the sternum.[28] Needless to say, the damage that can be caused by misdirection is frightening.

## CRANIAL DAMAGE

At points in the midline below the skull, the margin of safety between the traditional needling depth and penetration of the cervical cord or cerebellum was dangerously small,[77] although more recent editions of Chinese textbooks have reduced the depth and thus the danger.[28] Certain midline points on the skull itself are commonly used to induce relaxation. However, they are deemed forbidden points in children because of the danger of penetrating a fontanelle.

## INFECTION

### BACTERIAL

Bacterial infection is very rare with simple needling into normal tissue as the skin is self-cleansing. There is no need to use alcohol wipes;[78] indeed unless a full antibacterial alcohol cleansing is used, a brief wipe can destroy normal commensals and allow overgrowth of pathogenic bacteria. The only cases where bacterial infection is a problem are when indwelling needles are left in the skin and in the immunocompromised patient, particularly after radiotherapy.

### VIRAL

Viral infection, notably hepatitis B, is quite another matter. There have been several recorded outbreaks of hepatitis B in the West from lack of sterilization of acupuncture needles by non-medical therapists,[79-82] and the endemic nature of hepatitis in China may in part be due to the widespread use of unsterilized needles.[83] With a more general understanding of the need for sterilization, and the availability of cheap, disposable needles, this problem should become a thing of the past, but patients would be wise to check that their acupuncturist is following a correct practice. Use pre-sterilized, disposable needles and neither you nor your patients can be exposed to risk.

Patients also worry about transmission of the AIDS virus; perhaps needlessly, since there are no proven recorded cases.[84,85] There is unlikely to be any appreciable volume of blood transmitted. Unlike hepatitis where only a trace of serum is required, AIDS transmission is probably only possible with a hollow needle, that should not be used for acupuncture anyway.

The public assume that acupuncture is a totally complication-free therapy. In medical and dental hands they do not expect harm from the insertion of a needle. It is vital that we use acupuncture in a safe manner, avoiding the risks that are inherent in some traditional teaching, by thinking of the anatomy of any structure that we intend to puncture and bearing in mind that superficial needling is frequently as effective as deep stimulation.

**Training**

Simple as it is, like all practical therapies acupuncture should be observed and practised under supervision until confidence is reached. The easiest way of achieving this is to go on one of the introductory medical courses specifically aimed to teach doctors and dentists how to start treating patients safely in the surgery. Most of these basic courses are of good quality, short and inexpensive. The British Medical Acupuncture Society (BMAS) is happy to give advice about courses in Great Britain and has international contacts with equivalent medical societies throughout the world. Their address, and that of ICMART, the International Council for Medical Acupuncture and Related Techniques, are to be found at the end of this chapter. ICMART is a council of medical acupuncture societies (currently there are about 40 national societies with membership) that acts as a political voice to promote the medical use of acupuncture, and supports annual international symposia to encourage research and exchange of information.

There are large numbers of TCM-based courses run by non-medical associations of lay acupuncturists. For dentists I would first advise attending a medical acupuncture course that will relate the technique to your own professional Western medical knowledge. Far better to get a good grounding in the scientific use of acupuncture, and subsequently, if TCM or the historical aspects appeal, go on a proper TCM course in China. Then is the time to broaden your acupuncture base with useful traditional teaching, when you are more able to select and learn the beneficial parts of TCM, while enjoying the symmetrical beauty of traditional Chinese theory without becoming overwhelmed by its unfamiliar culture.

## Treatment techniques

This section is intended as a practical guide to dental acupuncture for beginners, bearing in mind that there is no substitute for attendance at a good practical and theoretical medical course. Remember also that as medical and dental practitioners we are expected to make as accurate a diagnosis as possible, and certainly to exclude any serious conditions, e.g. temporal arteritis as a cause of headache.

Inevitably other practitioners may have favourite points that I do not mention. As you gain experience you too will wish to try other points based on a rational approach to treatment as I have outlined above, particularly in problem patients. My aim is merely to give a reasonable chance of success in the typical patient.

### Point location

Whether you are convinced or not that acupuncture points naturally fall along meridians,[86,87] this should not influence your use of the effective, internationally agreed shorthand to describe accurate positioning of points. Each point is described by two letters standing for the meridian, followed by a number indicating the position on the meridian line. The anatomical descriptions are as follows, but the term 'inch' (25 mm) should be modified

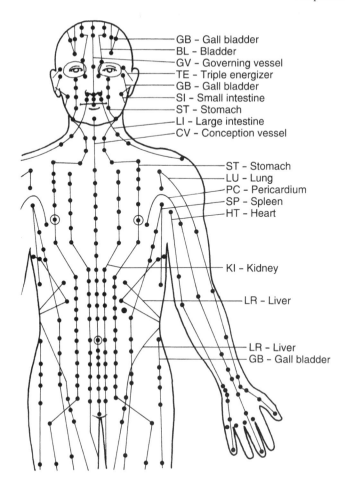

**Figure 6.5** Traditional acupuncture meridians of the upper part of the body

according to the size of the patient, such that the width of the four fingers at the level of the proximal interphalangeal joints is equal to three 'inches' for that patient. In the average adult it is indeed equal to 3 inches (75 mm), but in a child, the proportion is reduced. If in doubt about a position, remember that points are rarely over a bony prominence, but are frequently in a soft spot or hollow. Even if they are not trigger points, they are often tender. Described below, listed under their various meridians, are some of the common acupuncture points used in dentistry (Figure 6.5).

## Point description

### BLADDER MERIDIAN

BL.2 is above the inner canthus, in the hollow close to the inner end of the eyebrow. It is used for headache, facial paralysis and eye disease.

BL.10 is lateral to the trapezius muscle at the level of C1–2 interspace. It is used for headache (occipital), neck stiffness, sore throat and poor sleeping.

### CONCEPTION VESSEL

CV.17 is in the midline of the sternum, midway between the nipples with the subject lying flat on the back. It is used for hiccough, asthma and bronchitis. Needling should be horizontal to the skin, as a sternal foramen can occur here allowing unexpected penetration of the heart.

CV.22 is in the midline in the suprasternal fossa. It is used for sore throat, retching, hiccough, asthma and bronchitis. Use superficial needling only.

CV.23 is in the midline, midway between the top of the cricoid and the lower border of the jaw. It is used for sore throat.

### EXTRA POINTS

EX.1 is above the nose, midway between the eyebrows. It is used for frontal headache, vertigo and nasal disease.

EX.2 is in the hollow 1 'inch' behind the midpoint between the end of the eyebrow and the outer canthus of the eye. It is used for tooth extraction, facial neuralgia (ophthalmic), facial paralysis, migraine and eye disease.

EX.3 is in the supraorbital notch. It is used for frontal headache, facial paralysis and eye disease.

### GALL BLADDER MERIDIAN

GB.2 is anterior to the tragal notch of the ear, in a hollow formed on opening the mouth. It is used for TMJ pain, facial neuralgia (mandibular), facial paralysis and ear disease.

GB.3 is anterior to the ear on the superior border of the zygomatic arch. It is used for toothache, facial neuralgia (ophthalmic), facial paralysis and ear disease.

GB.14 is 1 'inch' above the centre of the eyebrow. It is used for headache (frontal), facial neuralgia (ophthalmic), facial paralysis and eye disease.

GB.20 is in the hollow below the occipital protuberance. It is used for headache, neck stiffness and vertigo.

GB.21 is a tender spot on the ridge of the shoulder about 2 'inches' from the nape of the neck. It is used for headache related to neck stiffness, and is a common trigger point. Needling should be horizontal to the skin, as the apex of the lung is close to the surface here, with risk of pneumothorax.

### GOVERNING VESSEL

GV.15 is in the midline, in the C1–2 interspace. It is used for headache related to neck stiffness, deafness and anxiety states. Do not needle deeply.

GV.20 is in the midline, on a line extended from the ear lobe through the ear apex. It is a relaxation point, and is thus helpful for any disease in which anxiety plays a part. Beware of needling through a fontanelle.

### KIDNEY MERIDIAN

KI.3 is midway between the medial maleolus and the Achilles tendon. It is used for toothache and sore throat.

### LARGE INTESTINE MERIDIAN

LI.4 is found by approximating the thumb and index finger; the point is in the highest spot of the muscle bulge so formed. It is an important strong point for the whole of the head, neck and arm, being particularly useful for headache, sore throat, toothache and tooth extraction. It also has an anti-allergic effect.

LI.11 is midway between the lateral epicondyle of the humerus and the end of the elbow crease when the arm is bent at a right angle. It is an anti-allergic point and is useful in skin disease, infection, and pain or paralysis of the arm and shoulder.

LI.20 is in the tiny hollow at the lower and outer point of the nares. It is painful to needle but is often effective in hay fever, sinusitis, blocked nose and snoring.

### LIVER MERIDIAN

LR.3 is at the top of the valley formed by the large and second toes. It is an important strong point for the lower half of the body, but acts as a strong distant point for the head. It is thus useful in headache. Additionally, it is an anti-hypertensive, anti-emetic and anti-epileptic point.

### LUNG MERIDIAN

LU.11 is on the outer edge of the thumb in the flesh just below the corner of the nail. It is used for sore throat and fever.

### PERICARDIUM MERIDIAN

PC.6 is 2 'inches' above the main wrist crease in a hollow between radius and ulna. It is an anti-nausea point and is also used for insomnia and hiccough.

### SMALL INTESTINE MERIDIAN

SI.17 is behind the angle of the mandible at the edge of sternomastoid. It is used for TMJ pain, salivary abnormalities, tonsillitis and sore throat.

SI.18 is in the hollow inferior to the zygomatic arch, directly below the outer canthus of the eye. It is used for facial neuralgia (maxillary), facial paralysis and toothache.

SI.19 is in the hollow formed anterior to the tragus of the ear when the jaw is opened. It is used in facial neuralgia (maxillary), facial paralysis and ear disease.

## SPLEEN MERIDIAN

SP.6 is a tender spot 3 'inches' above the medial maleolus, posterior to the border of the tibia. It is a hormonal point of particular use in menstrual abnormalities, and thus of help in premenstrual headache.

SP.10 is in the belly of the vastus medialis 2 'inches' above the patella. It is an anti-allergic point helpful in headache, skin disease and menstrual irregularity.

## STOMACH MERIDIAN

ST.2 is in the hollow of the infraorbital foramen. It is used in facial neuralgia (maxillary), facial paralysis, headache, sinusitis and eye disease.

ST.3 is at the level of the inferior border of the nose, directly below ST.2. It is used in facial neuralgia (maxillary), facial paralysis, lip or cheek pain, toothache and nosebleeds.

ST.4 is directly below ST.2 and 3, lateral to the corner of the mouth. It is used for facial neuralgia (mandibular), facial paralysis and salivation problems.

ST.5 is over the mandibular groove, anterior to the angle of the jaw. It is used for facial neuralgia (mandibular), facial paralysis, toothache and parotid salivary problems.

ST.6 is in the bulge of the masseter, felt when the jaw is clenched, above and anterior to the angle of the jaw. It is used for facial neuralgia (mandibular), facial paralysis, toothache, parotid salivary problems and spasm of the masseter.

ST.7 is anterior to the condyloid process of the mandible, in the hollow in the inferior border of the zygomatic arch. It is used for facial neuralgia (maxillary), facial paralysis, toothache and TMJ pain.

ST.9 is at the level of the thyroid cartilage on the anterior edge of sternomastoid. It is used for sore throat, gag reflex, hypertension and asthma.

ST.36 is in the hollow between the tibia and fibula, below the anterior crest of the tibia. It is used as a general tonic point, for nausea, gut disease and hypertension.

ST.44 is at the proximal end of the valley between the second and middle toes. It is used in toothache, tonsillitis and headache.

## TRIPLE ENERGIZER MERIDIAN

TE.16 is at the level of the angle of the jaw, on the posterior edge of sternomastoid. It is used for neck tension and deafness.

TE.17 is behind the ear lobe in the hollow between the mastoid process and the mandible. It is used for ear disease, facial paralysis and parotid salivary dysfunction. Needling should be superficial only.

TE.21 is in the hollow anterior to the upper notch of the ear, over the zygomatic arch. It is used for facial neuralgia (ophthalmic), facial paralysis and ear disease.

## Treatment modalities used in dentistry

Use a small number of points briefly for sensitive patients and more, with increased stimulation, for less strong responders. I have selected points using a combination of the methods previously described, so that although the following may appear as a cookbook listing of traditional points, most can be justified on a neurological basis

### TMJ PAIN

There have been quite a number of reports in which acupuncture has proved effective in the relief of TMJ pain; indeed it seems logical to try this cheap and pain-free option before attempting surgical treatment which can be expensive, hazardous and painful.[88-91]

General: LI.4, GB.20
Local: GB.2, SI.17, ST.7
Trigger point: Neck: sternomastoid, trapezius, platysma
　　　　　　　Behind mandible: lateral and medial pterygoids
　　　　　　　Under angle of jaw: posterior belly of digastric
　　　　　　　Under zygoma: deep layer of masseter

### DENTAL PAIN

Acupuncture has little place in the usual forms of dental pain, since this can be relieved so simply by conventional means, e.g. local anaesthetic. However, it can certainly be useful in particular cases and for post-extraction pain.[7, 92-96]

General: LI.4, ST.44, KI.3
Local: ST.6,7, TE.21
Ear: upper and lower tooth points on lobe
Trigger point: Under chin: anterior belly of digastric (lower incisors)
　　　　　　　Angle of jaw: masseter (all molars and premolars)
　　　　　　　Temporal: temporalis (all upper teeth)

### TOOTH EXTRACTION

There is little place for acupuncture as a replacement for conventional analgesia in extraction, except in special circumstances,[97-100] although the first use of acupuncture anaesthesia in China was for a dental extraction. There is, however, evidence that there is less postoperative pain, swelling, inflammation and infection when acupuncture is used.

General: LI.4
Local: ST.7, EX.2
Ear: upper or lower teeth

FACIAL NEURALGIAS

This includes post-herpetic and trigeminal neuralgias and atypical facial pain.[8,101–103] It may be necessary to needle contralaterally to the painful area and into the areas above and below it on the affected side so as to avoid needling directly into a neuralgic segment. I regard acupuncture as the treatment of choice for facial neuralgias, certainly in the first instance, since it has a high success rate (over 70% in some centres), is non-invasive and complication free, unlike most of the other treatment options. Carbamazepine and tricyclic antidepressants are commonly used drug treatments, both of which can be effective at damping down neuralgic pain. Do not stop or reduce these drugs while giving acupuncture, as both appear to enhance the benefit derived from the acupuncture treatment. Once treatment has proved effective, the drugs may be reduced very cautiously.

General: LI.4, ST.44, GV.20
Local: Mandibular: GB.2, ST.4,5,6
    Maxillary: SI.18,19, ST.2,3,7
    Ophthalmic: TE.21, GB.3,14, EX.2
Ear: shenmen, sympathetic, upper or lower teeth, cheek

### FACIAL PARALYSIS

The Chinese claim good success with this problem, although there is little work in the West to confirm their claims. Electrical stimulation is usually necessary.

General: GB.20, GV.20, LI.4
Local (depending on area of paralysis): GB.2,3,14, SI.18,19, TE.17,21, BL.2, EX.2, ST.2,3,4,5,7

### HEADACHE AND MIGRAINE

A number of controlled clinical trials have demonstrated the effectivity of acupuncture in headache and migraine.[104–110] Unlike most drug treatments, acupuncture is of long-term, prophylactic benefit, but can also be used effectively in acute episodes.

There are many causes of headache, some of which can also act as triggers for migraine. I have therefore suggested points for the different causes, which should be combined prophylactically with points for the area where headache is predominantly felt. During a headache, LI.4 alone often gives rapid relief.

General: LI.4, LR.3, GB.20, GV.20
Ear: shenmen, sympathetic, occiput, forehead

**Causes:**
*Tension*: GB.20,21, BL.10, TE.16, LI.4, LR.3, GV.15,20
*Myofascial*: trigger points, particularly in sternomastoid
*Allergic*: LI.4,11, SP.10
*Sinusitis*: LI.20, ST.2, BL.2, EX.1
*Eyes* (myopia): EX.2, GB.20
*Earache*: GB.2,20, TE.17,21, SI.19
*Premenstrual*: SP.6, GV.20
*Hypertension*: LR.3, ST.36, LI.4, SP.6, GV.20
*Migraine with nausea*: PC.6, LI.4, LR.3, GB.20, GV.20
*Cluster headache*: generally poor response

**Positions:**
Frontal: GB.14, Bl.2, EX.1,3
Temporal: EX.2
Occipital: GB.20
Top of head: GV.20

### DRY MOUTH OR OVER-SALIVATION

Surprisingly, the same points are used for both ends of the spectrum; there seems to be a rebalancing effect, just as traditional Chinese teaching suggests.

General: LI.4, PC.6, GV.20
Local: SI.17, ST.4,5,6, CV.23

### RETCHING OR EXCESSIVE GAG

A recent paper has found that acupressure at PC.6 is ineffective alone for retching.[111] However, acupuncture at other points may be useful,[112] or it may well be that sedative points are indicated initially, particularly GV.20 and LI.4.

General: PC.6, GV.20, LI.4
Local: CV.22,23, ST.9

### NAUSEA AND VOMITING

Over 30 controlled trials have now been published demonstrating that PC.6 acupuncture is a highly effective anti-nauseant in a variety of situations from the nausea of pregnancy,[113] through postoperative nausea,[114,115] to that associated with cancer chemotherapy.[116] This evidence is now so strong that not even the most virulent disbeliever in acupuncture could reasonably reject it. Much of the credit for this must go to Professor Dundee, who had already acquired expertise in the investigation of nausea and vomiting through work with many anti-emetic drugs. He set out to perform controlled trials of a high standard with acupuncture, acupressure and electrical stimulation at the PC.6 point. Despite attack from the medical hierarchy,[117] he maintained momentum with an objective series of trials, published in a variety of peer-reviewed medical journals. Although he died in 1991, his

Anaesthetic Department at the University in Belfast has retained an interest and work is still continuing.[118]

It has been shown that acupuncture is more effective for nausea than for vomiting, but as the distress felt by a patient is mainly because of the nausea, this still leaves acupuncture as a favourite with the patients. Ideally, acupuncture should be administered before the emetic stimulus occurs,[119] i.e. preoperatively before the premed, before getting out of bed in pregnancy and before boarding ship for sea sickness. The acupuncture can be prolonged in effect by acupressure maintained regularly by the patient.[120]

General: GV.20
Specific: PC.6, LR.3

HAY FEVER

Although many patients claim good, long-term relief from acupuncture, there is surprisingly little trial evidence for its benefits. However, a dummy acupuncture (needling at non-standard sites) controlled trial found that both standard and dummy acupuncture were equally effective (70%) in relieving hay fever.[121] So it may be that any point would do!

General: GV.20, LI.4, SP.10
Local: LI.20, EX.1

SORE THROAT

Used as an analgesic, acupuncture should prove effective, but there is also evidence that there is an increase in protective immunoglobulins and in white cell count, so an anti-infective action seems to be occurring.[122] This is unlikely to be of practical use in bacterial infection, since antibiotics are much faster and more guaranteed effective, but the longer lasting, untreatable, viral pharyngitis should certainly benefit from acupuncture.

General: LI.4, LU.11, KI.3
Local: SI.17, CV.23, BL.10
Ear: pharynx, tonsil

SNORING

I have personally found this symptom very responsive to acupuncture. Unfortunately, the points, LI.20, on either side of the nose, are rather uncomfortable to needle, but patients are very willing to put up with this as the results seem so good. I get particular praise from the spouse!

General: LI.4
Local: LI.20

## Conclusion

Used sensibly by doctors and dentists, acupuncture is an extremely safe method of treatment that has a surprisingly high level of success in the relief of facial pain, even where conventional medicine has failed to give benefit. It is worth trying also in non-painful facial disease, although the physiological rationale is sometimes less obvious. Even beginners can expect encouraging results, so do not be put off by the complicated traditional Chinese theory: use Western medical logic as I have described and have a go. Your patients will be delighted!

# References

1 Spoerel W E, Leung C Y. Acupuncture in a pain clinic. *Can Anaesth Soc J* 1974; **21(2):** 221–229.

2 Ma K W. The roots and development of Chinese acupuncture: from prehistory to early 20th century. *Acupunct Med* 1992; **10(Suppl):** 92–99.

3 Veith I. *The Yellow Emperor's Classic of Internal Medicine*. Berkeley: University of California Press, 1972.

4 Han J S, Terenius L. Neurochemical basis of acupuncture analgesia. *Ann Rev Pharmacol. Toxicol* 1982; **22:** 193–220.

5 Richardson P H, Vincent C A. Acupuncture for the treatment of pain; a review of evaluative research. *Pain* 1986; **24:** 15–40.

6 Penzer V, Matsumoto K. Acupressure in dental practice: magic at the tips of your fingers. *J Mass Dent Soc* 1985; **34(2):** 71–75.

7 Hansson P, Ekblom A. Transcutaneous electrical nerve stimulation (TENS) as compared to placebo TENS for the relief of acute oro-facial pain. *Pain* 1983; **15:** 157–165.

8 Merchant N. Facial pain: a review of 200 cases treated with acupuncture. *Acupunct Med* 1995; **13 (2):** 110–111.

9 Bowsher D. Physiology and pathophysiology of pain. *Acupunct Med* 1990; **7(1):** 17–20.

10 Kiser R S, Khatami M, Gatchel R J, *et al*. Acupuncture relief of chronic pain correlates with increased plasma met-enkephalin concentrations. *Lancet* 1983; **2:** 1394–1396.

11 Melzack R, Wall P D. Pain mechanisms: a new theory. *Science* 1965; **150:** 971–979.

12 Le Bars D, Villanueva L, Willer J C *et al*. Diffuse noxious inhibitory controls (DNIC) in animals and in man. *Acupunct Med* 1991; **9(2):** 47–56.

13 Bowsher D. The physiology of stimulation-produced analgesia. *Acupunct Med* 1991; **9(2):** 58–62.

14 Mayer D J, Price D D, Rafii A. Antagonism of acupuncture analgesia in man by the narcotic antagonist naloxone. *Brain Res* 1977; **121:** 368–372.

15 Cheng R S S, Pomeranz B. Electroacupuncture analgesia could be mediated by at least two pain-relieving mechanisms; endorphin and non-endorphin systems. *Life Sci* 1979; **25:** 1957–1962.

16 Clement-Jones V, McLaughlin L, Tomlin S *et al*. Increased $\beta$-endorphin but not met-enkephalin levels in human cerebrospinal fluid after acupuncture for recurrent pain. *Lancet* 1980; **2:** 946–949.

17 Clement-Jones V, Lowry P J, McLaughlin L *et al*. Acupuncture in heroin addicts: changes in met-enkephalin and $\beta$-endorphin in blood and cerebrospinal fluid. *Lancet* 1979; **2:** 380–383.

18 Kho H G, Van Edmond J, Zhuang C F *et al*. Acupuncture anaesthesia. Observations on its use for removal of thyroid adenoma and influence on recovery and morbidity in a Chinese hospital. *Anaesthesia* 1990; **45:** 480–486.

19 Abbate D, Santamaria A, Brambilla A *et al*. $\beta$-Endorphin and electroacupuncture. *Lancet* 1980; **2:** 1309.

20 Gongbai C. Acupuncture anaesthesia in neurosurgery. *Chinese Med J* 1981; **94(7):** 423–430.

21 Wong C K M. Acupuncture induced anaesthesia: fiction or fact? *Acupunct Med* 1993; **11(2):** 55–60.

22 Baldry P E. *Acupuncture, Trigger Points and Musculoskeletal Pain*. Edinburgh: Churchill Livingstone, 1989.
23 Travell J G, Simons D G. *Myofascial Pain and Dysfunction: The Trigger Point Manual*. Baltimore: Williams & Wilkins, 1983.
24 Travell J G, Simons D G. *Myofascial Pain and Dysfunction: The Trigger Point Manual. The Lower Extremities*. Baltimore: Williams & Wilkins,1992.
25 Melzack R, Stillwell D M, Fox E J. Trigger points and acupuncture points for pain: correlations and implications. *Pain* 1977; **3:** 3–23.
26 Liu Y K, Varela M, Oswald R. The correspondence between some motor points and acupuncture loci. *Am J Ch Med* 1977; **3:** 347–358.
27 Cheng X (ed). *Chinese Acupuncture and Moxibustion*. Beijing: Foreign Languages Press, 1987.
28 Beijing College of Traditional Chinese Medicine, Shanghai College of Traditional Chinese Medicine, Nanjing College of Traditional Chinese Medicine, and the Acupuncture Institute of Traditional Medicine. *Essentials of Chinese Acupuncture*. Beijing: Foreign Languages Press, 1980.
29 Mann F. *Textbook of Acupuncture*. London: Heinemann, 1987.
30 Brougham P. Short notes on ear acupuncture. *Acupunct Med* 1992; **10(1):** 32–35.
31 Magovern P. Koryo hand acupuncture: a versatile and potent acupuncture microsystem. *Acupunct Med* 1995; **13(1):** 10–14.
32 Gleditsch J. Oral acupuncture. *Acupunct Med* 1995; **13(1):** 15–19.
33 Yamamoto T. New scalp acupuncture. *Acupunct Med* 1989; **6:** 46–48.
34 Schjelderup V. ECIWO biology and bio-holographic acupuncture. *Acupunct Med* 1992; **10(1):** 29–31.
35 Gleditsch J. The 'very point' technique: a needle based point detection method. *Acupunct Med* 1995; **13(1):** 20–21.
36 Lapeer G L. Auriculotherapy in dentistry. *Cranio* 1986; **4(3):** 266–275.
37 Hsu E. The history and development of auriculotherapy. *Acupunct Med* 1992; **10(S):** 109–118.
38 Oleson T D, Kroening R J, Bresler D E. An experimental evaluation of auricular diagnosis: the somatotopic mapping of musculo-skeletal pain at ear points. *Pain* 1980; **89(2):** 217–229.
39 Guo Q, Wu S, Chen T. Clinical and experimental observation on treating cholelithiasis by ear point pressing. *Int J Clin Acup* 1991; **2(1):** 29–35.
40 Wen H L, Cheung S Y C. Treatment of drug addiction by acupuncture and electrical stimulation. *Asian J Med* 1973; **9:** 134–141.
41 Wen H L. Clinical experience and mechanism of acupuncture and electrical stimulation (AES) in the treatment of drug abuse. *Am J Ch Med* 1980; **8(4):** 349–353.
42 Patterson M. *Hooked? NET: The New Approach to Drug Cure*. London: Faber and Faber, 1986.
43 Allison G, Kravitz E. Auricular chondritis secondary to acupuncture. *New Engl J Med* 1975; **293:** 780.
44 Savage-Jones H. Auricular complications of acupuncture. *J Laryngol Otol* 1985; **99:** 1143–1145.
45 Lee R J, McIlwain J C. Subacute bacterial endocarditis following ear acupuncture. *Int J Cardiol* 1985; **7(1):** 62–63.
46 Jefferys D B, Smith S, Brennand-Roper D A *et al*. Acupuncture needles as a cause of bacterial endocarditis. *Br Med J* 1983; **287:** 326–327.
47 Redfearn T. Oh, what a surprise! *Acupunct Med* 1991; **9(1):** 2–3.
48 Gerard P S, Wilck E, Schiano T. Imaging implications in the evaluation of permanent needle acupuncture. *Clin Imaging* 1993; **17(1):** 36–40.
49 Imray T J, Hiramatsu Y. Radiographic manifestations of Japanese acupuncture. *Radiology* 1975; **115:** 625–626.
50 Nieda S, Abe T, Kuribayashi R *et al*. Cardiac trauma as complication of acupuncture treatment: a case report of cardiac tamponade resulting from a broken needle. *Jpn J Thorac Surg* 1973; **293:** 780.

51 Kusaba E. Surgical treatment of intramyocardial needles. *Nippon Kyobu Geka Gekkai Zassni* 1979; **27:** 1085–1090.

52 Hasegawa O, Shibuya K, Suzuki Y *et al.* Acupuncture needles, straying in the central nervous system and presenting neurological signs and symptoms. *Rinsho Shinkeigaku* 1990; **30(10):** 1109–1113.

53 Maruoka N, Kinoshita K, Wakisaka S. Cervical spinal cord injury caused by a broken acupuncture needle: a case report. *No ShinKei Geka* 1986; **14:** 785–787.

54 Kojima Y, Ono K, Ogino H *et al.* Migration of the needle of acupuncture into the cervical spinal canal. Report of four cases. *Chuba Nippon Seikeigeka Gakkai Zasshi* 1985; **23:** 292–294.

55 Lapeer G, Monga T N. Pain secondary to acupuncture therapy. *Cranio* 1988; **6(2):** 188–190.

56 Omura Y. Some historical aspects of acupuncture and important problems to be considered in acupuncture and electro-therapeutic research. *Acupunct Electrother Res* 1975; **1:** 3–44.

57 Brattberg G. Acupuncture treatments: a traffic hazard? *Am J Acup* 1986; **14(3):** 265–7.

58 Fujiwara H, Taniguchi K, Takeuchi J *et al.* The influence of low frequency acupuncture on a demand pacemaker. *Chest* 1980; **78(1):** 1285–1286.

59 Verma SK, Khamesra R. Recurrent fainting: an unusual reaction to acupuncture. *J Assoc Physicians India* 1989; **37(9):** 600.

60 Chen F, Hwang S, Lee H *et al.* Clinical study of syncope during acupuncture treatment. *Acup Electrother Res* 1990; **15:** 107–119.

61 Hayhoe S, Pitt E. Case reports: complications of acupuncture. *Acupunct Med* 1987; **4(2):** 15.

62 Lewis-Driver D J. Pneumothorax associated with acupuncture. *Med J Aust* 1973; **2:** 296.

63 Goldberg I. Pneumothorax associated with acupuncture. *Med J Aust* 1973; **1:** 941–942.

64 Waldman I . Pneumothorax from acupuncture. *New Engl J Med* 1974; **290:** 633.

65 Gray R, Maharajh G S, Hyland R. Pneumothorax resulting from acupuncture. *Can Assoc Radiol J* 1991; **42(2):** 139–140.

66 Huet R, Renard E, Blotman M J *et al.* Unrecognised pneumothorax after acupuncture in a female patient with anorexia nervosa. *Presse Med* 1990; **19(30):** 1415.

67 Schneider L B, Salzberg M R. Bilateral pneumothorax following acupuncture. *Ann Emerg Med* 1984; **13(8):** 643.

68 Corbett M, Sinclair M. Acu and pleuro-puncture. *New Engl J Med* 1974; **290:** 167–168.

69 Mazal D A, King T, Harvey J *et al.* Bilateral pneumothorax after acupuncture. *New Engl J Med* 1980; **302(24):** 1365–1366.

70 Ritter H G, Tarala R. Pneumothorax after acupuncture. *Br Med J* 1978; **277:** 602–603.

71 Bodner G, Topilsky M, Grief J. Pneumothorax as a complication of acupuncture in the treatment of bronchial asthma. *Ann Allergy* 1983; **51:** 401–403.

72 Kuiper J J. Pneumothorax as complication of acupuncture. *J Am Med Assoc* 1974; **229(11):** 1422.

73 Norheim A J, Fonnebo V. Adverse effects of acupuncture. *Lancet* 1995; **345:** 1576.

74 Halvorsen T B, Anda S S, Naess A B *et al.* Fatal cardiac tamponade after acupuncture through congenital sternal foramen (letter). *Lancet* 1995; **345:** 1175.

75 Schiff A F. A fatality due to acupuncture. *Med Times (Lond)* 1965; **93(6):** 630–631.

76 Liu Q, Deng Y C, Li L *et al.* Evaluation of acupuncture treatment for sensorineural deafness and deafmutism based on 20 years' experience. *Ch Med J* 1982; **95(1):** 21–24.

77 Academy of Traditional Chinese Medicine. *An Outline of Chinese Acupuncture*. Peking: Foreign Languages Press, 1975.

78 Dann T C. Routine skin preparation before injection: an unnecessary procedure. *Lancet* 1969; **1:** 96–98.

79 Communicable Diseases Surveillance Centre of the PHLS. Acupuncture associated hepatitis in the West Midlands in 1977. *Br Med J* 1977; **2:** 1610.

80 Boxall E H. Acupuncture hepatitis in the West Midlands, 1977. *J Med Virol* 1978; **2:** 377–379.

81 Kent G P, Brondum J, Keenlyside R A *et al.* A large outbreak of acupuncture associated hepatitis B. *Am J Epidemiol* 1988; **127:** 591–598.

82 Garcia-Bengoechea M, Cabriada J, Arriola J A *et al.* Hepatitis B caused by acupuncture and the same acupuncturist. *Med Clin Barc* 1985; **85(16):** 686.

83 Conn H. Acupuncture in epidemic HBV hepatitis: in China too? *Hepatology* 1988; **8(5):** 1176–1177.

84 Vittecoq D, Mettetal J F, Rouzioux C *et al.* Acute HIV infection after acupuncture treatments. *New Engl J Med* 1989; **320(4):** 250–251.

85 Castro KG, Lifson AR, White CR *et al.* Investigations of AIDS patients with no previously identified risk factors. *J Am Med Assoc* 1988; **259(9):** 1338–1342.

86 MacDonald A J R. Acupuncture analgesia and therapy – Part 1. *Acupunct Med* 1990; **7(1):** 8–12.

87 Buck C C. Propagated needle sensation. *J Ch Med* 1986; **22:** 15–16.

88 Ho V, Bradley P. Acupuncture for resistant temporo-mandibular joint pain dysfunction syndrome. *Acupunct Med* 1992; **10(2):** 53–55.

89 List T, Helkimo M. Acupuncture and occlusal splint therapy in the treatment of cranio-mandibular disorders. *Acta Odontol Scand* 1992; **50(6):** 375–385.

90 Raustia A M. Diagnosis and treatment of temporomandibular joint dysfunction. Advantage of computed tomography diagnosis. Stomatognathic treatment and acupuncture – a randomised trial. *Proc Finn Dent Soc* 1986; **82(S9–10):** 1–41.

91 Raustia A M, Pohjola R T, Virtanen K K. Acupuncture compared with stomatognathic treatment for TMJ dysfunction. Part 1: a randomised study. *J Pros Dent* 1985; **54(4):** 581–585.

92 Lao L, Bergman S, Anderson R *et al.* The effect of acupuncture on post-operative oral surgery pain: a pilot study. *Acupunct Med* 1994; **12(1):** 13–17.

93 Lapeer G L, Biedermann H J, Hemsted J J. Acupuncture analgesia for postoperative dental pain. *J Can Den Assoc* 1987; **6:** 479–480.

94 Scarsella S, Palattella A, Mariani P *et al.* Electroacupuncture treatment of post-operative pain in oral surgery. *Acupunct Med* 1994; **12(2):** 75–77.

95 Sung Y F, Kutner H H, Cerine F C *et al.* Comparison of the effects of acupuncture and codeine on postoperative dental pain. *Anaesth Analges* 1977; **56(4):** 473–478.

96 Ekblom A, Hansson P, Thomsson M *et al.* Increased postoperative pain and consumption of analgesics following acupuncture. *Pain* 1991; **44:** 241–247.

97 Thompson R. A dental elective to China 1990. *Acupunct Med* 1990; **8(2):** 70–71.

98 Hansson P, Ekblom A, Thomsson M *et al.* Is acupuncture sufficient as the sole analgesic in oral surgery? *Oral Surg* 1987; **64:** 283–286.

99 Sun S. Choice of anaesthesia in dental operations. *Med Inf Lond* 1991; **16(1):** 15–24.

100 Gu Z Q, Wang Y Q, Yin X R *et al.* Clinical research on tooth extraction under acupuncture anaesthesia. *Acta Acad Med Wuhan* 1985; **5(4):** 581–585.

101 Jenkins M. Trigeminal neuralgia: what does the patient need? *Acupunct Med* 1990; **8(2):** 65–67.

102 Craig J. Electroacupuncture for trigeminal neuralgia: a ten year review. *Acupunct Med* 1988; **5(1):** 35–36.

103 Hansen P E, Hersted Hansen J. Treatment of facial pain by acupuncture. *Acta Neurochir (Wisn)* 1981; **59:** 279.

104 Hesse J, Mogelvang B, Simonsen H. Acupuncture versus metoprolol in migraine prophylaxis: a randomised trial of trigger point inactivation. *J Intern Med* 1994; **235:** 451–456.

105 Vincent C A. A controlled trial of the treatment of migraine by acupuncture. *Clin J Pain* 1989; **5:** 305–312.

106 Dowson D, Lewith G, Machin D. The effects of acupuncture versus placebo in the treatment of headache. *Pain* 1985; **21:** 35–42.

107 Loh L, Nathan P W, Schott G D *et al.* Acupuncture versus medical treatment for migraine and muscle tension headaches. *J Neurol, Neurosurg, Psychiat* 1984; **47:** 333–337.

108 Børglum Jensen L, Tallgren A, Troest T *et al.* Effect of acupuncture on headache measured by reduction in number of attacks and use of drugs. *Scand J Dent Res* 1979; **87:** 373–380.

109 Børglum Jensen L, Melsen B, Børglum Jensen S. Effect of acupuncture on myogenic headache. *Scand J Dent Res* 1977; **85:** 456–470.

110 Johannsson A, Wenneberg B, Wagersten C *et al.* Acupuncture in treatment of facial muscular pain. *Acta Odontol Scand* 1991; **49(3):** 153–158.

111 Chate R A C. PC6 acupressure for dental nausea: a preliminary report of a prospective randomized double blind clinical trial, part 1. *Acupunt Med* 1997; **15**(1): 6–9.

112 Murata T, Himuro H, Tsubaki T *et al.* Application of acupuncture for dental practice. Suppression of choke reflex during dental treatment. *Fukuoka Shika Daigaku Gakkai Zasshi* 1986; **13(3):** 170–174.

113 Dundee J W, Sourial F B R, Ghaly R G *et al.* P6 Acupressure reduces morning sickness. *J Roy Soc Med* 1988; **81:** 456–457.

114 Dundee J W, Ghaly R G, Bill K M *et al.* Effect of stimulation of the P6 antiemetic point on postoperative nausea and vomiting. *Br J Anaesth* 1989; **63:** 612–618.

115 Dundee J W. Acupuncture and postoperative sickness. *Anaesthesia* 1991; **46:** 512.

116 Dundee J W, Ghaly R G, Fitzpatrick K T J *et al.* Acupuncture prophylaxis of cancer chemotherapy induced sickness. *J Roy Soc Med* 1989; **82:** 268–271.

117 Dundee J W, McMillan C M. Some problems encountered in the scientific evaluation of acupuncture antiemesis. *Acupunct Med* 1992; **10(1):** 2–8.

118 McConaghy P, Bland D, Swales H. Acupuncture in the management of postoperative nausea and vomiting in patients receiving morphine via a patient-controlled analgesia system. *Acupunct Med* 1996; **14(1):** 2–5.

119 Dundee J W, Ghaly R G. Does the timing of P6 acupuncture influence its efficacy as a post operative antiemetic? *Br J Anaesth* 1989; **63:** 630.

120 Dundee J W, Yang J. Prolongation of the antiemetic action of P6 acupuncture by acupressure in patients having cancer chemotherapy. *J Roy Soc Med* 1990; **82:** 360–362.

121 Williamson L, Yudkin P, Livingstone R *et al.* Hay fever treatment in general practice: a randomised controlled trial comparing standardised western acupuncture with sham acupuncture. *Acupunct Med* 1996; **14(1):** 6–10.

122 Bossy J. Acupuncture and immunity: basic and clinical aspects. *Acupunct Med* 1994; **12**(12): 60–62.

# Bibliography

Baldry P E. *Acupuncture, Trigger Points and Musculoskeletal Pain.* Edinburgh: Churchill Livingstone, 1989.

Beijing College of Traditional Chinese Medicine, Shanghai College of Traditional Chinese Medicine, Nanjing College of Traditional Chinese Medicine, and the Acupuncture Institute of Traditional Medicine. *Essentials of Chinese Acupuncture.* Beijing: Foreign Languages Press, 1980.

Lu G D, Needham J. *Celestial Lancets: A History and Rationale of Acupuncture and Moxa.* Cambridge University Press, 1980.

Mann F. *Textbook of Acupuncture.* London: Heinemann, 1987.

Pomeranz B, Stux G. *Scientific Bases of Acupuncture.* Berlin: Springer Verlag, 1991.

Stux G, Pomeranz B, *Basics of Acupuncture.* Berlin: Springer Verlag, 1991.

Travell J G, Simons D G. *Myofascial Pain and Dysfunction: The Trigger Point Manual.* Baltimore: Williams & Wilkins, 1983.

## Associations

Information on any aspect of acupuncture, including courses for doctors and dentists and the names of medical contacts in most countries worldwide, can be obtained from either of the top two addresses below.

International Council for Medical
  Acupuncture and Related Techniques
  (ICMART)
Rue de l'Amazone 62
1050 Brussels
Belgium
Tel: 0032 2 539 3900
Fax: 0032 2 539 3692

British Dental Acupuncture Society (BDAS)
26 Sheppenhall Grove
Aston
Nantwich
Cheshire CW5 8DF
UK
Tel: 01270 780418

British Medical Acupuncture Society
  (BMAS)
Newton House,
Newton Lane
Lower Whitley
Warrington
Cheshire WA4 4JA
UK
Tel: 01925 730727
Fax: 01925 730492

Complementary Practitioners without a medical or dental degree are eligible to join the following organizations; patients should therefore be advised to consult a GP before treatment.

British Acupuncture Council
Park House
206 Latimer Road
London. W10 6RE
UK
Tel: 0181 964 0222
Fax: 0181 964 0333

The European Federation of Modern Acupuncture
59 Telford Crescent
Leigh
Lancshire. WN7 5LY
UK
Tel: 01942 678092
Fax: 01942 515579

## Courses

A two-day Introductory Training Course in Acupuncture for Dental Practitioners is held annually in London or Sheffield, UK, organized by the BMAS (address above). Alternatively, dentists are welcome to attend their medical acupuncture courses for doctors. The BMAS and ICMART (address above) can also give details of many other courses and seminars suitable for doctor and dentists.

# Mercury toxicity

**Jack Levenson**

## Introduction

Mercury is number 80 in the periodic table of stable elements. It is a heavy, silver-white, poisonous, metallic element. It is liquid at room temperature, but evaporates easily with slight increases of temperature. It is ubiquitous, present in rocks, soils, plants, animals, fish, water and air.

The chemical abbreviation for mercury is Hg, abbreviated from hydrargyrum (*hydro* = water, *argyrum* = silver). It is commonly designated quicksilver (liquid silver).

In Roman mythology each god or goddess had their own metal, for example Mars the god of war, was connected with iron. The name mercury described the liquid and fast-running characteristics of the metal and was consequently linked to Mercurius, the god of trade and travel.

Mercury has been mined and used since ancient times in the Orient, Arabia and Europe. Some of the best known of these mines were in India, parts of the Roman Empire and at Almaden in Spain. Slaves worked the mines and suffered the consequences of exposure to mercury fumes. Early symptoms included mental and physical fatigue, difficulty in breathing, gastrointestinal pain and discomfort.

As exposure progressed, inflammation of the oral cavity followed, with swelling and bleeding of gums, bone destruction and loosening of teeth, accompanied by excess salivation and metallic taste. Later, mental symptoms predominated. The central nervous system is the predominant target for mercury, with irritability, moodiness, poor memory, anxiety, depression and involuntary shaking, followed by deterioration and death.

So even in ancient times the toxicity of mercury was well observed, indeed the Roman scientist Caius Plinius (AD 23–79) in his well-known 'Naturalis Historia' discussed the poisonous effects of this element. In more recent times mercury poisoning has been identified in a number of situations.

### Acrodynia (pink disease)

Pink disease was caused by the use of calomel, (mercurous chloride) in teething powders and ointments. Characteristic symptoms[1] were redness and swelling of the fingers, feet, nose and ears, loosening of the teeth, excess salivation, insomnia, sweating, diarrhoea, weakness and apathy, followed by more profuse sweating, photophobia and generalized rash. About 10% of the children died. Neither the occurrence of the disease nor its severity were dose related. Mercury in the aforementioned preparations also caused another common childhood ailment, fuming renal acidosis. Both of these conditions virtually disappeared after the withdrawal of teething powders in 1953. Some 1 in 500 children were affected. The disease had been prevalent for over 100 years before the cause was identified.

The term 'mad as a hatter' originates from the insanity that used to afflict the hatters in England and France who used mercury chloride in preparing felt.

## Minamata Bay

In 1953 a mysterious neurological condition appeared among the inhabitants of Minamata City, a Japanese fishing port located on Minamata Bay. The condition was first attributed, as most illnesses of unknown origin are, to a virus, but it was eventually shown to be due to environmental pollution by mercury.

The source was identified as a nearby factory that produced the plastic compound vinyl chloride from acetylene and hydrogen chloride, which passed through tubes containing a mercuric chloride catalyst. The waste catalyst was expelled into the bay, contaminating fish stocks.

Symptoms were mainly neurological. These included polyneuropathy, hearing defects, speech and visual difficulties and sometimes blindness, ataxia, tremor and mental disturbances. Post mortems showed gross damage to brain cells and nerve tissue.

Approximately 6% of children exposed *in utero*, via the mothers' consumption of fish, developed cerebral palsy. The incidence of cerebral palsy in unexposed populations would be expected to be in the region of 0.25%. 121 people were poisoned by the methyl mercury and 46 eventually died from the initial exposure.

## Methyl mercury

Iraq was the scene of the worst outbreaks of mercury poisoning and they were all initiated by eating bread and other products made from seed grain intended for planting.[2] These grains had been treated with methyl mercury to prevent fungal growth. There were three major incidents:

- 1956    100 reported cases of poisoning;
- 1960    over 1000 reported cases of poisoning;
- 1972    over 600 admitted to hospital, 450 died.

In Sweden, crop dusting with methyl mercury heavily contaminated food supplies. The government responded quickly by banning the activity. Eventually Sweden was to lead the world on the issues surrounding mercury in dental fillings.

These are some of the examples which have been reported and are mostly concerned with methyl mercury, which is considered to be more poisonous than inorganic mercury in its liquid form. However, vapour from mercury in its liquid form covers a far greater area and has a comparable poisoning potential to methyl mercury. Biological pathways are different though. Methyl mercury enters and disrupts cell mechanisms and can pass brain and placental barriers with ease. Hal Huggins, renowned pioneer of the anti-amalgam movement said: 'There is virtually no barrier in the body to methyl mercury.'

## Mercury vapour

Inorganic mercury vapour ionizes at body temperature and acts as a free radical, interfering with enzyme reactions, taking up cellular binding sites and blocking cell intercommunication.

Methods of mercury poisoning are largely academic. Various micro-organisms in the mouth can convert inorganic mercury vapour into methyl mercury.[3] Microbial flora of human faeces can methylate mercury as can most strains of Staphylococci, yeasts and other organisms in the human intestine.[4,5]

## Poisons

Given the very large human exposure to mercury, how poisonous is it? The University of Tennessee has a famous toxicity centre where they grade poisons based upon the least amount necessary to kill a human. Plutonium is the most deadly and is rated on the scale as 1900. Some other graded poisons are as follows:

- mercury, 1600;
- lead, 900;
- nickel, 600.

Mercury, except in severe allergic reactions, is not an instantly fatal poison. It is insidious in its action and accumulates in tissues and organs. This renders diagnosis more difficult. This is coupled with the fact that since the use of mercury by physicians has been drastically reduced in therapeutic medicine, the ability to diagnose mercury poisoning has shown a similar decline.

## History of mercury in medicine

It is thought that mercury was used as a medicine in India as early as 500 BC. Due to its bactericidal effects it was introduced as a drug by Arab physicians in the tenth century for the treatment of chronic skin disease. This therapy became the standard treatment covering a wide area due to the popularity of the medieval textbook, the 'Canon of Medicine' by Avicenna.

The use of mercury in medicine spread to Europe and by the 16th century was widely prescribed as an effective treatment for syphilis. By the 18th century as mercurial treatment became established in medical practice, so opposition to its use increased. The argument became a major topic for press and public. While the controversy raged in England, paradoxically it began to be used in the USA and even with intense minority opposition its use spread. Doctors were so convinced that mercury cured venereal disease that it was perceived to be a panacea for a variety of ailments.

Mercuric chloride was used as an antibacterial solution in disinfectant. This and other salts were used as purgatives and fungicides, as ointments in treatment of eye and skin diseases and in worm chocolate as treatment for intestinal parasites. Mercury increases urinary flow and found favour as a diuretic.

Even today, mercury is still used in skin lightening creams. They were banned in Nigeria as the mercury content can cause miscarriage and affect the brain and kidneys. Mercury is in some throat lozenges and is widely used as a fungicide and preservative in vaccines and contact lens sterilizing solutions.

CASE HISTORY

*A middle-aged female member of the optical profession presented for consultation after realizing that in handling sterilizing solutions for contact lenses containing the mercury compounds, thimerosol and methiolate, she was exposed to mercury daily. She had a number of amalgam fillings. Clinical history and tests clearly indicated mercury toxicity. Her fillings were removed with full protective procedures. She changed to a mercury-free sterilizing solution. Her symptoms cleared and it transpired that, prior to consultation, she had had a positive diagnosis of a pituitary tumour which she had not divulged. The tumour resolved after her exposure to mercury was removed. She became a convinced supporter of the anti-amalgam movement and never missed an opportunity to spread the word when lecturing professionally.*

## History of mercury in dentistry

During the early 1800s the only filling material available was gold. This was expensive and out of reach for the man in the street. Increasing sugar consumption resulted in more cavities in teeth and the search for less expensive restorative materials commenced.

Various materials were used experimentally. One such material was d'Arcet's metal[6] which consisted of 8 parts bismuth, 5 parts lead, 3 parts tin, and 1/10th part mercury to hasten the fusing process. The problem with this material was that it had to be melted and then poured into the cavity.

In 1812 Joseph Bell, a British chemist, introduced the forerunner of the modern amalgam filling. This consisted of a paste which was formed by filings from silver coins and mercury, which due to impurities in the coins tended to expand, sometimes resulting in a fractured tooth or an uneven bite.

Eventually a material with more satisfactory properties was introduced. This consisted in the main of filings of a mixture of silver, tin and copper, but other metals were often used. To this mixture was added an approximately equal amount of mercury. This was moulded into a paste, inserted into a prepared tooth cavity where it hardened and provided a tooth restorative of some permanence.

### AMERICAN DENTAL ASSOCIATION

Aggressive advertising by some practitioners in New York led to an increase in demand which in turn led to a reaction, which precipitated what has become known as the first amalgam war. The opponents were the American Society of Dental Surgeons (ASDS) founded by Dr C. A. Harris in 1840.

The society vigorously opposed the use of amalgam and in 1845 they passed a resolution 'pronouncing the use of all amalgams as malpractice'. They further demanded that their members sign the following pledge: 'I hereby certify it to be my opinion and firm conviction that any amalgam whatsoever, is unfit for the plugging of teeth or fangs and I pledge myself never, under any circumstances to make use of it in my practice as a dental surgeon, and furthermore as a member of the American Society of Dental Surgeons, I do subscribe and unite with them in this protest against the use of the same.'[6]

So, in effect, dental amalgam was banned for some 15 years. But an increasingly vociferous minority defied the ban. They had found a commercially viable material, inexpensive and easy to use, durable and with no apparent side-effects.

Economics won the day. The ASDA collapsed and a new organization, the American Dental Association (ADA), was founded to support the argument that mercury was locked into fillings and could not escape. Dentists found this easy to believe, conscience and commerce were satisfied and even though a number of case histories and anti-amalgam papers were published, the issue was largely forgotten until it again became a big issue – the second amalgam war – in the 1920s.

This was led by an outstanding German chemist Professor Alfred Stock. Stock published over 30 articles condemning the use of amalgams when his own medical condition cleared after amalgam removal. Most importantly he demonstrated, by a simple reproducible scientific experiment using copper sulphate and two metallic wires, that mercury vapour was released from amalgam fillings.[7] This gained him public and academic support. Records of the time show acceptance by the public: 'Then, as I say, there was Roger with 20 holes in his teeth to be stopped; and now I hear he has mercurial poisoning from these stuffings'('The Diary of Virginia Woolf', Vol. 2, p. 126).

World War II intervened and attention was diverted. Research continued after the war and began to polarize towards the amalgam-bearing population. It had become increasingly obvious that some doubts existed regarding the prevailing theory that amalgam was a stable compound. These doubts began to be expressed as concrete research programmes.

The question arose: 'What percentage of the amalgam-bearing population is affected?' Estimates from different researchers varied considerably. Djerassi and Berova in 1969 carried out a study of 240 test subjects which included 60 controls without amalgam fillings. The controls were subjected to the same series of patch tests – none of the controls had any positive reaction. They found 5.8% were allergic to their fillings where the fillings were under 5 years old, and 22.5% where the fillings were more than 5 years old.[8]

White and Brand carried out tests on dental students,[9] and the results were:

- freshmen, 5.2% positive;
- seniors, 10.8% positive.

At Baylor University, 171 volunteer dental students patch tested for hypersensitivity to mercuric chloride.[10] Students exhibiting allergic reactions had an average 9.5 amalgam restorations. Students with fillings 5 years or older had a positive reaction of 31.6%. Students with 10 or more amalgam restorations were 44.3% positive.

A 1973 study by the North American Contact Dermatitis Group consisted of 13 research dermatologists, in a definitive study on 1200 patients.[11] They patch tested the patients with ammoniated mercury. Results showed positive reactions in 8.3% females and 5.2% males. They concluded that 2% is sufficient to justify an antigen inclusion in a screening series.

Nebenfuhrer et al.[12] tested 1530 patients with routine allergy series that included mercury. Mercury allergy was found in 9.6% of those tested. Patch test results demonstrated that

- there was no reaction from patients without amalgam fillings;
- there was an increase in positive reactions dependent on two factors:
  (a) the length of time fillings had been in the mouth,
  (b) the number of fillings in the mouth.

If 1% of the population in the UK were hypersensitive to mercury it is estimated that this would represent 250 000 people. The figures show that a large number of the population may be affected. However, in many the reactions may be minor.

For the ADA, who had steadfastly maintained that mercury was locked into fillings and could not escape, this position became untenable. In 1984 a four-day workshop of historic significance was held, sponsored by the National Institute for Dental Research and hosted by the ADA in Chicago. In a consensus of opinion statement, with no references or research, they conceded that mercury did escape from amalgam fillings. This was a watershed, it added fuel to the third and hopefully the last amalgam war. It was started in Sweden by scientist Dr Mats Hanson, and independently by Dr Hal Huggins and Dr Olympic Pints in the USA. In Great Britain a conference held by the British Dental Society for Clinical Nutrition, entitled 'Hazards in Dentistry: The Mercury Debate', was held at King's College, Cambridge in July of 1985. This sparked off media interest and coincided with the publication of 'The Toxic Time Bomb' by Sam Ziff. Worldwide interest was escalating. The theory of 'amalgam stability' was no longer valid.

Once established that mercury vapour was released from amalgam fillings, scientific curiosity was aroused. This was no longer the domain of dentists. There was low-level chronic exposure to mercury. The mantle was taken up by corrosion chemists, biochemists, pathologists, neurologists, microbiologists and others concerned with the effects of mercury on biological systems. Two questions remained unanswered:

- the extent of low-level chronic exposure to mercury;
- the effect of low-level chronic exposure to mercury.


## The extent of low-level chronic exposure

Evidence in recent years has shown that mercury is continuously released from amalgam fillings and that the amount of vapour is increased when chewing, especially hot or acidic foods. Vimy and Lorscheider[13] analysed intra-oral air in 46 subjects, 35 of whom had amalgam restorations. Chewing stimulation in subjects with amalgams increased their mercury concentration 6-fold over unstimulated mercury levels, or a 54-fold increase over levels observed in control subjects. There were significant correlations between mercury vapour released into intra-oral air after chewing stimulation and the numbers and types of amalgam restorations.[13]

In a further programme these two researchers tested 35 subjects with amalgam occlusal restorations for intra-oral air mercury with a view to estimating the daily dose of mercury from dental amalgam. They showed that mecury concentration remained elevated during 30 min of continuous chewing and declined slowly over 90 min after cessation of chewing. They calculated that all subjects received an average daily mercury dose of approximately 20 micrograms ($\mu$g). Subjects with 12 or more occlusal amalgam surfaces were estimated to receive a daily dose of 29 $\mu$g of mercury, whereas in subjects with four or fewer occlusal amalgam surfaces the dose was 8 $\mu$g. These mercury doses from dental amalgam were as much as 18-fold the allowable daily limits established by some countries for mercury exposure from all sources in the environment. The results demonstrate that the amount of elemental mercury released from dental amalgam exceeds or compromises the major percentage of internationally accepted threshold limit values for environmental mercury exposure. These papers confirm the work of previous research.[14]

The fact that this cumulative poison is released into human systems on a daily basis, coupled with the fact that there are some 22 million fillings placed every year in an estimated 15 million patients, is probably one of the most important environmental health factors of this century.


### Chemistry and mechanism of action

Mercury has a high affinity for sulphydryl (thiol) groups, for chlorine, bromine, iodine and fluorine, and easily forms halogen salts. Mercurials, even in low concentrations, are capable of inactivating sulphydryl groups present in biologically active agents. These include proteins, enzymes and enzyme inhibitors, and allow mercurials to interfere with cellular metabolism. Mercury also combines with other ligands of physiological importance, such as carboxyl, phosphoryl, amine and amide groups. The binding with various groups results in cell membrane permeability, poor cellular nutrition and interference with enzyme reactions in the cell.

In the lungs mercury vapour tends to oxidize into free radicals, i.e. mercury ions. These ions are an electrically charged form of the element and will react quickly with haemoglobin, insulin, thyroxin, coenzyme A and other enzymes or proteins with a sulphydryl group – the sulphur amino acids.

When it reacts with haemoglobin, the result is chronic fatigue. When it reacts with insulin, the pancreas is stressed. When it binds to coenzyme A, which converts food to blood sugar, the result is hypoglycaemia. Coenzyme A is also necessary for the formation of haemoglobin.

When the mercury vapour enters the saliva in peoples' mouths and is swallowed, it will combine with hydrochloric acid, to form mercuric chloride, otherwise known as corrosive sublimate. In the past when this was taken as a purgative, it was found to damage the stomach walls and to destroy the glomerulus of the kidney. This also leaves the body deficient in hydrochloric acid, thus reducing the efficiency of the primary stage of digestion.

## Dental galvanism

The presence of different metals in the same tooth, or in different teeth, acts as a battery, producing an electric current with saliva as an electrolyte. This current with its attendant electromagnetic fields is inches from the brain and cranial nerves and it can produce a variety of disorders. Conditions which have been shown to improve when fillings with high electric readings are replaced include: Bell's palsy, migraine, trigeminal neuralgia, neuromuscular pathologies and epilepsy.

A significant number of patients have reported an increase in mental energy and an improvement in thought patterns when even one quadrant with high electrical readings is removed.[15]

When other metals such as gold or cheaper dental metals such as nickel are added to the equation there is a steep increase in the release of mercury vapour – from 4- to 10-fold and a consequent increase of corrosive debris.

Metals do not have to be in contact. If two dissimilar metals are placed in an electrolyte, by the laws of electrochemistry the less noble metal has to corrode. When you have a number of dissimilar metals there is a confusion of single and multiple corrosion products released with harmful potential.

These electrical currents are inches from the brain, itself an electrical organ, so it could be expected that the electricity and attendant electromagnetic fields would have an effect on the brain, the cranial nerves and the areas which they serve.

To obtain optimal health benefits fillings should be removed in a predetermined sequence, dependent on electrical readings and the presence of other metals.

CASE HISTORY

*This patient was a healthy female in her mid-thirties with 12 amalgam fillings and one porcelain crown with a metal base. She presented 2 months after crown insertion. She was suffering from palpitations and had gradually developed food allergies. Her health was deteriorating. She was clinging to her mother, suicidally depressed and unable to fill in the questionnaire. She had been advised by her GP to seek psychiatric help and treatment with beta blockers, tranquillizers and antidepressants.*

*The crown was removed but there was no change. The amalgam fillings were sequentially removed with full precautions. The patient was temporarily worse but recovery in her own words was 'astonishing'. She was back to normal in 2 months, and 6 years later is running her own company.*

**Mercury vapour pathways**

Mercury vapour is continuously released from amalgam fillings. The amount released increases with chewing, bruxism, hot, salty and acidic foods as well as toothbrushing. These peak values gradually diminish over the next 90 minutes, when most people tend to snack, raising to peak values again. There is a direct pathway from the mouth or oronasal cavity, to the brain via the valveless craniovertebral venous system. As there are no valves to direct the flow, distribution can move freely in any direction. Another pathway directly to the brain is by axonal transport along nerves.

Mercury vapour is inhaled into the lungs where it enters the arterial circulation and is deposited in various tissue and organs, particularly the kidneys. Vapour is absorbed by saliva and passes directly to the gastrointestinal tract. It spreads through the lymphatic system via the gingiva.

# The effect of low-level chronic exposure

## General symptoms of mercury toxicity

Symptoms of low-level chronic exposure to mercury vary enormously, depending on the inherent resilience of the individual. Symptoms may occur at the time of placement or when an old amalgam is removed. More often, however, the effects are insidious, taking perhaps 5 years or more to manifest themselves. This is an important feature as it goes part of the way in explaining why the release of mercury from fillings has not been generally accepted by the health professions as being implicated in disease. If a patient has fillings placed and 5 years later develops arthritis, migraine or is generally unwell, it is unlikely that a diagnostic correlation would be made by a physician.

Many lists of signs and symptoms are produced in the literature. They are exhaustive and could apply to many other conditions. Mercury may cause neurological, respiratory, cardiovascular and digestive disorders, interfere with collagen metabolism and be implicated in food, chemical and inhalant allergies,[16] Candida and other fungal proliferations.

Some features which are very common are chronic fatigue, joint and muscle pain, tingling in the limbs, tremor in hands, irritability, depression, metallic taste in the mouth, increased salivation, headaches and early vision deterioration.

## Mercury and the immune system

Despite anything medical science has achieved, the immune system is our main defence against disease. Immunology is a complex subject, but for the purposes of this presentation, simple general principles will suffice.

A central component of our protective system is the lymphocyte or white blood cell produced by lymphoid tissue in the body.[17] There are two main subdivisions of lymphocyte: the T cells, so named because their development is influenced by the thymus gland,[18–20] and B cells made from bone marrow. Of the 10 or more types of T cells, the most important are T4 and T8.

The T4s are called the T helper cells. Their function is to identify and label foreign bodies, much like a forester putting a cross on trees to be chopped down. Once marked they can be recognized by the B cells – the killer cells – which then carry out their function which is to engulf and destroy the foreign bodies.

If T4s are reduced or non-functioning, there will be reduced immune response to antigens,[18–22] i.e. a reduced response from B cells. This is what happens in AIDS. There are plenty of white cells to deal with infections but not enough T4s to mark the infecting agents.[23–25]

The T8s or T suppressor cells help to keep the B cells under control, i.e. to stop them attacking normal body cells. The correct amount of T8 cells and the ratio of T4:T8 is crucial; immune competence is dependent on total T cells and their ratio to one another. Reductions in total T cells and unbalanced ratios can result in autoimmune disorders such as systemic lupus erythematosus, multiple sclerosis, severe atopic eczema, inflammatory bowel disease and glomerulonenephritis.[25–32]

Smith, Kline and French laboratories specialize in T-cell evaluations. They state that the T lymphocyte percentage of total lymphocytes does not vary more than 10% and rarely more than 5% in an 8-week period. Ideally 70–80% of total lymphocytes are T lymphocytes.

In May 1984 the *Journal of Prosthetic Dentistry* published a preliminary report on 'The effect of dental amalgam and nickel alloys on T-lymphocytes' by David Eggleston, Associate Professor, Department of Restorative Dentistry, University of Southern California.[32] Three cases are cited, two involving dental amalgam and one a nickel restoration. What he did was to measure T cells, remove the restorations, remeasure T cells, replace restorations and once again measure T cells. In case one, 47% of lymphocytes were T lymphocytes. After removal of amalgams, 73% of the total were T lymphocytes. After reinsertion of amalgam fillings, total T cells dropped from 73% to 55%. Similar changes were observed in the other two patients.

In summarizing the report, Eggleston states: 'Preliminary data suggest that dental amalgam and dental nickel alloys can adversely affect the quantity of T lymphocytes. Human T lymphocytes can recognise specific antigens, execute effector functions, and regulate the type and intensity of virtually all cellular immune responses. Normal immune function depends on a proper quantity, quality and ratio of T lymphocyte helper and suppressor subsets.'

In a conference held in 1986 in New York, Eggleston confirmed that he had some 30 similar cases. So a number of studies confirm the effect of mercury on the immune system, the most recent examining alterations in immune response relative to brain MRI changes.[33]

Recent clinical trials on immune response to dental metals, carried out at the Chelsea and Westminster Medical School, will be published in due course.[34] These papers support the view that low-level exposure to mercury may adversely affect the defence mechanisms of the body.

# Research

Mats Hanson has compiled a bibliography of some 13,000 research papers published on mercury since 1965; and many more are in the pipeline. Since it became evident that mercury was released from dental fillings scientific research has broadened and been taken on board by a number of university departments, mainly in the USA, Canada and Sweden. Only the most important of these papers will be highlighted.

### Tracing mercury in tissues and organs

A combined programme of research which included the Department of Medicine, Radiology and Medical Physiology, was carried out at the University of Calgary, Alberta, Canada.[35] They placed amalgam fillings in 8 adult sheep. The amalgams used had a small tracer of radioactivity which guaranteed that the mercury could be easily located and also eliminated the need for a control, as there would be no radioactivity in mercury present in food or water.

The animals were allowed to live their normal lives for nearly a month, at which time a full body image scan was taken to see if and where mercury had accumulated. They discovered that mercury had accumulated in the jaw, lungs and gastrointestinal tract, and then migrated to liver and kidneys. Further research was carried out on monkeys, being closer to humans in metabolic terms.[36] The results were replicated, and once again mercury was found to accumulate in tissues and organs.

### Pathological and physiological effects

In 1990 the same team, which now included the Pathology Department, decided to see whether any pathology resulted from this mercury. As the kidney is one of the primary targets for mercury it was chosen for investigation.[37] After placing regular fillings in several sheep they found that within 30 days kidney function and its filtration capacity were reduced by 50%. A control group which had glass ionomer fillings placed showed no change in kidney function.

They also found a rise of sodium in the urine – one of the main functions of the kidney is to reabsorb sodium. Another indication of malfunction was a 68% decline in albumin excretion. This meant that kidney blood flow was reduced. A study of 10 humans showed that 1 year after fillings were removed urinary levels of albumin were significantly higher than levels 4 months prior to removal.[38]

### Retention of mercury

Recent human chelation studies have shown that mercury from amalgam fillings is retained and accumulates in the body. When using 2,3-dimercapto-1-propane sulphonic acid (DMPS) in one study, symptomatic amalgam-bearing patients were compared with controls and had a highly significant increase in urinary mercury. The mean value increased from 5.4 $\mu$g/l to 34.3

$\mu g/l.$[39] A similar study was able to show that two-thirds of the mercury excreted in the urine of those participants with dental amalgam came from their fillings.[40]

## Mercury and pregnancy

Further work was carried out by the Calgary team on five pregnant sheep.[41] Twelve amalgam fillings were placed containing radioactive mercury in the molars at 112 days' gestation. Mercury crossed the placenta in under 3 days and showed up in the blood, pituitary gland, liver, kidney and placenta of the fetus. By 33 days, around birth time, most fetal tissues had higher levels of mercury than the mother, particularly the liver, bone marrow, blood and brain. During lactation the mother sheep were found to have 8 times the amount of mercury in their milk than in their blood.

More recently, Gustav Drasch, Professor of Forensic Medicine at the University of Munich, has demonstrated a significant direct correlation between the number of amalgam fillings in the mother and the amount of mercury in the brain, liver and kidneys of stillborn children and dead fetuses.[42] Drasch concluded that the unrestricted application of amalgam for dental restorations in women before and during the child-bearing age should be reconsidered.

## Mercury and the gastrointestinal tract

Inorganic mercury is mainly excreted in faeces and urine and small amounts in sweat. Animal studies have demonstrated that in smaller doses the importance of the fecal pathway is increased, with 85% found in faeces. Human volunteers exposed to radioactive mercury vapour showed that 79% was excreted in the faeces.[43]

## Mercury and Candida

Mercury has been used in medicine as an antiseptic and as such it was used to inhibit bacterial activity. In the gastrointestinal (GI) tract, bacteria and yeasts compete for mucosal surfaces. There are some 3–5 lb (1.4–2.3 kg) of friendly and essential bacteria in the GI tract. Inhibition of these bacteria results in a surge in growth of the yeast fungus. Very often the Candida does not respond to antifungal treatment until amalgam fillings are replaced.

If digestion is incomplete, local reactions may be indigestion, heartburn, bloating and constipation, alternating with diarrhoea and imbalance of gut flora. Undigested food can be absorbed into the blood stream, causing an allergic response. The body always responds to an allergen with an increase in tissue fluid in an attempt to dilute that antigen. Normally white blood cells engulf invaders and destroy them internally. When mercury enters the cell, it responds by absorbing water until it bursts. The destructive elements within the cell are released into the blood stream and can produce allergic reactions. Alternatively, cells may divide with even more worrying implications. Even though diet may be adequate, the inability to process foods results in deficiencies of essential nutrients.

## Bacterial resistance

Universities of Georgia, Calgary and Tufts (Boston) collaborated in a study, using primates, which showed that a large proportion of common mouth and intestinal bacteria became resistant to mercury 2 weeks after placement of amalgam fillings.[44] Nearly all the mercury-resistant bacteria were also resistant to one or more antibiotics (e.g. tetracycline, ampicillin, streptomycin, erythromycin), despite the fact that the monkeys had not been exposed to antibiotics. Antibiotic-resistance can spread to other bacteria by strands of DNA material called plasmids.

A strong correlation between mercury and multiple antibiotic-resistant intestinal bacteria had been observed by researcher Anne Summers in 1981. But at that time it was believed that mercury could not be released from fillings. Mercury resistant bacteria recirculate mercury as vapour and block elimination. Antibiotic resistant bacteria – the super bugs – are a serious and escalating problem. It is time the possible causes are reconsidered.

## Mercury and the central nervous system

A joint research programme carried out by Professor David Eggleston of California and Professor Magnus Nylander of Sweden used neutron activation analysis on 83 autopsy cases from the Los Angeles coroner's office. They found a positive correlation between the number of surfaces of dental amalgam and mercury levels in brain tissue, irrespective of food sources.[45]

A similar study by Nylander[46] examined mercury levels in the central nervous system and kidneys on 34 autopsy cases. The results showed a statistically significant correlation between the number of amalgam surfaces and total mercury levels in occipital cortex and kidneys. Nylander[47] has also demonstrated surprisingly high post-mortem concentrations in the pituitary glands of dentists, out of all proportion to other areas of the brain. Stortbecker[48] explains, 'This is because the pituitary has an extra dose by direct transport from the nasal cavity'.

## Mercury and multiple sclerosis

Multiple sclerosis (MS) was first described by Charcot in the 1860s, which coincided with the introduction of and increasing use of amalgam fillings. Ingalls[49] demonstrated that areas of high incidence of MS showed high incidence of dental decay and repair with amalgams. The Swiss neurologist Basch[50] hypothesized that MS is a neuro-allergic ailment, the allergen being a heavy metal, probably mercury.

Britt Ahlsot-Westerland showed that mercury levels in the cerebrospinal fluid (CSF) of MS patients was 7–8 times higher than the controls, both groups having similar amounts of amalgam filling.[51]

Chang has shown that small amounts of mercury will cause a long-lasting impairment of the blood-brain barrier. He also showed that in nerve fibres in animals mercury was predominantly localized in the myelin sheath.[52]

CASE HISTORY

*This patient was a 35-year-old female diagnosed as suffering from MS in 1984. In addition to acute attacks of MS which caused her to lose the sight of one eye and suffer paralysis, she had chronic symptoms which included: headaches, lightheadedness, lack of concentration, fear of losing balance, constant fatigue, hypersensitivity all over her body, twitching of legs and a metallic taste.*

*Her amalgam fillings were carefully removed in 1990. Although she felt ill after each filling was removed, everything has cleared except the blurring of vision in the right eye. Since then she has had two babies, has started to play tennis again and now 6 years later continues to enjoy good health. So it would seem that mercury can mimic MS, exacerbate MS and in some cases possibly cause MS.*

## Mercury and Parkinson's disease

In an epidemiological case-control study of mercury body burden and idiopathic Parkinson's disease (IDP), subjects living in Singapore were measured for mercury levels in blood, urine and scalp hair. There were 54 cases of IPD and 95 matched controls. Subjects with Parkinson's disease had significantly higher mean levels of mercury than controls in all three areas.[53]

## Mercury and motor neuron disease

Motor neuron disease is a chronic neurodegenerative disease also known as amyotrophic lateral sclerosis (ALS). It is characterized by progressive atrophy and weakness of skeletal muscle, with small involuntary muscular contractions visible under the skin. Although clinical variants occur, the classical disease is readily identified by physical findings and electrophysiological studies. Pathologically there is atrophy and degeneration of selective motor neurons in the ventral spinal cord and the motor cortex.

Brown[54] reported 6 cases of ALS in farmers dusting seeds with methyl mercury. He stressed that the chronic form resulted from low-level chronic exposure. In the Iraq disaster, large groups of patients demonstrated neurological conditions similar to ALS.[55]

CASE HISTORY[56]

*This patient was a 29-year-old female teacher. In January 1984 a diagnosis of ALS was made at the Neurology Department, University Hospital, Umea, Sweden. No further appointment was made as the disease is pernicious and there is no known therapy. She had 34 tooth surfaces filled with dental amalgam. Her dentist replaced all amalgam fillings by March 1984. Five months after removal she returned to the same clinic where ALS had been diagnosed. She now felt extraordinarily healthy which was confirmed by the clinical report. 'The neurological status is completely without comment. The patient does not show any motor neuron disease of type ALS. She has been informed that she is, in neurological respect, fully healthy'. After 9 years the patient continues to enjoy good health.*

### Mercury and Alzheimer's disease

Public funds are sponsoring research programmes at the University of Kentucky. The Departments involved are Chemistry, Pathology, Neurology and the Sanders-Brown Centre on Ageing.

In a recent study on the brains of Alzeimher's disease (AD) autopsied cases, concentrations of trace elements were measured.[57] They consistently found the highest trace element to be mercury. In comparison with age-matched controls, the mercury content was found to be significantly higher. The mercury concentration was found in areas of the brain associated with memory. The study suggests that the elevation of mercury in AD is the most important imbalance the authors had observed. They further stated that this and their previous studies suggest that mercury toxicity could play a role in neuronal degeneration in AD.

Results were supported by Dr Boyd Haley who has shown that mercury specifically affects tubulin, which is responsible for the proper microtubule formation of brain neurons.[58] Both *in vitro* and *in vivo* experiments show effects which may produce neurofibrillar tangles, which are a recognized characteristic of AD and mean that brain communication systems may not connect.[59]

In further studies by Professor Vimy's Calgary team in conjunction with Boyd Haley, they have concluded that their studies are direct quantitative evidence for a connection between mercury exposure and neurodegeneration.[60]

### Mercury and infertility

This work was carried out at the Department of Gynaecology, University of Heidelberg. The chelating agent for mercury, DMPS, was given to women with hormonal irregularities, to remove mercury from the body. At the same time they investigated the blood for excessive levels of various pesticides. By far the most common problem was mercury contamination, which correlated directly with the number of fillings. Since recognizing and treating the environmental contamination burdens of the women, 70% became pregnant without the use of hormonal therapy.[61]

### Mercury and hair loss

From Heidelberg, 132 women were investigated for elevated mercury using the chelating agent, DMPS: 107 presented with alopecia (hair loss); 25 presented with hirsutism (excess hair growth), 49% showed elevated mercury and, of these, in 68% the condition disappeared after fillings were removed.[62]

### Safety of dental amalgam

No research has ever been produced to demonstrate the safety of amalgam fillings. No long-term studies have ever been carried out. There have been a number of reviews of published research papers, with questionable conclusions.

The latest comprehensive review was published by the British Dental Association in 1993, in which it was suggested that there was a need for further research.[63]

## Health improvement following mercury removal

Fredrick Bergland has reviewed case histories, published in scientific journals between 1944 and 1993, with oral and systemic symptoms.[64] Improvement rates varied between 80% and 100% after fillings were removed, and sometimes there was a temporary increase in symptoms, due to removal procedures. This encouraged other researchers and practitioners to evaluate results of amalgam filling removal on larger groups of patients. Results are shown in *Table 7.1*.

Over 500 patients in this survey were reported on by Mats Hanson. For some reason, one of the major findings has been omitted from the above. Over 90% of those presenting with 'joint and muscle aches and pains' were cured or improved.

As research escalated, media attention was alerted and a number of investigative television programmes and journalistic articles began to appear before an increasingly apprehensive public. While the ADA and BDA remained impassive, other countries took the initiative.

# World reaction to mercury fillings

## Sweden

In the early 1980s a Dental Mercury Patients' Association was formed by researcher Mats Hanson. It rapidly grew from 1000 members to some 18,000 today. As a result of their activities an expert panel commissioned by the government concluded in 1987 that mercury fillings were unsuitable from a toxicological point of view. On 18 February 1994 the Swedish Ministry of Health announced in a press release that the use of amalgam would be totally banned for children and adolescents up to age 19 by 1 July 1995 and for adults by 1997.

## Germany

In 1992 the German Ministry of Health, inspired by the Drasch paper[42] issued a pamphlet recommending that amalgam should be avoided for the following people:[65]

- children under 6 years old;
- individuals with kidney disease;
- pregnant women;
- any women of reproductive age.

**Table 7.1 Selected health symptom analysis of 1569 patients who eliminated mercury-containing dental fillings (From Bioprobe Newsletter, March 1993)**

The following represents a partial statistical symptom summary of 1569 patients who participated in six different studies evaluating the health effects of replacing mercury-containing dental fillings with non-mercury-containing dental fillings. The data were derived from the following studies: 762 Patient Adverse Reaction Reports submitted to the FDA by the individual patients; 519 patients in Sweden reported on by Mats Hanson, PhD; 100 patients in Denmark performed by Henrik Lichtenberg DDS; 80 patients in Canada performed by Pierre Larose DDS.; 86 patients in Colorado reported on by Robert L. Siblerud OD, MS, and 22 patients reported on by Alfred V. Zamm MD, FACA, FACP. The conbined total of all patients participating in the six studies was 1569.

| Per cent of total reporting | Symptom | No. reporting | No. improved or cured | Per cent of cure or improvement |
|---|---|---|---|---|
| 14 | Allergy | 221 | 196 | 89 |
| 5 | Anxiety | 86 | 80 | 93 |
| 5 | Bad temper | 81 | 68 | 89 |
| 6 | Bloating | 88 | 70 | 88 |
| 6 | Blood pressure problems | 99 | 53 | 54 |
| 5 | Chest pains | 79 | 69 | 87 |
| 22 | Depression | 347 | 315 | 91 |
| 22 | Dizziness | 343 | 301 | 88 |
| 45 | Fatigue | 705 | 606 | 86 |
| 15 | Gastrointestinal problems | 231 | 192 | 83 |
| 8 | Gum problems | 129 | 121 | 94 |
| 34 | Headaches | 531 | 460 | 87 |
| 3 | Migraine headaches | 45 | 39 | 87 |
| 12 | Insomnia | 187 | 146 | 78 |
| 10 | Irregular heartbeat | 159 | 139 | 87 |
| 8 | Irritability | 132 | 119 | 90 |
| 17 | Lack of concentration | 270 | 216 | 80 |
| 6 | Lack of energy | 91 | 88 | 97 |
| 17 | Memory loss | 265 | 193 | 73 |
| 17 | Metallic taste | 260 | 247 | 95 |
| 7 | Multiple sclerosis | 113 | 86 | 76 |
| 8 | Muscle tremor | 126 | 104 | 83 |
| 10 | Nervousness | 158 | 131 | 83 |
| 8 | Numbness anywhere | 118 | 97 | 82 |
| 20 | Skin disturbances | 310 | 251 | 81 |
| 9 | Sore throat | 149 | 128 | 86 |
| 6 | Tachycardia | 97 | 68 | 70 |
| 4 | Thyroid problems | 56 | 44 | 79 |
| 12 | Ulcers and sores in oral cavity | 189 | 162 | 86 |
| 7 | Urinary tract problems | 115 | 87 | 76 |
| 29 | Vision problems | 462 | 289 | 63 |

## Austria

The Austrian Minister of Health announced that the use of mercury fillings in children would be banned in 1996 and discontinued for all Austrians by the year 2000.[66]

## Canada

In January 1994 the Ontario Government demanded a report on mercury dental fillings, which is under way.

## World Health Organisation

In a document on environmental mercury,[67] their determinations regarding human daily retained intake of mercury from various sources are:

- Dental amalgam = 3.0–17.0 $\mu$g/day (mercury vapour);
- Fish and seafood = 2.3 $\mu$g/day (methylmercury);
- Other food = 0.3 $\mu$g/day (inorganic mercury);
- Air and water = negligible traces.

The committee also noted that 'a specific No-Observed-Effect Level (NOEL) cannot be established', meaning that no level of exposure to mercury vapour that can be considered harmless has been found.


# Mercury and the dentist

## Mercury regulations

Few people are aware of the stringent recommendations of mercury hygiene as documented by the Council on Dental Materials and Devices:

- store mercury in unbreakable, tightly sealed containers;
- perform all operations involving mercury over areas that have impervious and suitably lipped surfaces so as to confine and facilitate recovery of spilled mercury or amalgam;
- clean up any spilled mercury immediately – droplets may be picked up with narrow-bore tubing connected (via a wash-bottle trap) to the low-volume aspirator of the dental unit;
- use tightly closed capsules during amalgamation;
- use a no-touch technique for handling the amalgam;
- salvage all amalgam scrap and store it under used X-ray fixer;
- work in well-ventilated spaces;
- avoid carpeting dental operatories, as decontamination is not possible;
- eliminate the use of mercury-containing solutions;
- avoid heating mercury or amalgam;
- use water spray and suction when grinding dental amalgam;
- use conventional dental amalgam compacting procedures, manual and mechanical, but do not use ultrasonic amalgam condensers;
- perform yearly mercury determinations of all personnel regularly employed in dental offices;
- have periodic mercury vapour level determinations made in operatories.
- alert all personnel involved in handling of mercury, especially during training or indoctrination periods, of the potential hazard of mercury vapour and the necessity for observing good mercury hygiene practices.

The above recommendations provoked the comment from one dentist: 'It would seem that the only safe place for mercury is in the patient's mouth.' The degree of exposure to mercury would vary in different surgeries; however, it would seem from the literature that both dentists and their personnel are at risk.

Nylander[47] has demonstrated a high mercury content in the pituitary glands of dentists. Shapiro et al.[68] have demonstrated polyneuropathies in exposed dentists and state that these findings suggest that the use of mercury as a restorative material is a health risk for dentists.

Tests for methyl mercury carried out in the Department of Forensic Medicine in Glasgow on blood samples of 11 dentists working in University Conservation Departments and 17 controls for methyl mercury showed highly significant differences for total mercury and the ratio methyl/total mercury.[69]

The mortality rate from certain brain tumours (glioblastomas) among dentists and dental personnel is twice that of the remaining population. Mercury in amalgam is suspected to be the cause.[70]

Comprehensive studies conducted at Temple University show a statistically significant difference between dentists and the general population concerning cancer of the brain, cardiovascular disease, renal disease, non-malignant respiratory disease and suicide.[71]

Assuming the patient has had conventional medical investigations to exclude any life-threatening condition, and they have not responded to treatment, the experienced practitioner will:

- Take a comprehensive history.
- Check dental status of:
  Amalgam fillings, retrograde amalgams, crowns (particularly over amalgam cores), bridgework, implants, metal dentures, clasps on dentures, amalgam tattoos, posts and pins. Each individual filling should be tested for electrical activity using an instrument measuring either millivolts or microamps. Readings will indicate the extent of mercury vapour released, and the potential systemic effects of the electricity.
- Use special tests – urine tests and T-cell tests.

**Provocative urine tests**

Using a known mercury chelator, 2,3-dimercaptosuccinic acid (DMSA), a urine sample is taken. Three 100 mg capsules DMSA are taken and a further urine sample is taken 3 hours later; the samples are analysed for mercury and compared. The test is an indication of the body burden of mercury. In the surgery, electro-acupuncture (vegatest) may be used in conjunction with muscle testing (kinesiology) as an aid to diagnosis.

**Metal-specific memory t-cell test**

A new test has been established at the Chelsea and Westminster Hospital London after a research programme carried out by the author in conjunction with Dr Don Henderson and Dr Michelle Monteil of the Immunology Department.

The basis of the test is that lymphocytes are crucially involved in all immunological reactions. The test indicates a specific lymphocyte response to mercury and other dental metals such as silver, copper, nickel, gold, platinum, palladium, chrome and cobalt. This test determines *immunological memory* to dental and associated metals.

This is probably the best test available and should become standard procedure for patients. It may, however, give some false negatives and should be used in conjunction with the expertise of an experienced clinician.

#### WHAT DO WE MEAN BY IMMUNOLOGICAL MEMORY?

Take, for example, when a virus enters the body causing an infection, the immune system mounts a defence reaction and clears the infectious agent from the body. The next time the individual is exposed to the same organism, a more rapid and sometimes more powerful defence reaction occurs. This is because of the development of immunological memory. Such memory responses can be measured and a similar test system is used to determine immunological memory to dental and associated metals.

#### WHAT DOES IT MEAN TO HAVE IMMUNOLOGICAL MEMORY TO METALS?

Take, for example, individuals who develop a skin rash following contact with nickel. This is not a rare condition and using the test it can be shown that many people have immunological memory to nickel, but not all develop skin rashes on exposure to nickel. Those who do have a stronger immunological memory. Similarly, it has been shown that immunological memory to dental and associated metals (e.g. mercury) is not uncommon and that there are variations in the strength of the memory which can be graded similarly to nickel sensitivity. Currently, the process of determining the level of memory which causes reactions to dental and associated metals is being researched.

## Removal of amalgam fillings

Fillings should be removed in a predetermined sequence depending on electrical readings. Quadrants having the highest reading should be removed first. This is important when there are high differentials. Other considerations are also important and must be taken into account by the clinician.

### Priority order for amalgam removal

- Root canal-treated teeth with pins or screw-posts of non-precious metals and metal crowns with amalgam cores should be treated first.
- Next are amalgams in direct constant contact with gold. Often the amalgam can be removed while the gold inlays, the crown or the bridge, can be left. What to do with the gold can be decided later.
- Where there is direct intermittent biting contact between amalgam and gold in opposing teeth.
- Where there is direct contact between amalgam and other metals like partial chromium–cobalt dentures.
- Other teeth with root canal fillings of N2 and gutta-percha. The latter often contains cadmium. The filling materials and sealers generally contain an amazing array of highly toxic compounds.

- Retrograde amalgam fillings must be removed. These fillings can be seen on X-rays at the root apex.
- Most patients have several different types of amalgam fillings, and the ones containing the newer types of amalgam high in copper (non-gamma-2 amalgam) should be removed first. The priority order between different fillings can be based on the patient's own opinions or visible signs of corrosion and discoloration.
- Amalgam fillings in contact with gum tissue. It might be necessary to remove metal-impregnated gum tissue surgically.

### Pretreatment plan

Oral nutritional chelation therapy, dietary advice and supplementation should be started prior to treatment, together with other detoxification procedures to help flush mercury from the body. The pretreatment routine is varied, depending on presenting symptoms, particularly the efficiency of the digestive and elimination systems. Particularly efficacious vitamins and minerals include free radical scavengers such as vitamins A, C, E, selenium, copper, zinc and manganese.

When constipation is present, it must be treated. The patient should have a high-fibre diet, which often means eliminating most meat, fish and poultry. When patients are on this vegan-type diet, $B_{12}$, folic acid and zinc should be supplemented. Digestive enzymes are often useful, as is food-combining and herbal preparations.

Some patients may be allergic to the composite materials. This should be apparent from their history, such as reactions to other petrochemical derivatives, e.g. traffic exhaust fumes. The patient may be asked to suck a sample of proposed material for a few hours on consecutive days and monitor reactions. In extreme cases a complete blood count (CBC) is taken, a small filling placed without anaesthetic and a further CBC taken 2 days later. Provided that there has been no intervening illness, any changes of percentages of monocytes, eosinophils and basophils could be significant.

A course of homoeopathic dental amalgam or merc sol is helpful, but the practitioner should have some experience of homoeopathy. Charcoal tablets should also be used immediately before amalgam removal, to absorb mercury from any amalgam particles that may pass into the stomach.

### Protection of the patient during amalgam removal

The surgery should have good ventilation and an efficient filtration system. Where possible, rubber dam should be used in conjunction with efficient high-volume evacuation to protect the patient from the aerosol of water-coolant spray used with the high-speed cutting (see Figure 7.1). When drilling, the filling should be sectioned into chunks and elevated where possible. If any metal has been used as a restorative material, then all amalgams should be removed first. Patients should wear clothes covering as much skin as possible.

For sensitive patients, when drilling out amalgam cover the eyes with wrap-around goggles and use a Relative Analgesia nosepiece with tubing

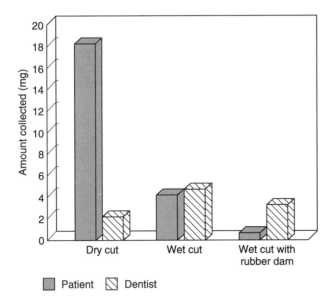

**Figure 7.1** Particulate inhalation during the removal of amalgam restorations (from Nimmo *et al.*,[76] by permission)

attached to extend out of operating area to protect against nose inhalation of mercury vapour. Some practitioners use oxygen flow.

Scheduling of appointments depends very much on the reaction of the patient after the first treatment. Patients should be monitored and supplementation varied as necessary.

Some dentists in Sweden, Denmark and Germany are using intravenous vitamin C as a detoxifying agent before, during and after removal of filling. The technique is fully described in a booklet called 'V-Tox Treatment'.[72]

## Post-treatment protocols

Removal of body mercury after removal of fillings is crucial, but often neglected. A reservoir of mercury has accumulated in the body over the years and needs to be flushed out. Methods depend on presenting symptoms, vitamin and mineral supplements such as vitamins A, C, E, $B_{12}$, folic acid, selenium, zinc, manganese, magnesium, amino acids, glutathione peroxidase, reduced glutathione, glutathione complex and glutamine, digestive enzymes, essential fatty acids and acidopholous. Homoeopathic remedies should be used and herbal remedies may be helpful.

Warm baths, low-heat saunas, acupuncture, massage, counselling and healing have all proved useful. Any remaining Candida, food allergies and digestive disorders usually become more amenable to treatment. Most patients who do not feel better retain hardened faecal matter containing trapped particles of mercury/amalgam and other combination of corroded metals.[43] Treat with high-fibre diets, added fibre, food-combining techniques where appropriate (Hay diet) and possibly colonic irrigation.

Green food supplements such as spirolina, chlorella, blue green algae and chlorophyll are rich in vitamins and minerals and bind to heavy metals, but provided that digestion and absorption are sound, the best source of nutrients is a good diet. Exercise and reduction of stress play their part in restoration of health.

**Chelation of mercury**

The effective chelating agents are 2,3-dimercaptosuccinic acid (DMSA) and 2,3-dimercapto-1-propanesulphonic Acid (DMPS).

DMSA is usually given orally at 10–30 mg/kg body weight per day for 5 days. DMPS may be taken orally 2–10 mg/kg body weight per day for 5-day course, or it may be used intravenously. Chelation will take other metals, particularly zinc, out of the body as well as heavy metals, and supplementation after chelation should be observed. Supplementation with glutathione should be avoided during chelation.[73]

Potassium and sodium citrates are also useful, especially in conjunction with DMSA, as they aid the passage of heavy metal chelates through the kidney. Chelation courses may have to be repeated a number of times, dependent on provocative urine tests. Research has highlighted the Humic Acids as an effective long-term natural chelation of heavy metals, including lead, cadmium and mercury.

# Conclusion

Mercury is continuously released from amalgam fillings, and numerous research investigations have clearly shown that mercury from this source provides the major contribution to body burden of mercury. The vapour has a direct pathway to the brain. It is inhaled into the lungs, oxidized to ionic mercury and binds to cell proteins.

Current research on the pathophysiological effects of amalgam has focused upon the immune system, renal system, oral and intestinal bacteria, reproductive system and the central nervous system. Research evidence does not support the notion of amalgam safety.[74]

Mercury crosses the placenta during pregnancy. This is particularly disturbing in the UK, as dentistry is free for pregnant and lactating women on the National Health Service.

**Mercury is the only cumulative vaporizing poison permanently implanted in the human body.**[75]

Due to changing conditions in the mouth there is a constant corrosion of dental materials. This means chemicals and metals are released into the body where they may cause untold damage. Investigation of potentially harmful dental materials must form part of any health programme.

# References

1 Jaro P. Mercury from dental amalgams: exposure and effects. *Int J Risk Safety Med* 1992; **3**: 14–16.

2 Bakir F, Damluji S F, Amin-Zaki L. Methyl mercury poisoning in Iraq. *Science* 1973; **181**: 230–241.

3 Heintze U, Edwardsson S, Derand T *et al*. Methylation of mercury from dental amalgam and mercuric chloride by oral streptococci in vitro. *Scand J Dent Res* 1983; **91**: 150–152.

4 Edwards T, McBride B C. Biosynthesis and degradation of methyl mercury in human faeces. *Nature* 1975; **253**: 462–464.

5 Rowland I R, Grasso P, Davies M J. The methylation of mercuric chloride by human intestinal bacteria. *Experientia* 1975; **31**: 1064–1065.

6 Goldwater I J. *A History of Quicksilver*, pp. 279–287. Baltimore: York Press, 1972.

7 Stock A. The hazards of mercury vapour. *Z Agnew Chem* 1926; **39**: 461–488.

8 Djerassi E, Berova N. The possibility of allergic reactions from silver amalgam restorations. *Int Dent J* 1969; **19(4)**: 481–488.

9 White R, Brand T R. Patch tests on dental students with amalgam fillings. *J Am Dent Assoc* 1976; **92**: 1204.

10 Miller E G, Perry W L, Wagner M J. *J Dent Res 64. Special Issue Abstracts.* p. 338 Abstract No. 1472. Dallas, Texas: Baylor College of Dentistry, March 1985.

11 North American Contact Dermatitis Group. Epidemiology of contact dermatitis in North America. *Arch Derm* 1973; **108**: 537–540.

12 Nebenfuhrer L, Korossy S, Erzebet V *et al*. Mercury allergy in Budapest. *Contact Derm* 1984; **10(2)**: 121–122.

13 Vimy M J, Lorscheider F L. Intra-oral air mercury released from dental amalgam. *J Dent Res* 1985; **64(B)**: 1069–1071.

14 Vimy M J, Lorscheider F L. Serial measurement of intra-oral mercury. Estimation of daily dose from amalgam. *J Dent Res* 1981; **60**: 1668–1671.

15 Levenson J G. Mercury, dental amalgam fillings and your health. *J Soc Environ Ther* June 1988; **8(2)**: 5.

16 Huggins H. *It's All in your Head*. New York: Avery Publishing Group Inc, 1993.

17 Guyton A C. *Function of the Human Body*, 2nd edn. p. 94. Philadelphia: W B Saunders Co, 1964.

18 Reinherz E L, Schlossen S F. Regulation of the immune response – inducer and suppressor T-lymphocyte subsets in human beings. *N Engl J Med* 1980; **303**: 370.

19 Auti F, Pandolphi E. The role of T-lymphocytes in the pathogenesis of primary immunodeficiencies. *Thymus* 1982; **4**: 257.

20 Legler D W, Arnold R R, Lynch D P *et al*. Immunodeficiency disease and implications for dental treatment. *J Am Dent Assoc* 1982; **105**: 803.

21 Reinherz E L, Schlossen S F. The differentiation and function of human T-lymphocytes. *Cell* 1980; **19**: 821.

22 Frazer I H, Mackay I R. T-lymphocyte sub-populations defined by two sets of monoclonal antibodies in chronic acute hepatitis and SLE. *Clin Exp Immunol* 1982; **50**: 107.

23 Oleske J, Minnefor A, Cooper R *et al*. Immune deficiency syndrome in children. *J Am Med Assoc* 1983; **249**: 2345–2349.

24 Sonnabend J, Witkin S S, Purtilo D T. AIDS. Opportunistic infections and malignancies in male homosexuals. A hypothesis of etiologic factors in pathogenesis. *J Am Med Assoc* 1983; **249**: 2370.

25 Chatenoud L, Bach M A. Abnormalities of T cell subsets in glomerulonephritis and systemic lupus erythematosus. *Kidney Int* 1981; **20**: 267.

26 Traugott U, Reinherz E L, Raine C S. Multiple sclerosis: distribution of T cell subsets with active chronic lesions. *Science* 1983; **219**: 308.

27 Leung D Y, Rhodes A R, Geha R S. Enumeration of T cell subsets of atopic dermatitis using monoclonal antibodies. *J Allergy Clin Immunol* 1981; **67**: 450.

28 Butler M, Atherton D, Levinsky R J. Qualitative and functional deficit of suppressor T cells in children with atopic eczema. *Clin Exp Immunol* 1982; **50:** 92.

29 Reinherz E L, Weiner H L, Hauser S L *et al.* Loss of suppressor T cells in active multiple sclerosis. *N Engl J Med* 1980; **303:** 125.

30 Morimoto C, Reinherz E L, Schlossman S F *et al.* Alterations in immunoregulatory T cell subsets in active SLE. *J Clin Invest* 1980; **66:** 1171.

31 Kohler P F, Vaughan J. The autoimmune diseases. *J Am Med Assoc* 1982; **248:** 2446.

32 Eggleston D W. Effect of dental amalgam and nickel alloys on T lymphocytes: preliminary report. *J Pros Dent* 1984; **51(5):** 617–623.

33 Tibbling L, Karl-ake T, Rodrica L *et al.* Immunological and brain MRI changes in patients with suspected metal intoxication. *Int J Occup Med Toxicol* 1995; **4(2):** 1–10.

34 Henderson D, Monte M, Levenson J. *Lymphocyte Responses to Dental Metals* (unpublished observations). Copies available from the British Soc. for Mercury Free Dentistry, 225 Old Brompton Road, London SW5 0EA.

35 Hahn L J, Kloiber R, Vimy M J *et al.* Dental 'silver' tooth fillings: a source of mercury revealed by whole-body image scan and tissue analysis. *FASEB J* Dec 1989; **3:** 2641–2646.

36 Danscher G, Horsted-Bindslevp, Rungby J. Traces of mercury in organs from primates with amalgam fillings. *Exp Mol Path* 1990; **52:** 291–299.

37 Vimy M J, Boyd N D, Benediktsson H *et al.* Glomerular filtration impairment by mercury released from dental silver fillings in sheep. *Physiologist* August 1990; 1010–1014.

38 Molin M Bergman B, Marklund S L *et al.* Mercury, selenium and glutathione peroxidase before and after amalgam removal in man. *Acta Odontol Scand* 1990; **48:** 189–202.

39 Godfrey M, Cambell N. Confirmation of mercury retention and toxicity DMPS. *J Adv Med* Spring 1994; **7(1):** 19–30.

40 Aposhian H V Bruce D C, Alter W *et al.* Urinary mercury after administration of 2,3 dimercapto-propane-L-sulphonic acid: correlation with dental amalgam score. *FASEB J* 1992; **6:** 2472–2476.

41 Vimy M J, Tacahashi Y, Lorscheider F L. Calgary Univ. Fac. of Med. Maternal-foetal distribution of mercury ($Hg^{203}$) released from dental amalgam fillings. *Am J Physiol* April 1990; **258:** R939–R945.

42 Drasch G, Schupp I, Hofl H *et al.* Mercury burden of human foetal and infant tissues. *Eur J Pediatr* 1994: **153:** 607–610.

43 Malmström C, Hanson M, Nylander M. Isterh Third Int. Conf. Trace elements in health and disease. Stockholm May 25–29, 1992.

44 Summers A O, Wireman J, Vimy M J *et al.* Mercury released from dental 'silver' fillings provokes an increase in mercury- and antibiotic-resistant bacteria in oral and intestinal floras of primates. *Antimic Agents Chemother* 1993: **37(4):** 825–834.

45 Eggleston D W, Nylander M. Correlation of dental amalgams with mercury in brain tissue. *J Pros Dent* Dec 1987; **58(6):** 704–706.

46 Nylander M, Friberg L, Lind B. Mercury concentration in human brain and kidneys in relation to exposure from dental amalgam fillings. *Swed Dent J* 1987; **11:** 179–187.

47 Nylander M. Mercury in the pituitary glands of dentist (letter). *Lancet* Feb 22 1986; 442.

48 Stortbecker P. *Mercury Poisoning from Dental Amalgam – A Hazard to the Human Brain.* Stortbecker Foundation, Akerbyvagen 282 S-18335 Taby/Stockholm, Sweden.

49 Ingalls T H. Epidemiology, etiology and prevention of multiple sclerosis. *J Forensic Med Path* March 1983; **4(1):** 55–61.

50 Basch E. Die multiple sklerose eine quecksilber allergie. *Arch Neurol Neurochir Psychiat* 1966; **98:** 1–18.

51 Ahlsot-Westerland B. Mercury in cerebrospinal fluid in MS. *Swed J Biol Med* 1989; **1:** 627.

52 Chang L W, Hartman H A. Electronic microscope and histochemical study on the localisation and distribution of mercury in the nervous system after mercury intoxication. *Exp Neurol* 1972; **35:** 122–137.

53 Ngim C H, Devathasan G. Epidemiological study on the association between body burden mercury level and idiopathic Parkinson's disease. *Neuroepidemiology* 1989; **8:** 128–141.

54 Brown I A. Chronic mercurialism. A cause of the clinical syndrome of ALS. *Arch Neurol Psychiat (Chicago)* 1954; **72:** 674–681.

55 Kantarjian A D. A syndrome clinically resembling ALS following chronic mercurialism. *Neurology* 1961; **11:** 639–644.

56 Redhe O, Pleva J. Recovery from ALS and from allergy after removal of dental amalgam fillings. *Int J Risk Safety Med* 1994; **4:** 229–236.

57 Wenstrup D, Ehmann W D, Markesbery W R. Trace Element imbalances in isolated subcellular fractions of Alzheimer's disease in brains. *Brain Res* 1990; **533:** 125–131.

58 Duhr E, Pendergraff C, Kasarskis *et al.* $Hg^{2+}$ Induces GTP–tubulin interactions in rat brain similar to those observed in Alzheimer's disease. *FASEB J* 1991; **5:** A456.

59 Palkiewicz P, Zwiers H, Lorscheider F L. ADP-ribosylation of brain neuronal proteins is altered by in vitro and in vivo exposure to inorganic mercury. *J Neurochem* 1994; **62:** 2049–2052.

60 Lorscheider F L. Paper presented at the *12th Int. Neurotoxicology Conf Univ Arkansas.* Med. Centre. Hot Spring 1994 Oct 30–Nov 2.

61 Gerhard I, Runnebaum B. Fertility disorders may result from heavy metal and pesticide contamination which limits effects of hormone therapy. *Z Gynäkologie* 1992; **14:** 593–602.

62 Klobusch J, Rabe T. Gerhard I *et al. Klinisches Labor* 1992; **38:** 469–476. Univ. Heidelberg, Dept. Gyn. and Fertility Disturbances.

63 Eley B, Cox S W. The release, absorption and possible health effects of mercury from dental amalagam: a review of recent findings [corrected and republished article originally printed in *Br Dent J* 1993; **175(5):** 161-168] *Br Dent J* 1993; **3:** 355–362.

64 Bergland F. *150 Years of Dental Amalgam.* Orlando FL, USA: Bioprobe Inc, 1995.

65 German Ministry of Health Zahnartzt. *Woche (DZW)* 1992; **8:** 1.

66 *FDI Dental World* 1993 March/April p. 6.

67 World Health Organisation. *Environmental Health Criteria 118: Inorganic Mercury.* Geneva: WHO, 1991.

68 Shapiro I M, Sumner A, Spitz L K *et al.* Neurophysiological and neuropsychological function in mercury exposed dentists. *Lancet* 1982; **1:** 1147–1150.

69 Cross J D, Dale I M, Goolvard J M A. Methyl mercury in blood of dentists (letter). *Lancet* 1978; **2:** 312–313.

70 Ahlbom A. La Env Med Karolinska Inst Swed. *Svenska Dag Bladet* 10 Sept 1985.

71 Orner G, Mumma R. *Mortality Study of Dentists.* Philadelphia: Temple Univ., 1976.

72 Hall G. *V-Tox Treatment.* Schadow Str 28, Dusseldorf, Germany 40212: Hall, 1995.

73 Pangborn J B. *Mechanisms of Detoxification and Procedures for Detoxification.* Chicago: Doctors Data Inc and Bionostics Inc. (708) 100.

74 Lorscheider F, Vimy M J, Summers A O. Mercury exposure from 'silver' tooth fillings: emerging evidence questions a traditional dental paradigm. *FASEB J* 1995; **9:** 504–508.

75 Levenson J G. *Controversy 1 Amalgam – Filler or Killer.* Lecture. Royal London Hospital, November 26, 1991.

76 Nimmo A, Werley M S, Martin J S *et al.* Particulate inhalation during the removal of amalgam restorations. *J Prosthet Dent* 1990; **63:** 228–233.

# Bibliography

Fasciana G S. *Are Your Dental Fillings Hurting You?* Springfield, Mass: Health Challenge Press, 1986.

Huggins H. *It's All in Your Head.* New York: Avery Publishing Group Inc, 1993.

Stortbecker P. *Mercury Poisoning from Dental Amalgam – A Hazard to the Human Brain.* Akerbyvagen 282, S-183 35 Taby/Stockholm, Sweden: Stortbecker Foundation for Research, 1985.

Taylor J. *The Complete Guide to Mercury Toxicity from Dental Fillings.* San Diego: Scripps Publishing, 1988.

Ziff S. *The Toxic Time Bomb.* Santa Fe: Aurora Press, 1985.

Ziff S, Ziff M. *Infertility and Birth Defects. Is Mercury from Silver Dental Fillings an Unsuspected Cause?* Orlando: Bioprobe, 1987.

Ziff S, Ziff M. *The Bioprobe Newsletter.* A bi-monthly review of research on mercury.

Ziff S, Ziff M. *Heavy Metal Bulletin.* Monica Kaupi, Lilla Aspuddsu 10, S-12649 Hagersten, Stockholm, Sweden. Quarterly publication.

Ziff S, Ziff M. *The What Doctors Don't Tell You Dental Handbook.* London: Wallace Press, 1996.

## Associations

IAOMT International
4222 Evergreen Lane
Anandale VA 22003
USA
Tel: 001 703 256 4441
Fax: 001 703 256 4441

IAOMT Europe
Schadowsrasse 28
D-40212 Dusseldorf
Germany
Tel: 0049 211 133 533
Fax: 0049 211 133 555

IAOMT Great Brtain
72 Harley Street
London W1N 1AE
UK
Tel: 0171 580 3168
Fax: 0171 436 0959

Australasian Society of Oral Medicine and
    Toxicology (ASOMAT)
P.O. Box A860,
Sydney 2000
Australia
Tel: 00 612 9867 1111
Fax: 00 612 0283 2230

British Society for Mercury Free Dentistry
225 Old Brompton Road
London SW5 0EA
UK
Tel: 0171 373 3655
Fax: 0171 373 3655

## Patient support groups

Australian Society of Dental Mercury
    Patients
PO Box 1288
Southport
Queensland 4215
Australia

Society for the Campaign Against Mercury
62 Highfield Road
Rock Hill
Bromsgrove
Worcestershire B61 7BD
UK
Tel: 01527 570 316

BBFU
Gorch-Frock Str 11
D-48527 Nordhorn
Germany
Tel: 00 49 59 213 5292
Fax: 00 49 59 213 5292

DAMS
6025 Osuna Blvd, Suite B
Albuquerque NM 87109
USA
Tel: 001 505 888 0111
Fax: 001 505 888 4554

## Courses

Courses and symposiums are held regularly by the IAOMT and The British Society for Mercury Free Dentistry. Details can be obtained from the relevant associations above.

# Hypnosis

**Geoff Graham**

## Introduction

Hypnosis is an altered state of consciousness, not very different from the normal consciousness, except that in hypnosis the imagination is greatly enhanced and the power to criticize is reduced. Because of these two facts suggestions are accepted more readily and acted upon more easily.

Many people who are hypnotized are not aware of being in a state of hypnosis and will often say 'I was not hypnotized'. Others may say 'I was just very relaxed'.

### Deep, medium and light trance

In a hypnotic trance the level attained can vary between people. Deep trance subjects are the only ones who really appreciate that they are being hypnotized. Everybody has their own ability to relate to what they are doing. For instance, some people like classical music and some do not. If you do not like classical music it is almost impossible to make you like it. Hypnosis is no different. It is very difficult to change someone from a light trance subject into a deep trance subject. Some people can go into a very deep trance, about 20% of the public, but others may only be able to experience some of the hypnotic phenomena and could be classed as medium trance subjects. These amount to about 50% of the public. Others may only achieve a light state of hypnosis and experience very few of the hypnotic phenomena. These will amount to about 30% of the public. Deep trance subjects can be treated and helped more easily, but medium and light trance subjects need more sophisticated techniques to help them. Patients with a poor trance capacity will probably respond better to neuro-linguistic programming (NLP) or some informal technique.

### Assessing hypnotic capacity

There are a number of ways of assessing what sort of hypnotic capacity a person will have. Before using formal hypnosis it is necessary to find out what sort of capacity the person is capable of. Spiegel's Capacity Test[1] is simple and quick to do and accurate for about 70% of the population.

Anyone who chooses can be helped, with hypnosis, to make significant changes to the way they live. The main proviso is that the person really wants help to change the way they feel or what they do. If a person does not want to change or is resistant to hypnosis, then you will not be able to hypnotize them. This can be a problem when treating children if they do not really want the treatment. Children are usually very easily hypnotized, but they will not stay in hypnosis if they do not want the treatment. If you are trying to do a filling for a child who does not want it, the child will break trance as soon as you pick up the drill.

## Stage hypnosis

Most people have seen a stage hypnotist who has put volunteers into a hypnotic trance. The hypnotist tells them that at a snap of the fingers they will open their eyes and act, for example, as if they are at work and that is what they do. This shows that the subjects can easily imagine they are at work and second that they can all respond to the suggestion of being at work without criticism. These facts confirm that in hypnosis the imagination is enhanced and the power to act to suggestion uncritically is strengthened. However, stage hypnotists can create problems with their acts.

First, they appear to show that the hypnotist has great power over the subjects. Remember that a stage hypnotist asks for volunteers and selects the best subjects from the audience, so all of them are deep trance subjects. Only 20% of people can respond in this way; the majority of people cannot. This gives the wrong impression to all medium and light trance subjects.

Second, because the stage hypnotist uses only deep trance subjects and uses them when they are in a deep trance, there is more chance that in the act the hypnotist may disturb some primal pain in that subject.

### Primal pain gate

Whenever something happens to a person that hurts them, the normal thing for them to do is to pretend that they are not hurting. They do this by various means of denial. To not feel the pain, they have to block it by putting what we call a primal gate up against the pain. When we hypnotize a deep trance patient, the very act of deep trance may often disturb this primal gate.[2,3]

This can also happen while giving a general anaesthetic or with relative analgesia (nitrous oxide). The patient may come out of a general anaesthetic crying. They are very rarely crying about what has just been happening to them, i.e. the operation, but they usually cry over something that happened in the past to hurt them. This can be something in the nature of, 'my dog got run over' or 'my baby has not been well'. Disturbing the primal gate will often result in the subject getting a headache and feeling uncomfortable during the trance. This uncomfortable feeling may occur some time later when the subject has gone home or at work some days after the show. They may not know what is bothering them, but may need help in the future to settle the trouble released by the trance. They may not want to be hypnotized again because it caused the problem in the first place. This is why professional hypnotists are reluctant to support stage hypnotism. They feel that hypnosis should not be lightly used for entertainment, but for professional help only.

Every hypnotized person should be questioned after experiencing a trance to make sure that their primal gates have not been disturbed. Questions like, 'How do you feel now?' or 'Do you feel good now?' will very quickly ascertain if any harm has been done. If the patient complains of having a headache which they did not have before the trance, then the hypnotist should investigate any negative feelings before the person leaves. These questions are not generally used at stage performances and most subjects if asked on stage would generally not admit to feeling bad anyway.

# Formal trance *v.* neuro-linguistic programming

### Formal trance

The first way of using hypnosis with dental patients is to use a formal trance induction and then use one of the many trance techniques to bring about a desirable change in that patient. This way is easier with deep trance patients, although the less capable they are of producing a deep trance the more sophisticated the technique has to be to bring about the change. Nevertheless, medium and light trance patients, can be helped by formal hypnosis. There are many ways to formally induce a trance in a person.

There are simple techniques, which are not time consuming, to find out how deep a patient can go with formal hypnosis. It is important to learn a number of techniques so that you can use one which suits the patient. This often takes some time to do, particularly if the hypnotist is just learning. Often a more experienced hypnotist will help someone to produce a deeper trance. With practice, however, the time taken to induce a trance is reduced and eventually it should take only a few minutes. With a formal trance there are two steps in helping a patient. The first is producing a trance state, the second step is then using one of the many techniques of help in the trance state to produce the desired change.

### Neuro-linguistic programming

The second way of using hypnosis with dental patients is to use an informal technique like neuro-linguistic programming (NLP). This is a technique which claims that it is possible to help anyone to produce a programme which should help them to do anything, with the only proviso that they want to do that particular thing. NLP uses the patient's senses for programming. It can be used with any trance depth patient, so it has an advantage over formal hypnosis, particularly when the person is either a light or medium trance subject. When using NLP, patients go into a spontaneous trance and no formal trance induction is necessary. This is time saving and trance depth is not necessary so it is more applicable to all patients. It is, however, more difficult to learn to be proficient when starting to practise NLP.

I believe it is better first to learn formal trance induction and treatment and then go on to NLP. In this way, with the formal techniques, you are practising some NLP without knowing it before you go on to the more subtle techniques of NLP. I would recommend that all hypnotists eventually make the transition into NLP, otherwise many patients will be unable to find help with hypnosis. Hypnosis then gets labelled as being 'no good'. It is not hypnosis at fault, but the hypnotist who is not experienced enough.

With NLP techniques you can reframe or collapse the fear by using a positive anchor. There are many other NLP techniques that one could research outside this chapter. The following two books explore NLP techniques in depth: 'The Happy Neurotic' and 'How to Change Your Life'. There are many more on the market.


## The mechanics of hypnosis

With all hypnosis, both formal and NLP, it is the patient who eventually makes the changes possible. Hypnosis is a quick and generally easy way of teaching the patient to make the changes in their behaviour that allow their life to be more comfortable and enjoyable. Hypnosis will achieve nothing if the person cannot use the techniques taught.

Having briefly explained above what hypnosis is and, equally important, what it is not, let me now try to explain how we use the state of hypnosis to bring about changes in our patients.

We have to accept that everything we think, feel, do or say is an interpretation by us of what we should think, feel, do or say. Nothing is the truth, there is no absolute truth. There is only the truth that each of us interprets as our truth. However most of us believe that our truth is *the truth*. For instance, most of us are quite happy to say the sun rises in the east and sets in the west. How do you feel about that statement? The sun does not rise or fall, it is the earth rotating on its axis, not the sun rising and falling. However, most of us like to think that everything revolves round us. It is this fact that causes a lot of mischief in the world.

Every interpretation that we make is largely based on learnt memories and memories are only interpretations. We are therefore making interpretations from interpretations and whenever we do this there is always a distortion. In the 1800s Kierkegaard, the Danish philosopher, described how whenever we translate 'What is' into language or thought, there is always a distortion of 'What is'. Our translated distortion then becomes our truth and we base whatever we think, feel, do or say on that distorted truth. It is always possible to change what we interpret and therefore change our truth, particularly when the new truth makes our lives more comfortable and happy. Hypnosis is the best way to make that change. Many patients become 'stuck' with their distorted truths and need to be shown how to get out of that 'stuck state'. Let us look at some of the distorted truths that some of our dental patients can get into.

# Distortions in dental phobics

### The 'pain maker'

Most dentists would like the patient to think of them as warm and approachable, but most phobic patients see the dentist as the 'pain maker' – a dark unapproachable character, perhaps with long sharp fingernails and a wicked grin. Both characters are the same person, the first interpreted by the dentist and the other by the phobic patient. Obviously these two people are going to have very different experiences of each other and what their roles are. If the dental phobic has their normal interpretation of the dentist, then there is no anaesthetic in the world that will stop that phobic patient from feeling pain. This is because they are programmed to receive pain from the pain maker.

There is a demonstration in which I take a hypnotized patient and place a coin on the back of their hand and then draw around the coin. I then press the coin lightly into the back of the patient's hand while I say, 'All the sensation in the hand is now moving into the coin'. I can then remove the coin and place it some distance from the patient. I can then stick a needle into the circle drawn on the back of that hand and the patient will feel nothing. The remarkable thing, however, is that when I then stick the coin with the needle the patient will complain of pain and probably withdraw their hand. I have done this demonstration with a very deep trance patient and when I stuck the coin the patient produced a spot of blood inside the circle on the back of their hand. I was doing this for a producer working for the BBC. He said, 'I'm getting out of here', when he saw the blood on the patient's hand, and I said, 'I am coming with you'. I have also touched the coin with a lighted cigarette and produced a burn in the circle on another patient's hand. We have no idea just how powerful the human mind really is.

The phobic patient with an interpretation of the dentist as the pain maker cannot have treatment without pain because they are doing to the dentist exactly what I did in the above demonstration. How do you anaesthetize a coin? What anaesthetic will numb a coin? Unless you change the patient's interpretation of the dentist as the pain maker you will have great difficulty in treating that patient. Hypnosis can change this interpretation, but I know of no other easy way of making that change. So for this reason alone hypnosis should be practised in dentistry and there are other reasons which I will describe later. I will also describe how to make these changes later in this chapter.

### The needle

What is the first thing the phobic patient says after they have proudly explained that they are a terrific coward when it comes to dentistry? They generally say, 'I hate the needle'. If they say this they have nearly always given the same attribute to the needle as I gave to the coin in my demonstration. If they have done that, then no surface anaesthetic will stop the needle from hurting.

You have to change the patient's interpretation of the needle to stop it from hurting. Hypnosis is the easiest way to do this. For them the needle is a giant size, designed to inflict the maximum pain. If you hand a dental needle to these patients the vast majority will say, 'I did not realize it was so small'.

### The drill

After the needle what is the next thing the phobic patient says? 'I hate the drill.' For them the drill is enormous, an elaborate instrument of torture. Once again if you give the phobic patient a turbine drill to hold while you run it they invariably say, 'I did not realize it was so small'. Unless you change that distorted interpretation, it will hurt if you use the drill, no matter how much anaesthetic you have given to the patient. Hypnosis can change that distorted interpretation. The phobic patient is also afraid of the sound of the drill. If you use the drill on a patient with this distorted interpretation, then the sound of the drill will hurt the patient, unless you change the distortion. Hypnosis can achieve that.

### The forceps

When I first started running workshops I used to take a trained subject along in case I had to demonstrate a phenomenon. I do not do that now because I have found I can always get someone from the participants to demonstrate my point. I was once talking about the power of the words we use on lay people. I turned to a lady in the audience and asked, 'What do you think of when I say forceps?' She looked at me and said, 'Crushed babies' heads'. I gasped and said, 'Why?' She replied that she had a book called 'Home Doctor' and it said the largest surgical instrument was a pair of obstetric forceps, hence when I said forceps she thought of crushed babies' heads. What sort of reaction do you think a patient with this distorted interpretation is going to have if you ask for a pair of forceps?

If you are going to crush babies' heads with your forceps, then the forceps have to be giant sized. Very different to the dentist's tool.

### The tooth

Most phobics who have to have a tooth removed ask, 'Have I got big roots doctor?' Their perception is of giant roots which require the use of giant forceps. I do not quite know how you get a tooth with giant roots in someone's jaw, but phobics have a distorted impression of how big their roots are going to be. Unless you can change that distorted interpretation before the phobic has to have a tooth removed, then you have a problem. Hypnosis can change that interpretation (see my patient's piece at the end of this chapter).

I am sure by now many must think of Geoff Graham as a distorted fanatic himself. But I ask you, 'Why do 50% of the British public never have dental treatment?' I think that the public must have a distorted perception of dentists if half the population never visit one. Hypnosis can change that. Why do dentists have a poor life expectancy? Why do so many either take early retirement or give up dentistry before their time, even when most of them are trained to do nothing else? Why do dentists have a poor record when we look at the suicide tables? Why do 45% of dentists have a higher blood pressure than the rest of the population when measured on an age basis? This may be because dentists are working in a very stressful environment. Hypnosis can help dentists to handle stress much better.

## Pain in dentistry

To explain and demonstrate exactly how much it is possible to change distorted interpretations I have had a surgical removal of one of my own teeth without any anaesthetic using self-hypnosis. I have a video of the operation and have had it broadcast on TV. I fractured the root of one of my teeth. The broken root had to come out. I had a gum flap lifted around three teeth. Bone was removed followed by the two halves of the root. The rough edges of the bone were then smoothed with a bone file and the gum stitched back into place. This was all done without any pain being experienced.

My strategy for this operation was that pain is an emotion to prevent us from harm. The root was fractured and useless as well as being infected; having it removed was getting rid of harm. As there was no harm being done, I did not need to feel pain. I made images in my head of the infected and useless tooth being expertly removed and the gum healing up, leaving my mouth free of root and infection. I told myself it would give me no problems either having it removed or afterwards. I imagined very vividly how good it would feel being rid of a useless root and how much more comfortable I would be when my mouth was free from infection. I had absolutely no expectation of pain or anxiety, so that was how it felt. I hope this explains how much we can distort what is happening to our detriment and if you can see that, then surely it is just as easy to use distortion for our benefit. Hypnosis is a wonderful way to achieve this.

A short time after I had had my own tooth removed, I was contacted by the surgeon who did my surgery about another of his patients. He had been asked to remove two roots from a lady who had some very bad experiences with both general and local anaesthetic. Following both her last general anaesthetic and last local anaesthetic, she ended up in the intensive care clinic with anaphylaxic shock and very nearly died. Her treatment card was marked with large red letters, 'Do not use any anaesthetic unless this patient's life is threatened'. This presented quite a problem for my surgeon friend. How was he to extract two roots from someone who could not have an analgesic or anaesthetic? He asked me if I could help.

I saw this lady and found she was quite a good hypnotic subject. She had used hypnosis before to have some small fillings done. I showed her the video of my own extraction and explained my strategy to have my tooth extracted without pain or anaesthetic. I explained that pain was an emotion to protect us from harm, and as the abscessed roots were badly infected, having them removed would do no harm, so she need not feel any pain doing that. She seemed to accept this, so we set up an appointment.

When we met I induced a trance state in this lady and told her that she was so relaxed that nothing would bother her and that as her roots were dead and useless, having them out would cause no discomfort. Notice my choice of words, 'no discomfort' instead of, 'no pain'. If you use the word pain, the patient will have to access the meaning of pain in her mind to know what pain means and if she does that she is much more likely to feel some pain. When she had settled down, I told the surgeon to go ahead with the first root extraction.

During this extraction the patient showed some signs of discomfort, so I questioned her afterwards, before we went on to do the other extraction. She said she was, 'loath to lose her teeth' which gave me a clue as to why she was feeling some discomfort. I had told her pain was an emotion to protect her from harm and if she was loath to lose her teeth, having them out was causing her harm, so then she would feel some discomfort. I explained to her that she had another root to extract, so if she did not want to feel that, she would have to want to have this extraction and that there would be no harm in having them out because the root was useless and infected.

At this point she accepted my statement uncritically because she was in a hypnotic state, so the surgeon was able to take the root out without the patient being aware of this being done. In fact she said, 'Hurry up and take it out' and the surgeon showed her that the root was actually out of her mouth. She smiled and said how wonderful the surgeon was in being able to extract these two roots without her feeling anything.

It is up to the patient to produce an absence of pain, not the hypnotist. I had chosen to give her a simple choice. She had to choose either to want to have her teeth out or to feel pain. She had chosen to want to have the teeth out.

## Rapport, pacing and leading

### Rapport

One of the most essential conditions we have to fulfil when communicating with anyone is to build rapport with that person. The quickest and easiest way to do that is to use the hypnotic procedure of pacing the patient. If we pace a person, then we rapidly build rapport and at the same time the patient goes into a spontaneous light informal hypnotic state.[4]

### LEADING

Leading means giving the person a way out of their difficulty and it is very effective after you have paced the person on more than one level. They will just follow your lead.

### VERBAL PATTERN

When a person leans towards a particular verbal pattern it is necessary to respond in the same pattern if you wish to establish rapport and keep the informal hypnotic state going. Leading the patient then becomes a mere formality.

## Pacing

To pace someone we have to get into the rhythm and flow of how that person thinks and processes their thoughts. When we do this we have a very powerful hypnotic procedure to assist us to make changes in that person. There are various levels of pacing which we should learn until pacing becomes second nature to us and we do it automatically. At first, people may think we are deliberately copying them but when pacing is automatic their unconscious mind begins to think, 'You are just like me and I can trust you'. They then do not realize that we are pacing them. I did a lot of pacing with the dental phobic patient who has given his experience at the end of this chapter.

### EMOTIONAL PACING

The first level of pacing is to meet the person on the same emotional level that they present with. This is necessary at the first interaction, otherwise the patient will switch off and it will take you at least 10 minutes, if you are lucky, to get them back. For instance, if the patient comes into your consulting rooms obviously nervous and frightened, it is no use trying to make them feel better by being jolly and happy to see them. They will just think 'It is all right for you being jolly and happy, I am the one about to have treatment, not you'. They will think on an unconscious level, 'You do not understand how frightened I feel, so I cannot trust you'.

You may say, 'I guess it is pretty frightening in here'. Their unconscious mind then thinks, 'You really understand me, I can trust you'. Whatever you have to do then will be easier.

### AGREEMENT PACING

The next level of pacing is agreement pacing. It is no good disagreeing with your patient at the first meeting otherwise they will not trust you at all. To disagree is to attack the patient and insult them (see the section on Talk strategies, below). If they say something that you cannot accept, then remember that the patient believes in what they are saying. That is unless they are just trying to wind you up, but this is unlikely if they are scared. They are generally too nervous to do that. If you disagree with their belief, you are insulting them. If what they are saying is really outrageous, you could say, 'I guess you really think that'. This is not directly disagreeing with them, but is indicating that you may have another idea about what they are saying. This may get you off the hook with a difficult patient.

### POSTURE PACING

This is done by you adopting a posture similar to your patient. If they sit down you sit down. If they cross their arms or legs you cross yours, but do it as if in a mirror image and try not to copy your patient exactly but do something similar. If you copy them exactly they may realize you are just copying them, but if you are clever and do something similar, once again their unconscious mind will notice you are just like them and they will trust you more.

## TONE AND TEMPO PACING

This means that you talk with your patient using the same tone and tempo as your patient when they talk to you. You also breathe at the same rate as your patient, breathing in when your patient breathes in and out when they breathe out. This is very important and very powerful as a level of pacing.

I remember a patient who came into my consulting room with a collar and bandage round her neck and with a tracheotomy tube sticking out of the bandage. She obviously had to have this to assist her breathing, because of an operation. She came for a new set of dentures and looked very frightened as she entered. She said she wanted new dentures, but was terrified of having an impression taken in case she choked and could not breathe. I do not know how one is unable to breathe when one has a tracheotomy tube in the neck. However, if she believes she may choke then that is her truth, so it is pointless to argue with her.

I began pacing her as soon as she came into my room. Following her saying she was afraid she would not be able to breathe because of her neck, I said, 'It must be very frightening for you with your complication'. As she sat in my dental chair I sat on my stool in front of her and quite away from her, so she could both see me and not feel trapped. I adopted a posture not unlike hers and began talking at the same tone and tempo that she was using. I also began to breathe at the same rate as she was breathing. After a few minutes spent pacing her on at least four levels I asked her if I might come over to her and show her how easy it would be for her to have the impression taken. This is leading the patient where she wants to go. She would want to have the impression taken easily. She accepted the lead and said she would like that.

I loaded an impression tray with material and approached her with it. As I did I deliberately began breathing a little louder, but still at her rate of breathing. I took the impression without any trouble and when I took it out of her mouth she thanked me and said, 'I know what you were doing, it was so kind of you'. I asked her what I was doing and she replied, 'You were breathing for me, weren't you'. Of course you cannot breathe for someone else, but if she thought I was breathing for her, then so far as she was concerned, I was. I said, 'I told you I would make it easy for you and I have'. This example just shows how powerful pacing and leading really can be.

## LANGUAGE PACING

This entails talking on the same level as the patient and particularly using the same sense of language.

### Visual language

If the patient is using visual language, then you must use visual pacing. For instance, if the patient says, 'The sky is a beautiful blue today', it is no good saying, 'And isn't it lovely and warm?' Blue is a colour and visual, warm is a feeling. Changing from seeing to feeling will upset the rapport and delay the ability to lead the patient to wherever you want to take them. It will also lighten the informal hypnotic state which results from correct pacing. The sort of language the patient will use if they are being visual is: Bright, Colourful, Clear or Seeing.

### Auditory language

Then the patient may be using auditory language, so you must reply in auditory language if you want to build rapport and deepen the informal hypnotic state. For instance, if the patient says, 'On my way here today the ambulance bells were ringing very loud'. It is no good saying, 'Did you witness an accident?' Bells are a sound but witnessing is seeing. You should answer by saying something like, 'Were the other cars making a commotion with their honking?' Or, 'Were people shouting?' The sort of words used in auditory language are: Sounds, Hear, Telling, Ring.

### Kinaesthetic language

Some patients may be talking in kinaesthetic language and it is necessary to reply to them using 'feeling' language. For instance if the patient comes into your consulting room and says something like, 'It's very cold today', it is no good replying, 'Is it overcast?' Cold is feeling, overcast is seeing. You could say, 'Do you prefer it cold or warm?' The sort of language used in kinaesthesia language is: Warm, Cold, Soothe, Gut feeling.

### Gustatory language

The person may use olfactory or gustatory language, then it is necessary to respond to taste or smell language. The sort of words used in olfactory or gustatory language are: Taste, Smell, Sniff, Distasteful.

### VALUES AND BELIEFS PACING

Yet another level of pacing is the values and beliefs pacing. Values and beliefs pacing is very like agreement pacing, but you should always remember that values and beliefs are 'the truth' to the patient who holds these values and beliefs. If you violate their values and beliefs at the first interaction with your patient, you will be very lucky if they ever trust or believe you again. So values and beliefs are held much stronger than mere agreement. Find out what the values and beliefs of the person you want to work with are, before you enter into any sort of pacing communication, otherwise you may never be able to help that person.

### CULTURAL PACING

Along with value and belief pacing must come cultural pacing. You must remember that different cultures hold different beliefs and values, so it helps if you are aware of the person's cultural background before you start trying to pace them.

### Content pacing

The last level of pacing I would like you to consider is content pacing. Many people do not listen and say something that has nothing to do with what has been going on in a communication situation.

For instance, at a lecture after the speaker has finished and the chairman asks for questions, it can happen that someone gets up on their feet and does not really ask a question at all, but wants to show the audience just how clever they really are. They offer their own opinion, often about something that has nothing to do with what the speaker was talking about. People at the lecture look round at the person and generally think, 'Why don't you keep quiet?'

You may be talking in a small group, enjoying each person giving their own opinion about some topic, when another person joins the group. Without listening first to what each of you are saying, the interloper starts to say something that has nothing to do with what you have been discussing and you all look round and think, 'Why don't you go away?'

So if some person starts to talk to you, for goodness sake have the courtesy to listen and reply to their topic if you can. If you cannot, then it is better to listen intelligently in silence.

Creating rapport by pacing someone, first of all creates a state of informal hypnosis in that person and second it enables you eventually to lead that person to wherever you want to take them. It can be likened to a gardener establishing a fertile soil to grow a bountiful harvest at some time in the future.

## Talk strategies when communicating

The next thing to remember when communicating is that there are various talk strategies. These can either cause the problems that exist between you to escalate or, by using different strategies, you can de-escalate the problems between the two of you. It is said that 80% of people talking to each other today use primitive talk strategies that are likely to escalate the problems in the world. If you do not agree with this statement look at a news broadcast on TV or read a newspaper and see how many confrontations occur in the world around us. Most of our leaders are attacking each other and creating situations where there is no way out. Marriages, partnerships and management are at risk because of negative talk strategies. It is possible to learn how to communicate with another human being without escalating the natural problems that exist between two different people with different beliefs and interpretations. This is most important if you wish to help dental patients who have different interpretations to dentists regarding their dental treatment. It is especially so if you are using an altered state of hypnosis to help them.

## SAD

When 80% of people are communicating in a way which will bring about an escalation in the problems between them, we think of this as a SAD way of communicating.

The S of SAD stands for Silence which communicates as sullen, angry silence. Whenever people meet with sullen silence their blood pressure rises and they often retaliate by attacking the silence.

The A of SAD denotes an Attack and along with attack comes judgement and advice. An attack is a human insult and results in various self-destruct mechanisms. This was clearly seen in Iran when the Iranians took the American Embassy staff as hostages. The American President was calling the Iranian leader a religious nut and he, in turn, was calling the American President an evil devil. If the negotiations had been left to these two, the hostages would still be hostages or dead by now, so it had to be taken out of their hands. The US President lost the next presidential election by a landslide and nobody believed in the Iranian leader afterwards.

I remember doing a workshop in London a few weeks before Margaret Thatcher was dethroned. I predicted that she would not stay in power for much longer because she was judging and advising almost everyone. Her judgement was in the form of an attack, but most judgements and advice are perceived as an attack, by the person being advised. Remember that when dealing with difficult dental patients it is no good attacking or judging them unless you want to get them to go somewhere else for treatment. If you attack them, you will destroy yourself in their eyes.

The D of SAD stands for Deceit, along with evading and lying. The trouble with lying is that once you start you have to keep it up until even you do not know what the lie is. All these facts seem fairly simple, but 80% of the population are using these techniques to communicate with one another. Any of these techniques will escalate the problems that exist between you and the world.

## IMPACT

If you wish to change or help someone, then you have to make an IMPACT on them. Both SAD and IMPACT are key words to help one remember how to communicate with another person.

The I of IMPACT stands for Information. If you wish to make a positive communication with anyone, it is essential to get as much information as possible about that person and yourself as soon as you can. You need to know where you and they are coming from, what your beliefs and truths are and how they differ.

Then you need to know how this information affects 'Me' and 'You' and each of your truths, before you can share feelings about 'Me' and 'You' without attacking or judging each other. So the M of IMPACT stands for Me.

The P of IMPACT stands for Positive. Is what you would like to communicate positive or is it negative? How is it positive or negative and what can you alter to make sure it is positive? If two people are stuck being negative, then if one can become positive and follow the other criteria in making the IMPACT, the one being negative is forced in the end to become more positive. So long as one person is making an IMPACT in any communication the other one has to change.

The A of IMPACT is for Adult and this is synonymous with maturity. Is what you are saying adult and mature and what are the real reasons behind your statements? Are those reasons adult and mature? If not, then what can you do about it? Many people try to fulfil childish needs when they are adult because their childish needs were never fulfilled. It is not possible to fulfil childish needs after you have reached adulthood. Most people who try this will be considered peculiar. Many people do not even recognize when they are acting childishly. If you can, then by you being adult, they have to change.

C stands for Creative. Are you being creative or destructive in your communications? If you find what you are saying is destructive, then look for ways to make it more creative. Most people like creative, positive adults and will want to be your friend. Nobody wants to be the friend of someone being negative and destructive. These criteria also apply to how a person communicates with themselves. If they are being negative and destructive they do not even like themselves, so they cannot expect anyone else to like them. Yet most people in this state are only too keen to complain, 'Nobody loves or appreciates me'.

The T of IMPACT stands for Translations. This is to remind us that whatever we think, feel, do or say is only a translation. There is no truth, yet most of us like to consider their translations to be 'the truth' and get angry if others do not believe them. This is no way to communicate with anyone and causes a lot of mischief in the world today. You will never make an IMPACT in your life unless you understand what has been discussed in this section labelled 'Talk strategies'. To learn more about this read William H Pemberton's book, *Sanity For Survival*.[5]

If you use rapport, pacing and leading combined with the talk strategies, as discussed above, you will have the person you are talking to go into an informal spontaneous hypnotic state. All your communication will be able to bring about change both in yourself and the person you are talking to.


## Behaviour therapy in dentistry

Behaviour therapy is most effective when there is a deep trance patient or at least a good medium trance patient. First of all it is necessary to establish rapport with the patient by the methods explained above. Then using the patient's imagination you use direct suggestion to relax them and make them more at ease. Following this it is easy to suggest a removal of their fear. You must remember that four-letter words are forbidden. Words like fear, pain, hurt are forbidden because to fully understand what these words mean the person being hypnotized must access their meaning, by which time it is too late. Once they have accessed their meaning of these words it is much more difficult to get them to change this meaning.

It is often useful to treat children by giving them a distraction technique. This can be done by asking the child patient what she or he likes doing in their fun time. If it is watching TV, then ask them what their favourite programme is. It is better if you know something about the programme, but not essential. You can always ask them what the programme is about and who the characters are. Having got them in an altered state of hypnotic consciousness, ask them to imagine they are at home watching their favourite programme. As soon as they can see the programme ask them to nod their head. You must always have feedback from the patient. Do not guess what they are doing and seeing. As soon as they nod their head, ask them to tell you what they are seeing in the programme. This will confirm that they can see it and by telling you what the characters are doing in the programme, it will deepen their trance and simplify your job.

You can then say something like, 'As long as you can see the programme, nothing I do will bother you. In fact you will know I am doing something in your mouth but you will hardly notice me'. In most cases this is all you need to do for fillings and the patient will feel nothing that bothers them. If they have a favourite game they like to play, then have them imagine they are playing the game and as soon as they tell you they are playing the game in their imagination then proceed as above. Adults will also like to partake of their favourite pastime while you service their teeth, but remember you cannot make someone do something they do not want to do. If you have a child who does not want fillings, they may be happy to watch an imaginary TV programme, but if you then try to do a filling the child will break trance and say, 'You are not going to drill my teeth'.

## Hypno-analysis in dentistry

Sometimes with very severe dental phobics it is necessary to find an answer to the question, 'Why is the patient so afraid?' I remember one of the most phobic dental patients I have ever treated was just such a case. I tried almost every technique in the book to relax him but to no avail. I then did some analysis to find out *why*. My patient just kept on saying that he had been to many dentists and with some he had run out of their rooms. He had an abscessed molar tooth which had to be removed. He had had the abscess treated with antibiotics many times, but he always felt that if he had it out somehow he would die.

I tried many hypno-analytical techniques unsuccessfully until I posed him the question while he was in trance. 'Is there a spirit in you that should not be there, preventing you from having your tooth out?' Much to my surprise and shock, I got the answer, 'Yes'. The next question I asked was, 'Can that spirit tell us who it is'. Once again and to my surprise, I got the answer, 'Yes'.

The spirit then went on to tell me he was a German officer in charge of removing the gold from Jewish prisoners before they went to the gas chambers during the war. He had been shot when the allies released the camp and his spirit went into my patient. The spirit was preventing my patient from having his tooth out because many of the Jewish people had died after having their gold teeth removed. The spirit was afraid that if my patient had his tooth out and died, then it would not have a host to live in.

After much persuasion I managed to get this spirit to leave my patient and move on to the next life, the natural progression after death. I have greatly shortened this story which took me at least five one-hour appointments to complete. However after my patient waved goodbye to the spirit he was able to have his tooth removed, but not without some difficulty. You may like to ask me, 'Do I believe this story and has this really happened?' My answer is, 'I have no idea if it really happened. What I do know is that subconsciously my patient believed this had happened and this belief was a dynamic force that was preventing him from having his tooth removed'.

Proof of the pudding was that he had the tooth removed after saying goodbye to the spirit. My patient had no conscious knowledge of this story, until after we had done this analysis and I am not even sure he believed it. It cured his phobia to let him have his tooth removed and that is all I know. Psychotherapy is telling a story. If the patient believes the story, they can change the way they are translating with their brain and make the necessary changes in their perception to be happy.[6]

## Case history

The following is a report from a dental phobic patient. It is in his own words and will show you why hypnosis should be used in dentistry. His name has been deliberately omitted.

*The following saga could be relevant to a few others and may indicate that help may not always start off in the most direct way. I can show how I went from a very long-established feeling of hopelessness to the incredible actuality of being released from my problem.*

*The problem was the terrible condition of my teeth and my mental blockage about taking action, even though I had entered my fifties.*

*I was born at Christmas-time just before the end of the 2nd World War. Some of my earliest memories were wondering why my lost baby teeth were replaced by quickly decaying 'permanent' ones. Normal people ended up with reasonable white rows. I cannot remember if there was a precise trigger to my not having early treatment, my dental condition was so obviously horrible that I extended 'avoidance' to supposed eccentricities of never smiling, covering my mouth with my hand when speaking or looking away.*

*I have never consulted a doctor since infancy and one brief, early trip to a dentist (under the motivation of enormous pain) left me with my prejudices intact, if not reinforced. Although I wished to be 'normal', years turned into decades with every birthday a reminder of my inaction.*

*There are several practising dentists in every High Street but for me they may as well have been on planet Mars. Going for treatment was like asking myself to walk blind-folded through a door with sudden unknown terrors on the other side. How could I expose my condition to a professional, used to ordinary requirements, without severe embarrassment?*

*Meanwhile, I had managed to follow a professional career but none of this helped and I reached a career cross-roads as I turned 50. I had the prospect of major advancement but could not face it as the need for extra social skills would create ever more embarrassment.*

*My glimmer of hope was having chanced upon Geoff Graham's books which appeared to have amazing relevance to my case. The really decisive moment was when I took the plunge into seeking a no-commitment, informal meeting with Geoff. I trusted that his counselling skills would take precedence over his dental skills initially. This indeed was the case and from our very first session I realized that everything would be done to give me reassurance, that my case was not unique and that my 'door' would be opened very carefully to let me pass through safely.*

*The therapy sessions with Geoff were different from any other experience but were very pleasant. I feel that in an incredible short number of weeks, if not days, I was able to make a smooth transition from pure therapy to handing him control to complete the treatment stage. By then I had changed my incorrect, deep-seated perceptions. The physical treatment was of course expertly done, bore no relationship to my preconceived horrors and resulted very quickly in my having a longed-for good dental appearance. I cannot put into words the sheer pleasure and satisfaction of simply being able to smile, to talk face to face and, not least, to enjoy foods which had been impossible for decades.*

*I also went on to take full advantage of my career opportunity.*

*This has happened recently and I still marvel that it happened at all. The process has also bolstered my self-esteem generally in all manner of other areas of my life. I am so grateful for the avenue which Geoff's approach gave me. I can only say that I could not have followed a 'conventional' route and do not know what would have happened with further passage of time. In simple layman's terms he broke the vicious circle of decay = avoidance = decay = etc.*

*In condensing a lifetime of experience into these few words I have necessarily skipped a vast amount of detail but I do have a final sentiment: If anyone feels that they have a problem they do not wish to expose to the normal system, please remember that you are not unique (billions of people continue to inhabit this planet). A little searching will find an alternative method to take you from hopelessness to happiness by breaking your own vicious circle.*

## Hypno-healing

We all possess a natural healing process in our body and mind that can be stimulated and accelerated by hypnotic suggestion. Our defence mechanisms can work with our regenerating systems and aid natural healing. However, occasionally this natural process works against itself and delays healing. In the latter case this can normally be changed by hypnotic suggestion.

A common time to observe this negative phenomenon is in the tissue reaction to burns and surgery. It is the oedema that occurs following surgery that often does more harm than the surgery itself. This oedematous swelling and subsequent tissue reaction can often be controlled by hypnotic suggestion, provided that the suggestions are made before the swelling or tissue reaction occurs. This will then allow the healing process to be greatly accelerated.

I had an apicectomy performed on one of my teeth and an observing dentist remarked that I would have a swollen face the next day. I told myself in trance that it would not swell and would heal naturally and quickly. There was no swelling and it did heal up remarkably quickly. Hypnotic suggestion may assist in mouth ulcer treatment, bruxism, trigeminal neuralgia and atypical facial pain, and reduce bleeding and the production of saliva.

It is possible to influence the autonomic nervous system to produce a stimulation of the sympathetic and parasympathetic systems. Hypno-healing is largely achieved through stimulation of the parasympathetic system to promote healing. Both systems work through the hypothalamus which can be influenced by hypnotic suggestion.

Sometimes healing is influenced by positive psychological processes in the mind, in this case accelerating healing or the reverse effect is also noticed when the mental processes are negative.

CASE HISTORY

*A young lady who fractured her spinal cord and was rendered paraplegic from the waist down felt responsible for doing this to herself. She felt so guilty she wanted to die. I found that, as a result of this, she was in constant pain everywhere in her body. Spinal specialists, physicians and psychiatrists could not understand how it could hurt below the level of fracture as she is paralysed and should be numb, nor could they help her with her pain. I saw her after 6 weeks of pain and gave her a number of reasons for living. Half an hour later she was completely free from pain. To a large extent she has been free from pain ever since. I have now seen her for a total of three one-hourly visits and her recovery is almost complete. Her son now recognizes her as the mother he knows and wants to be with, whereas before my treatment he just wanted to leave as soon as he entered the ward to see her.*

If a dental patient does not want to have the treatment done they will often suffer pain after that treatment. This goes to show that if you need to do something, it is very important to want to do that thing, especially if you want it to heal quickly and with no after-effects. If you do not, you suffer the consequences.

I hope this opens up another field in which hypnotic intervention can be of enormous use.

## Summary of uses of hypnosis in dentistry

To summarize the uses of hypnosis in dental practice, it can be most helpful in the following conditions:

- Stress management for the patient and for the dentist:
   Rapport building for achieving a good dentist/patient relationship. Improving dentist/staff relationships and dentist/spouse/friends relationships.
   Pacing and leading.
   Language patterns for de-escalating problems as opposed to escalating them.
   Teaching relaxing techniques and ego strengthening.
- Treatment of dental anxiety and phobias:
   The distortions in dentistry both in and out of hypnosis.
   How to avoid being rejected/sued by your patient/staff/friends.
   Patterns for a happy life.
   Desensitizing phobias and teaching new techniques with NLP to help make treatment less frightening for both dentist and patient.
- Hypnotic treatment of pain:
   Pain management in temporomandibular joint problems.
   Management of trigeminal neuralgia and phantom tooth pain.
   Help with atypical facial pain which has no physical apparent cause.

Pain control in surgery (fillings and extractions).
Production of analgesia.
- Hypnotic control of bleeding, saliva production and gagging.
- Help with tolerance of appliances, e.g. dentures, orthodontic appliances.
- Hypnotic treatment of bad habits, e.g. thumb sucking, tongue thrusting, smoking.
- Help with the treatment of mouth ulcers and gum disease by mind–body healing.
- Helping to promote healthy healing and reduction of post-operative swelling or pain.

## Conclusion

In this one chapter I have had to omit some of the uses of hypnosis in dentistry. To cover all the uses and techniques would take a whole book. I hope I have managed to show what hypnosis is, most importantly what it is not and why more dentists should consider using hypnosis in their dental practice. Hypnosis will help them build their practices and be in a position to help patients who otherwise would not be able to face dental treatment. Hypnosis should help a dentist to have a more relaxed and happy life and be more able to communicate with his patients, staff, lover, spouse or children.

## References

1 Spiegel H. *The Inner Source Hot*. New York: Rinehart and Winston, 1982.
2 Janov A. *The Primal Scream*. USA: Abacus, 1973.
3 Janov A. *Prisoners of Pain*. USA: Abacus, 1982.
4 Bagley D S 3rd, Reese E J. *Beyond Selling*. USA: Meta Publications, 1987.
5 Pemberton W. *Sanity for Survival*. USA: Pemberton, 1992.
6 Graham G. Hypno-analysis in dental practice. *Am J Clin Hyp* 1974; **16(3):** 178–187.

## Bibliography

Ambrose G J. *Hypnotherapy with Children*. UK: Staples, 1961.
Bandler R, Grinder J. *Frogs into Princes*. Utah: Real People Press, 1970.
Bandler R, Grinder J. *Trance Formations*. Utah: Real People Press, 1981.
Bandler R, Grinder J. *Reframing*. Utah: Real People Press, 1982.
Barber T X, Stanos N P, Chaves J F. *Hypnosis, Imagination and Human Potential*. New York: Pergamon Press, 1974.
Cheek D, Lecron L. *Clinical Hypnotherapy*. New York: Grune & Stratton, 1968.
Elman D. *Hypnotherapy*. Glendale, CA: Westwood Publishing Co, 1984.
Gardner G, Olness K. *Hypnosis and Hypnotherapy with Children*. New York: Grune & Stratton, 1996.
Graham G. *How to be the Parent You Never Had*. Newcastle upon Tyne: Real Options Press, 1986.
Graham G. *How To Change Your Life*. Newcastle upon Tyne: Real Options Press, 1990.
Heap M. *Hypnosis. Current, Clinical, Experimental and Forensic Practice*. London: Croome Helm, 1988.

Heap M, Dryden W. *Hypnotherapy: A Handbook*. Buckingham: Open University Press, 1991.
Janov A. *Prisoners of Pain*. USA: Abacus, 1982.
Janov A. *The Primal Scream*. USA: Abacus, 1973.
Kroger W S. *Clinical and Experimental Hypnosis in Medicine, Dentistry and Psychology*. USA: Lippincott, 1977.
Marks I M. *Fears and Phobias*. London: Heinemann, 1969.
Naish L N. *What is Hypnosis?* Milton Keynes: Open University Press, 1986.
Scott D L. *Modern Hospital Hypnosis: Especially for Anaesthetists*. UK: Lloyd Luke, 1979.
Shaw H L. *Hypnosis in Practice*. London: Baillière Tindall, 1977.
Waxman D. *Hartland's Medical and Dental Hypnosis*, 3rd edn. London: Baillière Tindall, 1989.
Wolberg L R. *Medical Hypnosis*, Vols 1 & 2. New York: Grune & Stratton, 1948.

## Associations

There is at least one professional hypnosis society in most countries round the world. Professional societies are all affiliated to the International Society of Hypnosis.

International Society of Hypnosis
Administrative Officer
Edward Wilson Building
Austin Hospital, Studley Road
Heidelberg, Victoria 3084
Australia
Tel: 00 613 9459 6499
Fax: 00 613 9459 6244

European Society of Hypnosis
Professor C. Hoogdin
Zoeterwoudsesingel 77
2313 EL Leiden
Netherlands
Tel: 003 171 514 4097
Fax: 003 171 512 4885

The professional British Societies are:

The British Society of Medical and Dental Hypnosis (BSMDH)
Hon Sec, Mrs Rhona Jackson
17 Keppel View Road
Kimberworth, Rotherham
South Yorkshire S61 2AR
UK
Tel: 01709 554558
Fax: 01709 554558

The British Society of Experimental and Clinical Hypnosis
Hon Sec, Mrs Phillis Alden
86 Scartho Road
Grimsby
NE Lincolnshire DN33 2BG
UK
Tel: 01472 873423
Fax: 01472 879238

The two professional societies in the USA are:

The American Society of Clinical Hypnosis
Suite 291, 2200 East Devon Avenue
Des Plaines
Illinois 600118-4534
USA
Tel: 001 847 297 3317
Fax: 001 847 297 7309
European Society of Hypnosis
Prof C Hoogdin

The American Society of Clinical and Experimental Hypnosis
Suite 304
3905 Vincennes Road,
Indianapolis, IN 46268
USA
Tel: 001 317 228 8073
Fax: 001 317 872 7133

Many of the other societies affiliated to the International Society of Hypnosis round the world are very active and most professional.

# Courses

Anyone wishing to learn the techniques of hypnosis is strongly advised to contact one of the professional societies who all run fully ethical courses in hypnosis. The courses and workshops are open to professionally qualified persons only. Other professional training courses leading to a Diploma in Hypnosis are run and organized by Michael Heap of Sheffield University. The courses run by BSMDH can lead to a Certificate of Accreditation in Hypnosis. Geoff Graham runs courses and workshops round the world as well as in the UK.

There are many courses organized by lay schools of hypnosis and many of these courses are sound and excellently run. However, there is generally no control over who may attend. This can be a drawback, as some of the participants may be unprofessional and some even unsuitable to be therapists. Normally the qualifications given by these lay schools are not professionally accepted by the Royal Colleges.

# Voice therapy

Angela Caine

## Introduction

The voice has traditionally been associated with music and the arts; a tool for creativity and communication skills. Outside working hours the dentist may enjoy singing in a choir, while during work he or she may realize that a mellow persuasive speaking voice can often influence treatment progress. However, it is unlikely that the dentist has considered the voice to be within the realm of dental treatment. It is even more unlikely that someone who sings out of tune or suffers recurring voice loss will consult a dentist. With the growing awareness of interdisciplinary treatment, that situation is going to change.

### Temporomandibular dysfunction

Amorino and Taddey[1] conducted the first survey on the incidence of voice problems among singers having temporomandibular dysfunction (TMD). The results of this survey showed that there is a significant relationship between TMD and voice dysfunction. In the future more and more dentists are likely to be consulted by professional voice users. It is important, therefore, that dentists understand the connections between voice and musculo-skeletal dysfunction. They should recognize dentally-related voice problems and when undertaking dental procedures not interfere with the patient's vocal skills and, as a result, the patient's confidence. A treatment plan that considers voice function may provide the means to access what every clinician aims to work with – the patient's own self-righting mechanism.

Crelin[2] discusses the actual extent of the vocal and respiratory tract. It takes up a large proportion of the head and neck, including both eustachian tubes and the tongue. These are both significant areas in dental and ortho-dontic treatment.

Many of the ligaments and muscles responsible for the forces involved in singing, swallowing, breathing or lifting heavy objects are also responsible for the forces which move the jaw, position the tongue, provide the rhythmic pump action to expel fluid from the eustachian tube or balance the head on the neck. In my experience of interdisciplinary work, the inclusion of the voice in assessment and treatment has shown that it can be:

- a diagnostic tool for balanced posture and alignment;
- a tool to re-programme facial muscles and prevent orthodontic regression;
- a developmental tool for posture;
- a developmental tool for growth of the dentition and facial bone structure.

## An interdisciplinary approach

Although an interdisciplinary approach is now widely accepted in clinical practice, the voice is not generally considered part of that approach. Research and clinical diagnosis in respect of tongue position, otitis media, cranial torque, malocclusion and orthodontic regression fail to take into account the weight and habitual use of the larynx which is suspended from the hyoid bone. Yet the tongue moves to articulate words and we listen to our own voices directly and internally through the eustachian tubes. The mouth opens and closes to speak, moving the joints and occasionally bringing the teeth together. The hyoid bone must move to swallow and chew, but it also moves to talk and sing.

## The vocal model

If voice is to be included as part of interdisciplinary diagnosis and treatment of musculoskeletal problems, one comprehensive model for the voice has to be established. This can then be applied for the purpose of clinical assessment. The training of the voice offers many different vocal models. There has been a tendency to divide training into the vocal functions of singing and speech which results in many speech teachers not being required to sing as part of their training and, conversely, singing teachers not being required to consider speech problems. Voice therapy often considers voice failure as a symptom of neurological, psychological or emotional problems, with little evidence in the literature of an interest in structural problems.

Functional anatomy on speech and singing courses is generally restricted to that directly concerned with voice production, exclusive of directly related structures like the jaw, the shoulder girdle and the cranium. In the absence of any integrated fundamental education for the voice specialist, loopholes exist where anyone who can play the piano and has a qualification in general music can teach singing.

## Changing our belief system

This is not an attractive scenario for the clinician, who wants specific guidelines with which to work. Dentists, like most of the population, may be nervous of their *own* powers of speech and singing. It is generally believed that some people are born with a 'good' voice; that the 'good' voice is coincidental and if you have one you are able to sing. Those who can sing are then classed as 'musical'. Good voices, like varicose veins, are thought to run in families. The voice can only be used in assessment and diagnosis by stepping out of this concept and discovering clear and simple guidelines for the recognition of structural problems concomitant with a dysfunctioning voice. Those guidelines must apply to all voices if they are to provide simple and clear information for the dentist which can be used to assess the need for specific treatment. Then dental patients who are also experiencing voice problems can be selected for cross-referral with other clinicians.

THEORETICAL CASE STUDY

*A dental patient with a TMD problem is questioned about whether they can sing and the dentist discovers that the patient habitually sings out of tune. Muscle spasm in the suprahyoid system can limit vocal pitch and interfere with articulation and resonance, resulting in a seriously 'out of tune' voice.[1] Similarly in a pelvic distortion described by chiropractors as a Category 1 or 2, compensatory muscle spasm can be expected in sternocleidomastoid and the suprahyoid system, resulting in the same voice problem, with the addition that distortion in the pelvis will also mean the singer is constantly running out of breath.*

*This voice will only improve when the dental and skeletal clinicians discover a combined order of treatment which releases the spasm in both the suprahyoids and the psoas/iliac systems. A broader and more integrated assessment of all head and neck problems may help to select the order of correction. The voice may eventually answer the question: Where do we begin treatment? With dental input? With skeletal input?*

## Natural characteristics

The physical prerequisites for singing and talking, the *anatomical* constituents, are not chance endowments limited to a few individuals. Every person possesses the physical means to talk and sing. It is not because the organ of phonation is missing that people cannot sing, but that the natural inborn facility is being obstructed or interfered with. The vocal model you are invited to consider as a diagnostic tool is based on the biomechanics of all functions of the larynx, acknowledging that its primary function is to breathe. Its potential for sophisticated articulation of language and pitch in speech and singing is responsible for all significant modifications to the head and neck over the last 500,000 years.

## The larynx

### The suspension of the larynx from the cranium

The larynx consists of two large articulated cartilages between the trachea and the pharynx. They enclose and support a system of folds which regulate the size of the air passage. Fink and Demarest[3] describe the larynx suspension as 'a system which binds the supports and the folds of the larynx into a working unit'. This suspension divides into a *main* suspensory system, supporting hyoid bone, thyroid and cricoid cartilages, and a *subsidiary* system, supporting the arytenoid cartilages.

Figure 9.1 illustrates the linkage between the cranium and the arytenoid cartilages which control laryngeal plication (folding) of the *vocal* fold itself. The normal head weighs more than 10 lb (4.5 kg). In upright posture, two-thirds of the weight of the head is in front of the pivot where the head

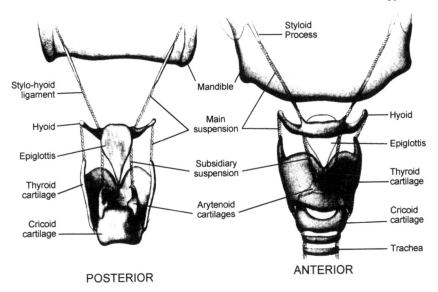

**Figure 9.1** Suspension of the larynx from the cranium (From Fink and Demarest,[3] by permission)

balances on the neck by means of the atlanto-occipital joint. As the weight of the head falls forward and down, balance is maintained by the occipital muscles which provide 'fingertip' control. The styloid process is a projection from beneath the petrous section of the temporal bone. The styloid process helps support the hyoid bone, the weight of the tongue, the mandible, pharynx, larynx and trachea.

Bibby and Preston[4] discovered that in a natural upright posture the temporomandibular and atlanto-occipital joints provide a reciprocal proprioception between them which influences the position of the hyoid bone by influencing the position of the mandible and C3. This assists the maintenance of the cross-sectional area of the vocal tract, i.e. the widening of the throat. Figure 9.1 shows how the larynx is affected by the position of the head. In the event of a habitual tilt of the head to one side or an anterior/posterior misalignment, the jaw and hyoid bone would also eventually reciprocally tilt or misalign.

### Functions of the larynx

The primary functions of the larynx are:

- breathing (inspiration and expiration);
- swallowing;
- effort closure (bracing in physical strength);
- phonation (singing and speech).

Three of these – breathing, swallowing and physical strength – are already part of an assessment and diagnosis of musculoskeletal efficiency. The following issues appear regularly on introductory questionnaires for patients:

'Is the patient a mouth breather or a nose breather?' and 'Is there a natural swallow, or a deviate swallow?' Applied kinesiology is used to test the strength of different muscular pathways by resisting force. This indirectly tests the efficiency of effort closure. If three out of four laryngeal functions affect and are affected by musculoskeletal dysfunction, it would appear illogical that the fourth function is independent of it.

### BREATHING

Inspiration and expiration are dependent on the excursion (down-spring) of the larynx, which explains the necessity for a suspensory mechanism. The larynx pulls down when we breathe in. When we stop breathing in, it returns to the position of least effort. This generates a continuous rhythmic movement of the hyoid bone which is co-ordinated with the rhythm of breathing.

### Plication

The dynamic rationale of all functional laryngeal anatomy is plication. Plication is the process by which internal surfaces of the larynx fold or unfold to control airflow. The vocal chords are one of these folds. Different functions initiate different folding patterns, all of which couple with the vertical respiratory excursion of the larynx. During inspiration the larynx descends and the hyoid bone descends and tilts downwards anteriorly. Because the coupling is affected by elastic ligaments, elastic recoil automatically reverses the process during expiration.

### SWALLOWING

Swallowing is vital to existence. It must be strong enough to force food far enough down into the gut for peristalsis to take over the ingestion process and also far enough to prevent its entry into the lungs via the trachea. During swallowing the epiglottis closes the larynx. This closure, when coughing, is able to withstand pressures from above that may be twice as high as the peak pressures applied from below in effort closure. This is managed by the folding processes within the larynx along with vigorous upward movement of the hyoid, larynx, trachea, pharynx and oesophagus. This complicated multiplicity of devices is necessary to ensure that no scraps of food remain lodged at the entrance to the larynx.

In the development of upright posture and articulate speech in *Homo sapiens* the common passageway for air and food has increased to such a length that the risk of choking to death has been considerably increased. But most consonants would be impossible to articulate without this long upright pharynx according to Edmund Crelin.[5] This illustrates the strength of the evolutionary selection process in favour of sophisticated human speech.

### EFFORT CLOSURE

The folds of the larynx systematically overlap to form a plug which blocks the passage of subglottal air. At the same time the laryngeal entrance is foreshortened by approximation of the thyroid cartilage and hyoid bone.

This further compresses the laryngeal folds, and stops the breathing and the rhythmic excursion of the hyoid bone. The whole rib cage is thus effectively braced and becomes a pressurized 'brick' which gives purchase to the postural system in lifting weights.

PHONATION – SINGING AND SPEAKING

### Vocal folds

The folding within the larynx resembles the folding of a bellows. Closing the bellows increases angularity of the fold surface, unfolding does the opposite. The sounding of the voice is dependent on this 'bellows' folding system. The fine tuning of singing and speech requires a precise and extreme angularity at the internal surface of the laryngeal fold, coupled with the flexibility which allows a 'wave' motion to be produced. Two opposing folds provide a pattern of resistance which can open and close the glottis. In phonation, the internal edges of the vocal fold are vibrated by the following actions:

- one end of the vocal fold attachment is immobilized, which is achieved by rotation and sliding together of the arytenoid cartilages (see *Figure 9.1*);
- the cricothyroid muscle regulates the tension of the vocal fold by stabilizing the position of the adducted arytenoid cartilages;
- the out-breath is used to excite the appropriate vibration in the vocal folds.

Van den Berg[6] states that 'Pressure energy from compressed subglottic air is transferred to the vocal folds and forces them apart; potential energy of air compression is converted to kinetic energy of fold motion'. The vocal folds are tensed to resist the subglottic air by the subluxation of the arytenoid cartilages. The cricoarytenoid muscle forces the cartilages together in such a way that they bend, producing a recoil which springs them apart when the muscle relaxes. In the development of an extended pitch range, there is an additional rotation and translation at the cricothyroid joint. The two possibilities of increasing vocal fold tension are rotation and translation. This is brought about by the arrangement in two directions of the cricothyroid muscle fibres.

### Rhythm

All functions of the larynx are rhythmic and dependent upon the rhythm of breathing. This rhythm is generated by the downward excursion and subsequent recoil of the larynx. This rhythmic excursion is also reflected in the uniquely rhythmic suspension of the whole larynx, tongue, mandible, hyoid and trachea from the styloid process of the temporal bone. The voice sounds at the extremity of this downward excursion by the combined action of the out-breath and the energy of the recoil itself.

*Experiment 1   Take a tennis ball, and bounce, catch – bounce, catch – a few times. To ensure that your breathing is responding to and co-ordinating with the rhythm of the ball, bend your knees as you bounce it. Now say a vowel loudly as you bounce the ball: for example AH! OH! OO! etc. You will discover that the voice automatically sounds at the moment the ball rebounds from striking the floor.*

This is a demonstration of how the voice *begins* to speak a sentence or sing a phrase. After the sound has been initiated, it must continue throughout the phrase, from vowel sound to vowel sound, uninterrupted by the articulation of consonants. This complex movement is facilitated by coordinating the rhythms of speech or singing with the rhythmic excursion of the suspensory muscle system of the larynx.

*Experiment 2    Put your thumb and finger around your own larynx and move it about to feel its suspension. Now say your name loudly and feel the movement that occurs.*

Imagine how much movement is required to recite a speech to a large audience. If sung, pitch is to be extended into the range required to sing Mozart or Puccini, and the suspension must also be flexible enough to facilitate translation between thyroid and cricoid cartilages.

## Voice development

### The fetus

The small articulating bones of the tympanum of the ear (stapes, incus and malleus) ossify in the embryo at 6–7 weeks, and the primitive tongue, palate, pharynx and larynx are present at 7–8 weeks; so all the necessary mechanics for listening are present long before stimulation of those processes by the outside world. Vocal stimulation begins with the fetus listening to the mother from *inside;* the first cries are a response to the mother's voice. This early fetal development is the template for efficient function of the voice, in either speech or singing, throughout life. The ear (listening) is the primary control, followed by the posture of the tongue (see the section on Balanced facial development, below). The tongue is part voluntary (the extrinsic muscles) and part involuntary (the intrinsic muscles) and the latter can only be controlled indirectly. Although starting and stopping the voice is a voluntary act, control of the sound itself is only affected by listening, the imagination and the action of the tongue.

### THE EAR

A sound 'reference library' is collected throughout life by the following processes:

- sounds of the outside world through the external auditory meatus;
- our own vocal sounds directly from the pharynx, through the eustachian tubes;
- bone conduction.

## THE TONGUE

The tongue:

- is central to breast feeding, nose and mouth breathing, swallowing, development of the facial bones and development of the nasopharynx;
- is a determining factor in the shift of the larynx from the infant position; where the epiglottis can lock into the soft palate, to the adult position where the larynx lies between the 6th and 7th vertebrae;
- supports and maintains the development of language skills during the transition period between approximately 1 year and 6 years of age, when shifting vocal and articulatory mechanics can interfere with articulate speech;
- is the main articulator in adult speech and singing – its efficiency affects all communication skills and therefore, to a great extent, personal confidence;
- its position determines the position of the mandible;[7]
- its position affects postural balance and co-ordination.[8]

### The infant

Breast feeding strengthens all the muscles of the tongue and co-ordinates several fundamental rhythms in mother and child: the rhythm of breathing, cranial rhythm and the rhythm of sucking. All of the tongue lies in the oral cavity during this early sucking period, the hyoid bone high enough in the oropharynx for the soft palate and epiglottis to lock together to facilitate obligate nose breathing. This ensures that the baby can suck and breathe at the same time. The tongue then 'pumps' the soft palate, which encourages steady, even breathing. The co-ordination of rhythms in mother and baby can be further strengthened by the mother singing lullabies to the baby as it feeds.

Vocally and cranially, the human infant resembles the infant chimpanzee and can make only vowels and babbling noises; articulation is restricted by the high position of the larynx. The relatively oversized tongue stimulates the nipple and also the growth and development of the maxilla. This prepares the palatal arch for the developing dentition.

### The toddler

Speech patterns and recognizable tunes are starting to formalize by about 1 year of age. Of course the child will only speak and sing if it *hears* speaking and singing. Examples should include adults, children, strangers, parents and friends; natural voices coming out of all the people who can be reached out to and touched. The face, head and neck muscles are exercised by reading aloud, word games, stories and experimenting with different languages and dialects. Poetry, songs and nursery rhymes are most easily copied and fun is a vital ingredient for encouraging these activities.

From birth to about 2 years of age, the infant is also learning how to be upright on two feet and developing the muscle strength to cope with that. The stages of rolling and crawling develop cross-patterns in arms and legs.

The toddler experiments with balancing and this selects specific muscle patterns for control of upright posture in standing, sitting, movement, etc. First teeth are appearing during this period of change from infant to toddler in a palate already rhythmically massaged into continuous widening by the tongue and by developing speech and singing. The upright trunk in sitting, reaching with arms for climbing possibilities and the rotation of the head on the neck to find the next place to cling, all provide a gravitational stimulus for:

- the shift of the larynx and tongue to their adult position level with the 6th–7th cervical vertebrae;
- a deeper excursion of the hyoid bone down the pharynx;
- tongue strength to be concentrated on development of the *posterior* maxilla, to make room for the molar teeth.

During the period of toddling and balancing, the tongue moves inferiorly to form a muscular anterior laryngopharynx (front wall of the throat) where vowels can be articulated. This period of shift for larynx and tongue is completed between 5 and 6 years of age.[5] Deciduous dentition begins at approximately 6 months and changes to mixed dentition at approximately 6 years.[7] Because of the evolutionary policy of economy it is reasonable to assume that this is not coincidental, but that development of the child's voice and that of the deciduous dentition inter-depend on each other. The development of the voice can be directly influenced and may between 2 and 6 years of age indirectly stimulate the development of a satisfactory cranial and mandibular base for positioning the teeth.

### The adolescent

The position of the larynx is stable from approximately 6 years of age until the onset of puberty, when the thyroid and cricoid cartilages enlarge. The blood supply to the tissue lining of the pharynx and larynx is influenced by either the female hormone oestrogen or the male hormone testosterone, which charge the voice with an emotional and sexual response. The vocal fold itself acquires the characteristics of the genitalia to erect and less air is required to activate phonation in the adult than in the child. Less air, but a more sensitive vocal fold produces the true adult voice, with all its emotional and expressive range. Vocal instability during this balancing of the relationship between air pressure and the voice in puberty is generally referred to as the 'breaking' of the voice. Contrary to general opinion this occurs in both male and female voices.

THE TONGUE

When the tongue is in its adult position, it forms a right angle between the anterior and posterior halves. The posterior section of the tongue forms the front wall of the throat and co-ordinates with the walls of the pharynx to modify vowel sounds. The anterior horizontal section of the tongue (which in nose breathing is suspended at the back of the mouth by the styloglossus muscle) can spring forward and backward from its suspension to articulate consonants, as illustrated in Figure 9.2.

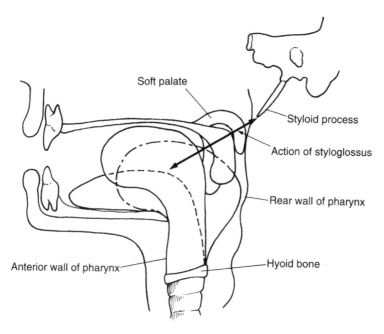

**Figure 9.2** Articulation possibilities in the adult

Crelin[5] experimented with a latex rubber pharynx moulded from casts taken from cadavers. He was able to produce the vowels used in all languages by suspending the latex rubber pharynx and changing its shape by means of wires positioned at the relevant muscle attachments (*Figure 9.3*). He was thus able to disprove the generally held theory that vowels are shaped in the oral cavity, by cheek and lip muscles, with the tongue lying in the floor of the mouth.

## Upright posture

*Homo sapiens* developed an upright posture and thereby gained a sophisticated communication system. The head of the previous upright biped, *Homo erectus*, was entirely forward of the spine, its position determined by the weight and size of the large mandible which was necessary for holding and tearing food. The vocal tract in *Homo erectus* was straight, but positioned at an angle which prioritized a forward tongue posture for chewing. The right angle in the tongue, which accompanied upright posture, allowed the tongue to pull back as well as move forward from its fundamental nose-breathing position and articulate complex bunches of consonants. Consonants are articulated against the hard palate, the alveolar ridge and the back of the pharynx. They are also articulated against and in co-ordination with the soft palate. All of this movement is co-ordinated with the vowels being shaped by the fixed end of the tongue forming the muscular anterior wall of the pharynx, as in *Figure 9.2*. The evolutionary modifications to the larynx

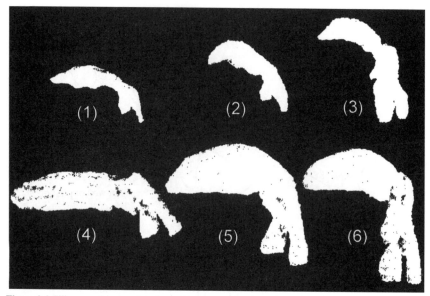

**Figure 9.3** Silicone rubber casts of vocal tracts arranged to show that the development of ontogeny is a resumé of the evolution or phylogeny of the hominid tract from 500 000 to 1 000 000 years ago: (1) 2-year-old child; (2) 4-year-old child; (3) 6-year-old child; (4) Australopithecine hominid; (5) Homo erectus; (6) Homo sapiens (From Crelin,[5] by permission)

which accompanied the reduction in the size of the mandible, the development of the cerebral cortex and the sophistication of speech are illustrated in Figure 9.3.

The 'modern' vocal tract evolved between 500 000 and 1 million years ago, facilitating all the sounds of articulate speech. This phylogenetic event is recapitulated in the development of every present-day human between birth and 6 years of age. Although the right angle of the tongue is achieved at 6 years of age, the larger skeletal frame and larynx of the adult are necessary before the voice finally matures physically, intellectually, neurologically and sexually by approximately 25 years of age. By a unique evolutionary arrangement, the voice is functionally efficient, with all the articulatory mechanism available by the time the child is 6 years old. Between then and 25 years the voice absorbs and reflects all life's experience of adult development. It is this rounded maturity which actually makes the 'good voice' and builds into it the communication skills generally considered to be coincidental.

## Balanced facial development

### Facial muscles

Muscles influence the position and movement of bones. The facial muscles are viewed slightly differently in the different disciplines: osteopathy and chiropractic, dentistry and orthodontics, voice and speech, health and beauty. The understanding of facial muscle function is also obscured by the association of the facial muscles with expression and emotion. This is part involuntary and part a natural desire to appear attractive, which centres attention on the face as reflecting the personality.

Breathing, speech, singing, chewing and swallowing all move the face, but the *primary* function of the face musculature is nose breathing. If the face and tongue muscles are developed with this priority of nose breathing, then facial muscle balance will also develop naturally for speech, chewing, swallowing and facial expression and, as a result of this, beauty.

## TONGUE POSTURE

Tongue posture is central to both nose breathing and facial balance.[8] There are two basic postures of the tongue:

- suspended against the back of the hard palate;
- lying in the floor of the mouth against the lower teeth.

These two basic postures of the tongue divide the facial muscles into two groups. Group A facial muscles are associated with a backward position of the tongue against the hard palate and nasal breathing. Group B facial muscles are associated with a forward positioning of the tongue in the floor of the mouth and the chewing of food.

## GROUP A FACIAL MUSCLES

Group A facial muscles radiate from the centre of the face. They all insert into moveable tissue. As the cranial rhythm dips the vomer and flares the zygomatic processes of the temporal bones, cranial flexion is enhanced at the mid-line sutures of the facial bones by the action of zygomaticus major and minor, quadratus labii superior and buccinator. The lateral action of all these muscles encourages the cranium to widen in the facial area and flares the nostrils. This reduces pressure throughout the nasal cavities and maxillary sinuses, and as a result the reduced pressure aids inspiration. The air can then be warmed, cleaned and sterilized before the contraction of the diaphragm and opening of the glottis of the larynx pulls it into the lungs. Imagination and emotion can extend this action into what we describe as 'bursting into laughter – bursting into tears'.

## GROUP B FACIAL MUSCLES

Group B facial muscles act in the vertical plane to chew. They originate in bone and insert into bone and they have more bulk and less delicacy than group A. Medial and posterior temporalis snap the teeth together and masseter applies a vertical force to crush food against the molar facets (aided by lateral movement from the pterygoid muscles). These muscles generally have no function in breathing, speech, singing or swallowing. An exception is the anterior temporalis which in speech and singing suspends the mandible in a position which gives the tongue independence in articulation.[9]

Group B muscles are activated by the tongue taking up a forward position to push food between the teeth when orbicularis oris closes the lips. Orbicularis oris is not strictly a facial muscle but a sphincter to close the anterior end of the gut. The lips must be closed to chew, but closing is not necessary for nose breathing. With the lips open it is only possible to chew things that stick to the teeth – like chewing gum. When tongue action is efficiently balanced and the tongue suspended at the back of the mouth, it is the seal between tongue and soft palate which determines whether you breathe through the nose or whether the lips are open or closed.

Pressing the lips together in an effort to ensure nose breathing merely interferes with facial muscle balance and narrows the nostrils. Scowling, sulking and other facial expressions generally associated with introversion are involuntary expressions of group B. Overdevelopment of group B generally achieves a dull impassivity of expression. When an orthotic appliance is fitted in the mouth, care must be taken to stimulate group A. The appliance can become 'food' and initiate group B. It can also be seen as an 'unhappy' event. An exercise programme may be necessary to maintain the efficiency of group A while the orthotic is worn.

*Experiment 3   Press your lips tightly together. Remain like this for the count of 5. Now try to smile and discover how you have restricted facial expression. Breathe through your nose. You can only 'hoover' in air, narrowing the nostrils because the whole face has become involved in the action of closing and protecting the anterior sphincter of the gut. If you tighten your anal sphincter and maintain the tension, you will discover the same sphincteral support in the gluteal muscles.*

### Nasopharynx and oropharynx

Facial balance results in the mouth gently and effortlessly resting closed with equal fullness in upper and lower lips.[9] The nasopharynx is suspended anteriorly from the nasal septum and medial pterygoid plates, and posteriorly from the pharyngeal tubercle of the occipital bone. As its suspension is mainly from bone attachments, its position is stable. The oropharynx is a tube which is open anteriorly, where it is attached to the pterygoid raphe. The position of the pterygoid raphe is determined by the action of the facial muscles (the anterior attachment of the pterygoid raphe is the buccinator muscle). The position and size of the oropharynx is therefore more flexible than that of the nasopharynx. With contraction of orbicularis oris in response to food entering the mouth, contraction of buccinator will flatten the cheeks and pull the pterygoid raphe forward, reducing the oropharyngeal space and the danger of food accidentally passing into it. This reduces the risk of choking, given that there is a common passage for air and food. Buccinator, in co-ordination with the tongue, has a role in both group A and group B facial muscles.

Relaxation of orbicularis oris changes the role of contraction of the buccinator muscle, as is shown in *Figure 9.4*. The pterygoid raphe is pulled posteriorly, increasing the oropharyngeal space in order to facilitate swallowing, talking, singing and any greater demand on the breathing system. Any activity which demands maximum efficiency in breathing, rhythmic

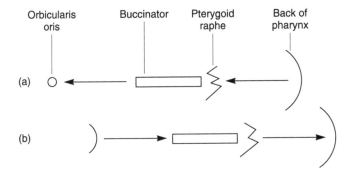

**Figure 9.4** Role of buccinator in (a) chewing and (b) talking and singing

co-ordination and power needs to prioritize facial muscle group A. An apparently smiling face is the mark of the successful runner, singer, wind player, dancer, etc. It is also the face which is generally considered to be most attractive. Its open, welcoming quality inspires a similar quality in the faces it meets and the easily opening mouth is always ready to communicate to make other people feel comfortable and secure.

## The extrinsic frame

The extrinsic muscles of the larynx function as a co-ordinated system of strap muscles that add transitory stresses and background support to the main and subsidiary systems which are shown in *Figure 9.1*. This external suspensory 'frame' acts as a shock absorber between physical movement and excursion of the larynx. Thus Fred Astaire could simultaneously sing and dance; his body executing intricate movements, his feet tap-dancing, while his voice effortlessly sang, his breathing stable. The extrinsic frame supports and stabilizes the hyoid bone, and through it, acts to balance and co-ordinate any movement of the vocal tract which is in opposition to movement of the mandible and of the head and neck. For instance, as the head turns to look over one shoulder the rhythmic excursion of the hyoid bone must be maintained for efficient breathing. If an extended pitch range is called for when turning the head, additional translation and rotation at the crico-thyroid joint must be supported. The muscles which support this balancing act of the hyoid bone during movement of the whole upper body are shown in *Figure 9.5*. They are:

- the stylohyoid muscles and ligaments, which are common to both the main suspension of the larynx and the extrinsic frame – they provide lateral and vertical support and together with the stylomandibular ligament influence the position of the hyoid bone relative to the mandible;
- the anterior and posterior digastric muscles which connect the hyoid bone to the mandible and the mastoid process of the temporal bone, respectively;

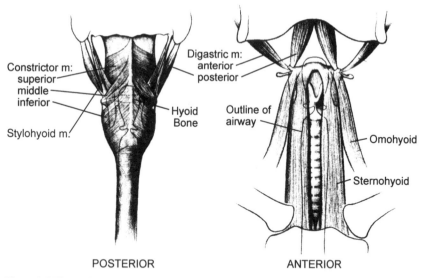

Constrictor m:
superior
middle
inferior

Stylohyoid m.

Digastric m:
anterior
posterior

Hyoid
Bone

Outline of
airway

Omohyoid

Sternohyoid

POSTERIOR                    ANTERIOR

**Figure 9.5** The extrinsic laryngeal strap muscles (From Fink and Demarest,[3] by permission)

- the omohyoid muscle which connects the hyoid bone to the scapular and thus brings it under the stabilizing influence of strong posterior muscles of the trunk;
- the sternohyoid muscle stabilizes the hyoid bone, larynx and trachea inferiorly and brings them under the influence of the strong anterior muscles of the trunk.

The extrinsic frame is connected to bony attachments on the mandible, the scapula, the sternum and the cranium. An active pathway can be traced from the vocal fold to these bony attachments. The arytenoid cartilages are adducted and subluxed by the activity of the intrinsic laryngeal muscles to control vocal fold tension. This motion is regulated by the main and subsidiary suspensions, the subsidiary suspension supporting the arytenoid. The main and subsidiary suspensions are then attached to the skeletal system via the extrinsic 'frame' of strap muscles.

### The Alexander technique

Evidence for the influence of the extrinsic frame on voice function comes from a variety of disciplines. In 1932 F. M. Alexander[10] discovered that the relationship of his head and neck affected his voice. He went on to improve his voice and his whole quality of life by attending to the balance of the head at the atlanto-occipital joint and from that developed the Alexander technique. He probably made the first connection between skeletal structure and laryngeal function. Sonninen[11] and Zenker and Zenker[12] proposed that '...the strap muscles (the extrinsic frame of the larynx) also assist in regulating the tension in the vocal folds'.

## Stammering

Further connections between structure and voice did not appear again until Caine *et al.*[13] examined 36 stammerers and found that they all had severe structural problems. Current voice pathology is reluctant to consider that musculoskeletal problems might influence the voice. The poor posture, rhythm and co-ordination which often accompany stammering is looked upon as symptomatic of the lack of confidence caused by stammering.

Since the work by Caine and colleagues, increasing interest among dentists and orthodontists has led to parents being questioned about speech problems *other* than tongue thrust occurring in children brought in for treatment. In all cases where speech problems exist, the child needs to be recommended not just for orthodontic treatment, but cranial correction as well. Therefore any successful treatment plan for stammering must include assessment for structural correction as well as help with changes of attitude and self-image. If a stammer is observed the dentist can assume there will be particular problems of skeletal misalignment and function.

## Singers and temporomandibular dysfunction

Tension in the jaw muscles or an unnaturally high hyoid is usually diagnosed in singers as tension due to either performance stress or fear of musical inadequacy. Nervous singers *do* run out of breath. But which is the symptom and which the cause? Are they really nervous about their lack of musical ability? Or are they nervous as a result of an instinctive feeling that the voice will let them down? Is this due to sensory feedback from inefficiency in the laryngeal strap muscles in the presence of malocclusion or cranial torque?

Amorino and Taddey[1] discovered that the singers with TMD who filled in their questionnaire had breathing problems when singing, dissatisfaction with voice quality, limited pitch range and little confidence. Of the singers I have worked with as a voice teacher, some of whom were performers and some students, almost 50% were found to have structural defects which affected the extrinsic frame. The quality of singing in this 50% did not improve until treatment began to correct jaw and skeletal problems. Singers not satisfied with achievement of potential were variously found to be suffering dysfunction in molar/tongue reference, lack of molar support, insufficient maxillary dimension, skeletal instability, unbalanced excursion of the hyoid bone, an uneven translation of the mandible in the glenoid fossa or unequal weight-bearing on two feet. Structural correction *always* reduced singing effort, extended pitch range in singing and increased resonance. This resulted in increased singing confidence. From structural correction a domino effect then led to performance without stress.

## Structural dysfunction

Fonder,[14] Alexander,[10] Rocabado,[15] Gelb[16] and Selye[17] are just some of the distinguished clinicians who have linked structural dysfunction with collapse of the posture of the cervical vertebrae and the concomitant problems of forward head posture, forward shoulder posture, collapsed tongue and facial muscle function. Their evidence supports the theory that as muscles compensate to support and protect the dysfunctioning structure from further damage, they transmit tension and misalignment from the extrinsic frame, through the main and subsidiary suspensions of the larynx, to imbalance the action of the arytenoid cartilages, causing the voice to dysfunction.

Voice function can therefore be affected by dysfunction in any of the structures which provide attachment for the extrinsic laryngeal frame such as:

- malocclusion of the teeth;
- lack of molar support;
- tongue thrust;
- temporomandibular joint dysfunction;
- cranial torque.

### THEORETICAL CASE STUDY

*A voice problem may be symptomatic of musculoskeletal dysfunction. A typical application of this 'pathway' from cause to symptom might be in the case of a child with articulation difficulties and general reluctance to communicate. If there is for instance severe cranial torque, the temporal bones will unbalance the larynx suspension by misalignment at the styloid process, thus interfering with the balanced excursion of the hyoid bone on inspiration and its subsequent recoil in expiration. Spasm in digastric muscle to prevent further cranial distortion will raise the hyoid bone and restrict the excursion further, also restricting the articulatory movement and speed of the tongue.*

*The child would experience this restriction in speech and may 'try too hard' in order to overcome it, causing perhaps a stammer or at least diffi-culty with multiple consonants. Because of the tilting of the hyoid bone, the tongue could fail to make a seal with the soft palate at the back of the mouth. The escape of air would then create a speech problem – 'S' would sound like the 'Ll' in the Welsh prefix - 'Llan...'. Panic at not being able to speak properly initiates further panic. The cranial torque may also cause problems with breathing and rhythm, so singing may not be good. This child is then unlikely to be offered a chance to play a musical instrument. Because intelligence is largely judged on the basis of reading ability, the symptomatic voice problem, when reading aloud, may be judged as a lack of intelligence and the child can be deprived of appropriate education by problems which are not perceived to be causative and which could easily be treated.*

*Because the dentist does not ask about the voice, the school teacher does not ask about the teeth, and the games teacher does not ask about either, the voice problem may be treated by a speech therapist without reference to co-ordina-tion, posture or dentition. The voice problem is only symptomatic, and because of lack of development in the other areas, the voice treatment will probably regress.*

# The voice as a diagnostic tool

Are the other functions of the larynx affected by structural problems affecting the extrinsic laryngeal muscular frame?

Dysfunction in breathing, swallowing and effort closure may be life-threatening. Voice problems are not life-threatening; they limit potential by limiting communication skills. Therefore, it is quite impossible for voice problems to be ignored. A dysfunctioning voice interferes with *all* human interaction. The croaking voice while on the telephone, singing a song or buying the bread initiates immediate response. That voice can express a cry for help as powerful as one from the person who falls in the river, provided that we can learn to interpret the real problem behind the voice and not become distracted by the cry itself. Evolution may have provided one simple and instantly recognizable method to report on a variety of systems which could affect survival.

If the voice is used as a diagnostic tool, potential pathological systems affecting laryngeal function can be diagnosed and maintained in a healthy state by preventive clinical treatment. These symptoms include:

- temporomandibular joint function;
- cranial torque;
- postural balance;
- breathing;
- swallowing;
- eustachian tube evacuation;
- facial function;
- tongue posture;
- co-ordination;
- potential voice skills.

## The voice in assessment

Most people have sung as children, but some have failed to develop adult singing through lack of opportunity. In my experience everyone can sing a nursery rhyme or similar song from childhood. For some reason that I have not yet discovered, on being invited to sing 'anything at all' it is always 'Baa, baa black sheep'.

Dentistry is generally considered to be entirely mechanical and devoid of self-expression. Singing, on the other hand, is seen as a means of expression and nothing whatsoever to do with mechanics! You must get your patient to sing using whatever guile you may and if necessary enlisting the help of other members of your staff. When the patient does sing it is easy to *see* the following problems:

- the tongue flat in the mouth for 'EE' and 'EH' vowels';
- the cheeks shaping the vowels 'OO' and 'OH';
- tongue and jaw functioning together;
- priority for facial muscle group B;
- a deviating mandible;
- limited excursion of the mandible;
- postural instability.

You can easily *hear* these problems:

- sharp intakes of breath;
- a shrill high-pitched voice;
- articulation problems – a stammer, hesitation, difficulty with some sounds.

Although the latter problem may not appear in the singing, it will certainly be exposed by any conversation about the selection of something to sing. The information gained from discussing and singing this little song will expose habitual patterns of use and indicate where muscle reprogramming is necessary to stabilize corrective treatment. None of this information will be discovered from a written questionnaire.

### Mouth breathing

Many people who breathe through the nose when not using the voice believe that singing, reading aloud or using the voice over a distance, requires a switch from nose breathing to mouth breathing: 'I need to take a good breath before I begin.' A sharp intake of breath through the mouth initiates the 'fight or flight' emergency breathing system, elevating the hyoid bone. A patient who mouth breathes to use the voice and who is also a professional voice user (e.g. a school teacher or a singer) will interfere regularly and powerfully with any dental realignment treatment programme. Although more breath may be needed to sing, nose breathing is always maintained as the fundamental system. Extra air is taken in through the mouth, supplementary to nose breathing, by reflex modification of the tongue/soft palate seal.

### The balance board

A high hyoid bone with restricted excursion (see the section on the Extrinsic frame, above) limits the ability to reproduce speech rhythms. Reading a poem aloud reveals problems with rhythm and thus with hyoid bone and tongue position. If the poem is read while standing on a balance board, ability to balance, leg length, tongue posture, head posture and general co-ordination can also be observed. A balance board exposes our natural ability to cope with being upright in a situation which changes moment by moment. When the patient combines personal experience of balancing with reading a poem or singing, this moment-by-moment co-ordination exposes any inefficiency of the extrinsic frame.

*Experiment 4    First stand the patient against a postural grid and write down your observations. Next, stand them on a simple balance board (see the note on equipment in the Appendix). Last, stand them on a balance board while they are reading a poem or singing a song. Write down your observations at each stage.*

Each stage demands a little more efficiency in co-ordination. Compensatory muscle systems become very efficient in maintaining postural stability over a long period and are thus difficult to discover. However, muscles must be reprogrammed for efficient function along with structural correction if regression is not to occur. Singing a song or reading a poem on a balance board defeats the most subtle and entrenched compensation system which, once observed, can be reprogrammed to gain real efficiency levels rather than patient-perceived efficiency levels.

## The voice as a tool to reprogramme muscles

As the extrinsic frame realigns with correction of the cranium or mandible, the hyoid bone will be released and its excursion extended. The voice will then respond better to the rhythm of singing and language patterns.

The patient can be encouraged to participate actively in this process by undertaking a voice and body exercise programme specifically designed to re-educate upright posture and facial balance. This would involve singing and reciting while using body balls, therabands and balance boards (see Appendix) to introduce rhythm and stretch into the body and into the whole vocal/respiratory tract. The tongue can be repositioned by reading and singing in dialect and foreign languages and by learning to understand, recognize and use facial muscle group A. All this can be made fun, as well as giving the patient a measure of control in the treatment.

### Voice and body exercises

Caine[18] has developed a programme of exercises for voice and body to correct tongue thrust. A natural tongue position is one in which sufficient permanent tone is maintained on the styloglossus muscle to allow *all* vowels to be articulated in the pharynx and nose breathing to be maintained as a fundamental system (see section on Balanced facial development, above) even when talking or singing. Mouth breathing should *always* be a supplementary system.

It is the experience of this author that many dentists and orthodontists only class a tongue protruding between the teeth as 'tongue thrust'. A tongue which is not striking the maxilla with its total width or which articulates generally forward of the alveolar ridge has sufficiently poor articulatory mechanics to allow regress of good functional orthodontic work.

Voice and body exercises using balance boards are also described by Caine.[9] The patient is given exercises which use the voice and body together, maybe using equipment such as a body ball or a balance board. This encourages the patient to take responsibility for bringing about his or her own share of musculoskeletal correction and opens a dialogue with the clinician for reporting and discussing progress. The exercises are designed so that even people who have never sung before and are terrified of 'music' will be able to enjoy singing. Throughout musculoskeletal treatment these exercises can be a reference for postural improvement.

### Self-righting

We all have natural self-righting mechanisms, but we access them most readily when we feel positive about the improvement offered by the treatment plan. Structural or postural improvement is often slow – a fixed appliance can be difficult to cope with on a daily basis at work or school and constant muscular pain is debilitating. Singing produces a feeling of well-being which in itself helps to access self-righting mechanisms. If the patient is doing daily exercises which are fun and makes them feel good, as well as speeding up correction, he or she is also likely to monitor progress, rather than passively wait for things to happen.

The interest engendered by getting involved, plus the dialogue throughout with the clinician, can initiate a process in which the patient can learn much more about the cause of his or her problem, the process of correction and how to manage that correction to best advantage. The exercises provide an area for the patient to stabilize or self-right themselves. This would be an extension of patient education to include positive participation in treatment.

## The voice as a developmental tool

If the development of deciduous dentition and the voice are interdependent, it follows that orthodontic treatment in children cannot be successful if the vocal tract is underdeveloped and functionally inefficient. It also follows that by achieving efficient laryngeal function, development of a stable dentition will be assisted. Middle ear infection is currently a difficult problem to clear. Voice work which exercises rhythm and develops effortless postural balance also strengthens the pump action which evacuates the eustachian tubes. There is a direct connection between the vocal tract and the eustachian tubes. Singing and bouncing, whether sitting on a big bouncy ball or playing hopscotch, all develop healthy ears, nose and throat, as well as postural balance, while skipping with a rope directly increases the pump action of the eustachian tubes.

Skipping, bouncing and singing games bounce the larynx and tongue into their adult positions. Climbing, jumping about, hopping from foot to foot, while having fun and not thinking about it, stimulates natural postural reflexes. It is vital that lots of this natural bouncing and balancing takes place before children's posture is determined for them by riding bikes, sitting at desks and computers and playing musical instruments. They should also be encouraged to sing, chatter and tell stories with actions and making faces so as to stimulate the whole respiratory tract.[18] Then the facial bone structure will continue to develop forward in spite of the increasing visual stimulus which all children have to deal with by about 5 years of age.

Unfortunately, most parents do not recognize orthodontic problems except cosmetically. Often, mixed dentition will have begun by the time problems are obvious. Patient education should include invitations to bring children in young enough for the clinician to detect co-ordinative development problems between dentition, posture and voice. Children who become patients need the same balancing and 'Baa, baa black sheep' tests as adults. If early postural and vocal stimulation have been missed, all the developmental 'windows' must be reopened when orthodontic treatment begins. Otherwise vocal or postural underdevelopment will work against, and may even regress, treatment.

## Conclusion

Parents need to be made aware of the connections between voice, posture and developing dentition. They can then encourage activities in which the voice and body act together to develop good tongue posture, an expansive palate and a dentition that naturally occludes. They also need to be made aware of the importance of singing throughout school life, and especially singing with the tongue suspended where it can spring backwards as well as forwards. Nose-breathing efficiency and facial muscle balance will then be encouraged, whether sitting at a computer or playing sport.

A balanced tongue that articulates against a fully developed palate, which it has shaped for such a purpose between the ages of 2 and 6, facilitates efficient nose breathing and good vocal mechanics for life, *if the musculoskeletal system maintains its symmetry*. Conversely, in the presence of structural misalignment, none of the mechanics associated with a balanced tongue *can* be efficient because the body is unstable. It may be that in the presence of structural symmetry the tongue, in nose breathing and speech, will go on developing palate width for life. The voice, when singing and speaking rhythmically across its whole range, is the tool by which the tongue will maintain the muscular tone to facilitate this. But musculoskeletal misalignment interferes dramatically with this possibility. If misalignment is before the age of 6 years, good vocal mechanics will not develop fully. If the misalignment is later, the mechanics can be *heard* to dysfunction.

Speech has, during the last 500,000 years, superseded chewing. Simpson[19] states: 'Language has become far more than a means of communication in man. It is also one of the principal means of thought, memory, problem solving and other mental activities.' Recently a very experienced dentist who was watching small children shift the tongue to its natural nose-breathing position by singing said: 'We must come to accept that the mandible is undergoing a change in function. It is no longer designed for chewing, but to support a system of sophisticated, articulated speech.'

Crelin[5] states that, 'Ultimately, articulate speech led to a complicated spoken and written language, abstract thought, the fifth symphony and the theory of relativity'. If this view of evolutionary progress is acceptable it would indicate that any orthodontic treatment should take account of the long-term effects on the voice. The value of a beautiful smile is somewhat mitigated by the inability to communicate efficiently because the tongue/palate relationship is underdeveloped through the early extraction of teeth for overcrowding. On the other hand, if a system so powerful exists within the musculoskeletal structure, it seems sensible to access that power for development, corrective treatment and subsequent maintenance of that structure.

# References

1 Amorino S, Taddey J J. Temporo-mandibular disorders and the singing voice. *Nat Assoc of Singing Teachers J* 1993; **50(1):** 3–14.
2 Crelin E S. Development of the upper respiratory tract. *Clin Symp* 1976; **28(3):** plate 10; CIBA.
3 Fink R B, Demarest R J. *Laryngeal Biomechanics*. London: Harvard University Press, 1978.
4 Bibby R E, Preston C B. The hyoid triangle. *Am J Orthodon* 1981: **80(1):** 92–97.
5 Crelin E S. *The Human Vocal Tract, Anatomy, Development and Evolution*. Atlanta: Vantage Press, 1987.
6 Van den Berg J. Myoelastic-aerodynamic theory of voice production. *J Speech Hearing Res* 1958, **1:** 227–244.
7 Hiatt J L, Gartner PG. *Textbook of Head and Neck Anatomy*. Baltimore: Williams and Wilkins, 1987.
8 Garliner D. *Myofunctional Therapy in Dental Practice*, 3rd edn. Florida: Coral Gables, 1974.
9 Caine A. *The Voice Workbook* (with audio work tape). London: Hodder and Stoughton, 1991.
10 Alexander F M. *The Use of the Self*, 1988 edn. London: Victor Gollancz, 1932.
11 Sonninen A. The external frame function in the control of pitch in the human voice. *Ann NY Acad Sci* 1968; **155:** 68–90.
12 Zenker W, Zenker A. Über die Regelung der Stimmlippenanspannung durch von Aussem Eingreifende Mechanismen (On the regulation of the vocal folds through the extrinsic suspension mechanism). *Folia Phoniatrica* 1960; **12:** 1–36.
13 Caine A, Cardew E, Stimson N. Structural predispositions in the etiology of stammering. *Proc IFA World Congress on Fluency Disorders*. Munich, August 1994.
14 Fonder A C. *Dental Distress Syndrome*. Rock Falls, USA: Medical-Dental Arts, 1990.
15 Rocabado M, Annette Z. *Musculoskeletal Approach to Maxillofacial Pain*. Philadelphia: Lippincott, 1991.
16 Gelb H. *Clinical Management of Head Neck and TMJ Pain and Dysfunction*, 2nd edn. Philadelphia: W B Saunders Co, 1985.
17 Selye H. *Stress without Distress*. New York: Lippincott, 1974.
18 Caine A. *Lost Your Tongue? A Voice and Body Exercise Programme with Audio Tapes*. Southampton: The Voice Workshop, 1993.
19 Simpson G G. The biological nature of man. *In* Washburne S L, Jaye P C (eds). *Perspective on Human Evolution*. New York: Rinehart and Winston, 1968.

# Bibliography

Alexander F M. *The Use of the Self*, 1988 edn. London: Victor Gollancz, 1932.
Caine A. *The Voice Workbook* (with audio work tape). London: Hodder and Stoughton, 1991.
Crelin E S. *Functional Anatomy of the Newborn*. New Haven: Yale University Press, 1973.
Crelin E S. *The Human Vocal Tract, Anatomy, Development and Evolution*. Atlanta: Vantage Press, 1987.

# Appendix

## Equipment to use with voice and body exercises.

A BALANCE BOARD

This is a circular board with a hemisphere underneath. The balancing surface should be large enough to stand with the feet as far apart as in normal upright posture. The hemisphere height should be not more than 8 cm. The feet must be kept parallel on the board and the knees not braced. It is helpful to stand on the board with bare feet. There should be a period for just balancing before beginning any reading or singing.

A ROCKER BOARD

This is a square board with two curved rockers underneath, so that it can be 'walked' side to side by the flexibility of ankles, knees and hip joints while a poem is read aloud or a song sung. It improves breathing by releasing leg flexors which have become postural muscles as part of a compensatory muscle pattern. By fixing the legs for instance, the psoas muscle, which inserts into the lumbar section of the diaphragm, can be co-opted to increase inspiration, causing hyperventilation.

BODY BALLS

These are large inflatable balls which will support the weight of the body. They are used to sit on and bounce to the rhythm of singing and poetry. They can also be used to lie over, either forwards or backwards, to allow the spine to stretch to its maximum length. They are available in all sizes from that suitable for the 3 year old, to the size and strength which supports a large adult male bouncing to a poem or a song.

THERABAND

Stretch band, often used in aerobics. It can be obtained in different strengths and is used to give joints a greater range of movement. It is important to remember that muscle reprogramming is not so much about 'building' and 'powering' but more about flexibility and facility.

SKIPPING ROPE

A normal skipping rope can be used.
Body balls and theraband are available from:

EPSAN Sports and Therapy (UK) Ltd
Unit 4
The Grinnall Business Centre
Sandy Lane
Stourport on Severn, DY13 9QB
UK
Tel: 01299 829213
Fax: 01299 829214

The Voice Workshop
436 Winchester Road
Southampton SO16 7DH
UK
Tel: 01703 390555
Fax: 01703 390555

Balance boards and rocker boards are available from:

Multiturn
10 Merdon Ave
Chandlers Ford
Eastleigh
Hampshire SO53 1ES
UK
Tel: 01489 789068

# Courses

For details of the tongue training programme contact:

The Voice Workshop
436 Winchester Road
Southampton SO16 7DH
UK
Tel: 01703 390555
Fax: 01703 390555

# Holistic practice

## Stuart Ferraris

*Stuart graduated from the University of Stellenbosch, South Africa, in 1976. He spent the next two years as a dental officer in the navy. His free time was spent flying, sailing and starting his own practice 100 miles north of Cape Town.*

*During this time he built a 45-foot sailing boat that he launched in 1979. He then left the navy to give full-time commitment to his private practice. In 1981, having finished the boat and sold his practice, he set sail with spouse and friends to South America.*

*'Bella del Mare' being equipped with a dental surgery, was well used in many ports of call. The main route included St Helena, Rio de Janeiro, the Caribbean, Bermuda and Holyhead. They had spent two years afloat when his first daughter arrived, so 'Bella' came to Menai Bridge, his wife's home town, where he once again settled into general practice.*

*In March 1984, while preparing 'Bella' for the summer season, a gas explosion destroyed the boat and nearly Stuart himself. A year later he returned to work, albeit a little compromised. Among other wounds he was left with a brachial plexus injury. This meant he could not lift his right arm and had no function of biceps, deltoid and spinatus muscles. An arm splint allowed him to maintain his hand in a useful position; so life continued.*

*The chiropractic profession, and a passion for new ideas in complementary medicine, gave new hope to a condemned arm and other injuries. Now, although only slightly compromised, he practises as a holistic dentist and lectures nationally and internationally on this subject. A colleague recently said to him, 'Stuart, you are going so far down the alternative path, you are sure to meet yourself coming back the other way'.*

*Stuart's philosophy is that there are many cures to support healing and a lot of fun in the sphere of complementary dentistry. He says one should maintain an open mind, but not so open that everything falls out. [Editor]*

## Introduction

Using complementary therapies is fun and rewarding. The fun is in the diversity and team involvement. The reward is being able to view patients' oral health in a broader perspective and being able to improve their general health management.

We can all use complementary therapies in our practice, but like anything new, we need the time and energy to learn. This gives an added dimension to the postgraduate programmes we maintain to support the orthodox therapies we use every day.

Many people become concerned when questions are raised about their routines, perhaps due to fear of change. We instinctively enjoy routine and habit; it helps us feel more secure, but is often the barrier to introducing new concepts to our practice. The reward for overcoming this fear can be the freedom of thought that allows us to advance.

Routine preventive care relies on basic principles. What is needed is good hygiene and a healthy diet, the same diet that protects teeth and gums, protects against heart disease and cancer. Oral hygiene is based on reducing the number of micro-organisms, not on reducing their quality, which is controlled by the body's health balance. These same concepts used in oral hygiene apply to the whole body. The basis of holistic care relies on the natural principle of reducing the number of noxious stimuli and encouraging the body's own health balance.

Understanding comes with knowledge and leads to an enhanced perception and greater insight. Thomas Edison once said: 'Our journey through life, exploring knowledge and gaining experience, often leads us back to the place where we first started. When we get there we often find it hard to recognise as the same place.' With knowledge and experience we view things differently.

Orthodox medicine is not complacent and is continually searching for answers. It is often unsurpassed in its ability to deal effectively with acute ailments. Yet there is a degree of disillusionment felt by many, especially those plagued with chronic conditions. Much of this shortfall may be effectively addressed by natural medicine.

Dentistry has always embraced innovation. It has contributed a lot to health care, from anaesthetics[1] to natural medicine.[2] What we should be careful to avoid in dentistry, like all specialities, is the temptation to narrow our perspective. The well-being of every cell is shared and influenced by the fate of all the others. It is said that each cell is a hologram of the entire individual. By reminding ourselves of this, we can easily shift our focused concept of the oral environment to a broader concept of health and disease. The oral environment and the individual's general environment are inseparable.

## Terminology

Complementary therapies have come to embrace a host of meanings. In this text, they will be considered as the therapies of natural medicine used to complement the restorative therapies we traditionally practise as orthodox dentistry.

Holistic care is used to convey the unbiased use of all therapies, orthodox and complementary. When delivered in a compassionate and caring way, it will restore and support the long-term health of the patient.

The term psychophysiology can be taken to include all aspects of the person. These include the physical, biological, emotional and spiritual components that make up the vital functioning person, as well as its interaction with the environment.

Holism, derived from the Greek word 'holos' for 'whole', is a philosophy in which the person, their body and their mind are considered as an individual entity.[3] In German, the word 'health' is derived from the Old High German root word for 'whole', being 'wohl',[4] which implies that all parts are present, properly arranged, and properly functioning in harmonious balance.[5]

Health is commonly viewed as the absence of disease, pain or defect. Health should rather be the presence of something. It should be a positive definition – that which makes us whole, with all parts in proper arrangement, functioning in harmonious balance.

## Philosophy

What is appealing about complementary therapies is that they are person orientated. They lack many of the side-effects associated with orthodox medicine. As one patient has put it: 'Drugs do not have side-effects. They have many effects on the body, most of them undesirable. These are remedied by yet another drug. Eventually the patient suffers from the affliction of poly-pharmacy all for the benefit of the original drug. Later when the person is ill, it is difficult to lay the blame at a specific source. Does the orthodox world look at natural medicine? That would be like changing religions.'

This view may be a little harsh, yet for us as health practitioners it may be a good warning. A more holistic approach, using natural medicine alongside routine orthodox practices, may help us to come across as more sensitive to our patients' needs.

Orthodox medicine can often be drug orientated and invasive by nature. This comment is not meant to be contentious, but rather to highlight what is a growing perception, and probably the main reason why so many people are seeking 'alternative' care. It is helpful for us to acknowledge this change and to improve the image of orthodox medicine by placing it within a holistic environment. Orthodox medicine has a lot to offer to both the patient and the professional. We must therefore provide the best of both orthodox and natural medicine in a holistic approach to patient care.

Health care should mean caring in the traditional sense. The patients need to be listened to and viewed in all their complexity, not partitioned for the convenience of treatment and research. Even the concepts of spiritual, emotional, mental and physical[6] are boundaries used for ease of description. The holistic practitioner should always be reminded of this concept. The patient in front of you, seeking your guidance, knows only the boundaries laid down by education. As a functioning being there are no boundaries, only 'pauses', where the flow of life may be supported, challenged and modified, but the movement persists as a necessity of life itself. This process is similar to the law of energy, which may move from one form to another, but remains flowing within a constant balance.

Aristotle (384–322 BC) addressed the ethics of balance, which formed the basis of Greek medicine.[7] He felt that to achieve health and happiness, we must use all our abilities and capabilities. For this to be achieved he suggested that three forms of happiness had to be present at the same time and in balance. These are:

- a life of pleasure and enjoyment;
- a life as a free and responsible citizen;
- a life as a thinker and philosopher.

It is particularly easy in our profession to be wooed into the fragmented treatment of our patients. For us it is a challenge to be aware of the psycho-physiology that connects the rest of the person with the oral cavity.

The concepts of holistic health should become fundamental to the practitioner. We are better at teaching a philosophy that we live and breathe ourselves. We feel more confident when our health is under our personal control. Our patient rapport is improved by the health credibility factor. Very few will feel confident with treatment from a colleague with oral health that is poorly maintained. It is important to lead by example.

Health is the responsibility of the individual. In order to maintain better health, the patient must be encouraged to take control. Kirsten Olsen[8] says: 'The holistic health movement is about taking charge of your healthcare lifestyle. It means self-knowledge and an active sense of accountability for one's own well-being. Knowing yourself and what it takes for you to be well, helps you to live your daily life in a health-enhancing way.'

We can facilitate the healing of our patients, yet we still rely totally on the patient's inherent healing capacity to do the work. It is the respect for the patients' capacity to heal that will make us better health care providers. Voltaire (1697–1778) said: 'The art of medicine consists of amusing the patient while nature cures the disease.'

## Setting the environment

To run a holistic practice it is necessary to create an environment conducive to the type of natural therapies that you intend to practise. It is necessary to consider the preparation of the patient, the ambience of the practice and the attitude of the team of which you are all contributing members.

### Psychological preparation of the patient

We need to consider the psychological preparation of the patient, even before they see the health care professional. Rossi,[9] in his book *The Psychobiology of Mind–Body Healing* covers much of the research in this field. He discusses 'the power of optimism', 'the belief in cure' and 'the placebo'. These concepts are related to the limbic-hypothalamic system of the brain, the function of which is to modulate the biological activity of the autonomic nervous system in response to mental suggestion and beliefs. Research by Evans[10] shows a remarkably consistent degree of placebo response, averaging 55% of the therapeutic effect of all the analgesics studied. These include morphine, codeine and aspirin. The power of psychological healing must therefore be a very important part of all health programmes.

#### PRACTICE AMBIENCE

We try to develop a good rapport by adapting ourselves and staff to the individual needs of each patient. There are, however, areas of the practice that have to cut a more average path. These range from décor to the smell of the practice. It is hoped that these will be enjoyed by most patients and at least tolerated by the rest.

The rapport and 'mind–body healing' mentioned above, can be influenced by many factors. These include the literature generated by the practice, the telephone personality of the staff and treatment of the patient on arrival at the practice. The décor and setting have much to contribute. The 'feel good' factor can contribute to the initiation of healing. How many patients, on arrival in your surgery, have said something like the following to you? 'Doctor, the pain that was making my life unbearable for the last three days has almost gone since calling you this morning.'

Paintings, flowers, soft music and personal photographs are useful. They lend a homely atmosphere to the environment. If well designed, the balance of clinical efficiency will be retained, yet the austerity that can be associated with the clinical setting is softened.

### Colour

Colour can be a useful influence on healing.[11] Violet can be therapeutic for nervous and mental disorders, while blue is useful for teething. Yellow is associated with cures for skin troubles. With the rising number of allergies associated with latex gloves, perhaps we should have yellow light shining on us over the hand basin.

White is definitely associated with sterility and the clinical environment. While this may appeal to some, many of us are concerned with emotions when visiting the practice. The softer pastel shades of green, violet and yellow are often favourites, being associated with general healing and warmth. While blue is useful, it needs careful thought, for it can be considered a little cold. Blue uniforms, for example, are often quite acceptable and smart. Blue décor, paradoxically, needs to be well chosen, if it is to avoid the cool emotional message and effect.

### Crystals

Crystals have gained the attention of many patients. We know that crystals were used in early radios to set the vibrational frequency. It is believed that vibrations, or energy, from the crystals, have many effects on the living system. Everything in life and of the earth has its own frequency. This is described by Christine Moore[12] in her editorial column of *Homoeopathy International*. These range from the soothing calming qualities of rose quartz to the healing qualities of moss agate and amethyst. Soozi Holbeche[13] in her book *The Power of Gems and Crystals* gives a wealth of background on this subject. There do not appear to be any clinical trials to validate these effects as is often the case in branches of natural medicine. This does not in itself prove the concept ineffectual, but rather that no one has as yet done the necessary work. Whatever one's feelings on this issue, the crystals are held and enjoyed by patients and can only assist with the background ambience of a caring environment.

### Aromatherapy

Aromatherapy uses the smells of natural herbs and flowers as therapeutic agents to treat differing pathologies. These agents are reduced to essential oils and applied to the skin as massage techniques or simply inhaled.

Smell is one of the most easily remembered senses. The smell of the dental office, especially for the patient, is very characteristic. The historical use of oil of cloves takes much of the blame for this. Dentists were therefore using aromatherapy long before it became popular. All we now need to do is camouflage the environment with other essential oils associated with more pleasant memories. Valerie Ann Worwood[14] gives an excellent overview of essential oils and their uses. Oils such as lavender are useful in the reception and the surgery because of their calming properties. A cotton wool roll, with a subtle fragrance of lavender placed below the patient's nose, acts to please and calm the patient during the dental procedure. Rubber dam can be useful for holding the cotton wool roll in place.

Lemon oil, with its refreshing properties, may be used in the staff area to keep the team alert! The immune system gains useful stimulation from oils such as tea-tree, cinnamon and thyme. Aromatherapy oils can be used directly as 'disinfectants', for treatment of ulcers and lacerations or in root canals and cavities. The oils are diluted in a carrier oil, depending on the application needed, as the pure oils may irritate.

Some of the conditions treated with aromatherapy oils are listed below:[15]

Abscess: bergamot, lavender
Allergies: camomile, melissa
Anxiety: camomile, jasmine, lavender
Conjunctivitis: lavender, rose (compress)
Fainting: basil, black pepper, camomile
Gingivitis: camomile, myrrh
Glossitis: bergamot, geranium
Halitosis: lavender, peppermint
Herpes: bergamot, eucalyptus
Migraine: basil, eucalyptus, rosemary
Oedema: juniper, patchouli
Otitis: basil, camomile, lavender
Teething: camomile
Throat infections: eucalyptus, geranium
Toothache: camomile, peppermint
Ulcers: bergamot, geranium, juniper

### Music

Music has an important influence on our lives. It can enhance the relaxation of our patients, yet if the wrong type of music is playing it can increase their irritability and anxiety (refer to the Coffea patient in Chapter 1). It is important to reach a consensus between the team and the patients as to which music is chosen to form the background ambience of the practice. Popular classical music of a relaxing nature is the usual choice.

It is often a good idea to invite the patient to bring their own music. This can be played through earphones while they are being treated. The privacy of their own world of music can often be as relaxing to the patient as intravenous sedation. It can also be piped for general listening and provide variety for the rest of the team.

## PACING AND LISTENING

We must be sensitive to the beliefs of our patients and use these beliefs to support their psychological preparation. A useful concept in this area is known as 'pacing'. This means figuratively to get in step with another person. The concept of communication is to share the same language with another person. The dentist and patient need to communicate at all levels, which includes empathy of body language, word and voice. Pacing plays an important role in hypnosis and neuro-linguistic programming. Hypnosis is an important tool in the holistic practice and is covered fully earlier in the book.

Empathic listening is another important concept in good communication and the technique is well covered by Dr Stephen Covey.[16] Aaron Moss[17] discusses many specific applications for using hypnosis, from alleviating bruxism to eliminating the gag reflex.

## STRESS MANAGEMENT

While stress management is well documented as useful to the harmony and health of the practice team, it is also an important consideration in a holistic approach to a patient's health. Prolonged stress can depress the immune system. Dr E.L. Rossi[18] describes the sequence and the mechanism of stress and the mind–gene connection in psycho-immunology. This is based on scientific research and especially the breakthrough work of Kiecolt-Glaser and Glaser[19] in 1991.

When dealing with stress, whether it is the 'impossible person' or a seemingly impossible challenge, Marcia Sutton[20] suggests following the basic management rule, 'either change the stressors, or change your approach'. Dr Sutton also discusses how to gain a holistic control over stress. This includes getting to know and value yourself, diet, exercise and relaxation. She emphasizes the importance of balance between Eu(good) and Dis(harmful) stress.

Dental practices need to come to terms with stress. The team that learns effectively to manage all resources, will not only be successful, but also relaxed and stress-free. Dr Stephen Covey[21] describes the seven habits of highly effective people. These are:

- personal vision;
- being proactive;
- personal management;
- interpersonal management;
- empathic communication;
- creative co-operation;
- balanced self-renewal.

This is good advice towards gaining and maintaining emotional and financial health.

The lifestyle stressors, including emotional, environmental, postural and nutritional stress, need be completely understood to achieve a positive attitude and proactivity that gets results. One of the stresses in our lives, dental disease, can be corrected most often by mechanical therapies. As dentists we have an important role to play in reducing the stress levels of our patients. Holistic practice, with an understanding of lifestyle stresses, will gain successful results more quickly with less relapse.

### LAUGHTER

'A merry heart doeth good like a medicine: but a broken spirit drieth the bones.' – King Solomon, *Proverbs* 17:22

Laughter is important to individual and collective health and therefore a valuable asset to dental practice. Robert Holden,[22] who established the first NHS Laughter Clinic in Great Britain, feels that laughter 'is the best medicine'. He describes one benefit of laughter as its 'internal massage' effect. This creates healthy stimulation as the body is manipulated and exercised, while during the afterglow of mirth, the body becomes relaxed and soothed. His other theories on the benefits of laughter are supported by Dr Robert Willix,[23] who explains that happiness strengthens the immune system, while stress, depression and unhappiness weaken it. Stress generates a flash flood of free radicals. So laugh with your team, laugh with your patients and most of all laugh with yourself.

### The team

A positive staff attitude is essential in running any practice. The team morale and motivation need to be supportive of the practice philosophy. Education is all-important. It is necessary to involve all staff with good in-house communication through combined courses, shared literature and meetings. It is rewarding to see how enthusiastically the staff enjoy the opportunity to be part of holistic health.

Understanding each other's individual needs is fundamental to team morale and enables rapport to develop between the team and the patients. Ron Hubbard[24] describes the balance needed between affinity, reality and communication in order to achieve good understanding.

If the front desk staff are given time, they have the opportunity to communicate the practice philosophy to the patient. The philosophy is then reinforced by the team in the clinical environment. In this way the patient is better informed and is more aware of the practice supporting their health goals.

It is necessary to involve the staff in complementary therapies, both in theory and in practice. Staff should be encouraged to use complementary therapies at home. They should be given the opportunity to experience treatment from the complementary practitioners used by the practice.

This will help the staff to communicate their concepts more clearly to the patient.

It is often the caring way in which the rest of the team supports the patient, that makes the greatest impression. The nurse who holds the patient's hand or places a reassuring arm around the shoulder wins hearts for the practice. Other gestures that are appreciated are a warm towel placed around the patient's neck and a light blanket draped over the patient. This is especially useful during long appointments, where the patient's core temperature may drop more easily than that of the working team.

Clothing is also an important consideration. A consistent theme of dress can help to communicate the team concept to both the patient and the practice. The colour and nature of dress should communicate a comfortable balance between clinical efficiency and a relaxed happy atmosphere.

# The patient

The patient seeking a complementary practitioner is usually well informed. These patients are not easily side-lined by 'science'. They are ready to accept an orthodox solution only if the practitioner can give an opinion based on an overview of both orthodox and natural medicine.

The patient may arrive for a consultation having read or heard of a complementary therapy they feel would benefit their needs. This patient has more than likely been disillusioned with the health care they have received to date. The fact that they come seeking a homoeopathic or hypnosis solution does not imply that they will only settle for such a treatment. By listening to the patient, the practitioner often discovers that their real needs have not been met by previous health advisors. These patients respond well to a caring approach with a well-presented treatment plan. If it can encompass a truly holistic philosophy they will remain happy, loyal and healthy members of your practice.

It is essential to take a comprehensive general and medical history. The occasional patient may ask why a dentist needs to have knowledge of non-dental medical matters. This is a useful opportunity to communicate the philosophy of holistic health on which the practice is based.

The examination, while including teeth charting, radiographs and general examination of hard and soft tissues, should also assess the dental stress the patient is experiencing. Dental stress could include the various materials used in the mouth with their associated allergen,[25] toxic, hormone mimicking,[26] galvanic and ionizing[27] effects. It can also include biomechanical factors such as occlusal imbalances and habits.

It may be necessary to carry out special tests, such as the memory lymphocyte immuno-stimulation assay (MELISA)[28] test for metal sensitivity, the Dentocult saliva test[29] to evaluate patients for caries prognosis or perhaps to refer the patient for further opinions. A network of good complementary and orthodox practitioners for referral purposes is essential to meet the needs of a comprehensive holistic approach. First-hand experience with these practitioners, by the dentist and staff, is useful to improve the confidence and rapport with the patient.

### Referrals

As dentists, we are an important link in the health management business. We are needed by other practitioners, including our medical colleagues. It is up to us to improve our relationship and communicate the areas of useful referral.

There is a growing desire among complementary practitioners to seek out an informed dentist to whom they can refer their patients. The main reason for this growing co-operation is their philosophy of 'wholeness'. They are aware of the influence of dental balance on health.

## Common tools used holistically

### General concepts

In the clinical setting, some of our day-to-day tools lend themselves favourably to the holistic practice. For example, the use of mounted study models is a more holistic approach to orthognathic function than hand-held models. They convey the message of the teeth functioning in relation to the joints.

Using electronic endoguides avoids the over-use of radiographic exposure. Further attention to radiation can be given by ensuring that appropriate filters are fitted to X-ray equipment, that fast X-rays and lead aprons are used and that all associated equipment is kept at maximum efficiency and well maintained. The holistic practitioner should consider using automatic developing, as research indicates that film results are consistently better than manual processing.[30] Computer-assisted radiovisiography can give further benefits in reducing radiographic exposure.

As a more general concept, the use of rubber dam provides for greater patient comfort and protection. Listed below is a selection of conventional instruments that the dentist may use to advantage when running a holistic practice.

### Local anaesthesia

There is a paradox with local anaesthesia in that most patients are scared of needles, yet it is the needle that can deliver pain-free dentistry. Painless injections can gain the practice a wonderful reputation. The holistic practitioner is addressing the psyche by laying old fears to rest and preventing new fears from developing. They owe it to their patients and practice to learn to deliver painless injections.

Many patients do not enjoy the effect of adrenaline that traditionally accompanies local anaesthesia. It can be an additional benefit to patient rapport if the practitioner either identifies these patients or develops the routine of using local anaesthesia without adrenergic vasoconstrictors. Homoeopathic medicines can help to reduce physical and psychological effects of local anaesthetics.

## Intra-oral cameras

The intra-oral camera is an excellent aid in communication. The practitioner has the opportunity to provide far more explicit details of the patient's condition. This leads to greater patient involvement in the decision-making process. It gives the patient more insight into the nature of the treatment, leads to appreciation of the complexity involved and enhances what is termed, in the market place, added value. This leads to greater job satisfaction for the dental team.

## Computers

Computers are becoming a way of life. They can be of major benefit in the modern practice. Their function can range from the simple PC, for word-processing, to a major role in patient treatment. Computerized treatment cards can tie in with the use of intra-oral cameras. They can produce comprehensive treatment plans which are essential for proper patient communication and understanding.

### COMPUTER PROGRAMS

Computer programs are available to help the holistic practice. They can be used to aid homoeopathic constitutional diagnosis and nutritional analysis. Whether such enhanced technical support is substantiated in the general dental practice is a question of operator preference, the size of the practice and patient needs.

While still associated with computer technology, it is useful to mention instruments such as Vega[31] and the 'Listen System' from Biotech. This technology is used to tap into the body's natural 'computer' via acupuncture points.[32] Practitioners use these instruments to diagnose allergies, nutritional deficiencies and body energy status, relating dental ailments to the greater pathophysiological picture. They give guidance as to useful homoeopathic and nutritional needs. They may indicate which restorative materials are best tolerated by the patient. These instruments can be used to detect where possible allergies may be significant in influencing a treatment plan.

They use the concept of energy meridians linking the individual teeth to many other body systems (*Table 10.1*). These relationships are worth bearing in mind when considering a diagnosis based on all the information gathered from your patient. The condition of each tooth, either from abnormal occlusal loading, high amalgam galvanism or an inadequate root treatment, could cause an interruption in the healthy flow of energy along an energy meridian. This would then be expressed as 'dis-ease' in a related organ, which is not associated with teeth in an orthodox sense.

## Laser

Soft and hard laser treatments are proving more popular as various systems are created for the dental office. Surgical lasers are used for cutting and can cause tissue damage, yet they have their therapeutic usefulness. Soft lasers are more gentle and use energy from the visible and invisible end of the light

**Table 10.1 The teeth and the body: energetic inter-relations**

| | | | | | | | | | | | |
|---|---|---|---|---|---|---|---|---|---|---|---|
| **Endocrine glands** | Pituitary gland Anterior lobe | Para-thyroid | Thyroid | Thymus | Pituitary gland | Pineal gland | Pineal gland | Pituitary gland | Thymus | Para-thyroid/Thyroid | Pituitary gland Anterior lobe |
| **Sensory organs** | Ear, Tongue | Tongue | Nose | Nose | Eye | Nose | Nose | Eye | Nose | Nose | Ear, Tongue |
| **Sinuses** | | Maxillary sinus | Ethmoidal cells | Ethmoidal cells | | Sphenoidal sinus, Frontal sinus | | | Ethmoidal cells | Ethmoidal cells | |
| **Vertebrae** | C1 C2 C7 TH1 TH5 TH6 TH7 S1 S2 | C1 C2 TH11 TH12 L1 | C1 C2 C5 C6 C7 TH3 TH4 L4 L5 | C1 C2 C5 C6 C7 TH3 TH4 TH2 L4 L5 | C1 C2 TH8 TH9 TH10 | C1 C2 L2 L3 S3 S4 S5 | C2 C1 L3 L2 S5 S4 S3 | C2 C1 TH8 TH9 TH10 | C2 C1 C7 C6 C5 TH4 TH3 TH2 L4 L5 | C2 C1 C7 C6 TH4 TH3 L5 L4 | C2 C1 C7 TH1 TH7 TH6 TH5 S2 S1 |
| **Organs** | Heart, Duodenum, Jejunum ileum | Spleen, Oesophagus, Stomach | Pancreas, Oesophagus, Stomach | Lung, Large intestine | Liver, Biliary ducts | Kidney, Bladder, Rectum, Anal canal | Kidney, Bladder, Rectum, Anal canal | Liver, Biliary ducts | Lung, Large intestine | Pancreas, Oesophagus, Stomach | Heart, Duodenum, Terminal ileum |
| **Teeth number** | 28  Left | 27 | 26 | 24 25 | 23 | 21 22 | 12 11 | 13 | 15 14 | 17 16 | 18  Right |
| **Teeth number** | 38  Left | 37 | 36 | 34 35 | 33 | 31 32 | 42 41 | 43 | 45 44 | 47 46 | 48  Right |
| **Organs** | Jejunum, Ileum, Heart | Oesophagus, Stomach, Spleen, Pancreas | Large intestine, Lung | Oesophagus, Stomach, Spleen, Pancreas | Liver, Biliary ducts | Rectum, Anal canal, Bladder, Kidney | Rectum, Anal canal, Bladder, Kidney | Liver, Biliary ducts | Oesophagus, Stomach, Spleen, Pancreas | Large intestine, Lung | Terminal ileum, Heart |
| **Vertebrae** | C1 C7 TH1 TH5 TH6 TH7 S1 S2 | C1 C2 TH11 TH12 L1 | C1 C2 C5 C6 C7 TH3 TH4 L4 L5 | C2 C1 TH12 TH11 L1 | C2 C1 L3 L2 S5 S4 S3 | C1 C2 L2 L3 S3 S4 S5 | C1 C2 L2 L3 S3 S4 S5 | C2 C1 TH8–9 TH10 | C2 C1 TH11 TH12 L1 | C1 C2 C5 C6 C7 TH3 TH4 L4 L5 | C1 C7 TH1 TH5 TH6 TH7 S1 S2 |
| **Sinuses** | | Maxillary sinuses | Ethmoid cells | Maxillary sinuses | Sphenoid sinus | Frontal sinus | Frontal sinus | Sphenoid sinus | Maxillary sinuses | Ethmoid cells | |
| **Sensory organs** | Ear, Tongue | Tongue | Nose | Tongue | Eye | Nose | Nose | Eye | Tongue | Nose | Ear, Tongue |
| **Endocrine glands** | | | | | Gonad | Adrenal gland | Adrenal gland | Gonad | | | |

spectrum to stimulate cellular activity, so enhancing the body's reparative and defence mechanisms.

Soft lasers, like many treatments both orthodox and natural, rely on the basic and inert property of living tissue to move in the direction of health, if given the right activation. Soft laser energy can also be used to stimulate acupuncture points and ease trigger point symptoms.

The most popular applications for soft laser treatment in the dental office are for relief of localized pain and stimulation of diseased tissue towards healing.[33] Pain control includes such diverse applications as apical lesions, temporomandibular joint (TMJ) and associated muscles. Lesions that respond well range from intra-oral ulcers to surgical wound healing. Cold sore and herpes lesions respond very well to soft laser treatment.

### COLD SORES

If treated with soft laser in the prodromal phase, experience indicates that the majority of cold sores will resolve before full expression, just as effectively as treatment with Acyclovir. Soft laser has the added benefit of resolving the full-blown lesion faster than its normal healing time, even if therapy is started after onset. Patients appreciate this service and refer others to the practice. Neither of these two solutions will prevent the recurrence of herpes activity, but the appropriate nutritional programme may prevent the cold sores reappearing. The immune support given by nutrition has wide applications in dental health.

### TENS technology

Electrofrequency instruments that use transcutaneous electrical nerve stimulation (TENS)[34] technology can be useful to ease tension headaches, reduce TMJ pain and may be adapted for use as electro-anaesthesia. This is a form of electro-acupuncture and can be put to great advantage in the dental office. For the holistic practitioner it can reduce the need for local anaesthetic, adrenaline and analgesics.

## Holistic tools used in dental practice

In addition to those conventional tools listed above, the holistic dental practitioner should have a wide repertoire of techniques for diagnosis and treatment, that can effectively bring the whole patient to a state of harmonious balance. Some of the techniques available are mentioned below.

### The body computer in diagnosis and therapy

Many believe it is possible to access the 'computer' knowledge of the body, without the aid of outside technology, by using the patient's own 'body computer'. Kinesiology and acupuncture are examples of this concept. Both these modalities are discussed in other chapters. Contact reflex analysis is one development using the muscle-testing concept of kinesiology and acupuncture reflex points.

### Contact reflex analysis

Contact reflex analysis (CRA) is a simple natural method of analysing the body's structural, emotional and nutritional needs using applied kinesiology and knowlege of reflex areas around the body. In dental practice, CRA can be a useful aid to the differential diagnosis, for example, of the sensitive tooth. This is done by 'therapy localizing' the test area, called a 'reflex' area, against a strong muscle. Usually the patient's arm muscle is used. When a healthy reflex is touched, the arm muscle will remain strong. When the reflex is unhealthy, the muscle will weaken and give way.

CRA has been developed over the last 30 years by Dr Versendaal,[35] in conjunction with a clinical nutritionist, a dentist and a haematologist. Its application is diverse, being initially used in nutritional and chiropractic applications and now also in more dental and neuro-emotional applications.

CRA is useful in scanning for possible chiropractic imbalances that may underlie a dental problem. This is particularly helpful in matters relating to the TMJ. It is then possible to refer the patient for further chiropractic assessment, if indicated.

When a typical CRA reflex is weak, it indicates that the body is working hard to correct an imbalance underlying a disease. Treatment can be given mechanically or the reflex may indicate that tissue breakdown needs nutritional support to aid healing. The following case history demonstrates one area in which CRA can play a useful role.

CASE HISTORY

*Gillian, a 56-year-old patient, presented for an emergency consultation. Although a patient of the practice, she had not made a visit for 12 months. Her symptoms were of background discomfort in the lower right posterior quadrant, with acute unbearable temperature sensitivity of the first molar, particularly to cold. Radiographic and clinical examination of the teeth in the affected quadrant were non-contributory. Gillian could not even bear the air drying to check the occlusal contacts and almost rose to the ceiling with each blast of air. There was a small burnish mark on the amalgam restoration of the first molar and this was confirmed by the articulation paper as an occlusal contact. Bearing in mind that she had not had any dentistry done in over a year, this was a little perplexing. It could be an incipient cusp fracture. A CRA test was used. This revealed that the premature contact on the molar was the result of a neck vertebral misalignment. On further questioning, Gillian did remember bumping her head in her garden shed and noticed a little stiffness in her neck on waking in the ensuing week, but really did not connect this with her toothache. Her neck was then adjusted and rechecked with CRA. Her tooth was then checked, after she had been asked to swallow and make tooth contact in her usual way. The interesting observation is that she did not flinch when the tooth was dried by the air syringe. She confirmed that the sensitivity had gone, except for a very slight awareness only. On follow-up, she confirmed that all was well provided she kept up her neck exercises. At no time was a drill used to solve this patient's premature contact. All that was needed was to restore her skeletal alignment and CRA proved an invaluable tool.*

When a practitioner is comfortable with the use of CRA, it becomes a daily indispensable aid to the holistic practice. As with all techniques used for our patients, it is essential that correct and adequate training is achieved

## Body reference maps

Muscle and joint function should be assessed as part of the general dental examination. The range of mandibular movement, joint discomfort and noises should be recorded. The relationship of the occlusal plane to the other facial planes and facial asymmetries, such as nose alignment and lip shape, are taken into account.

A grid map on a wall or door can be very useful to assess postural balance. With the patient first standing against the grid, an assessment of eye, ear, occlussal and shoulder levels can be recorded. Any tendency to be leaning to right or left is also noted. Then the patient can stand at right angles to the grid. This will give a quick record of profile posture.

Posture can have a fundamental bearing on the outcome of any treatment plan. Liaison with a practitioner using the Alexander technique[36] and a basic understanding of the influence of posture on neurological patterns and facial development will be very helpful to the holistic dentist.

This information is noted together with clinical history-taking. If findings suggest major balance and functional discrepancies (e.g. restricted jaw opening with highly toned muscles, facial plane malalignment, neck or back pain), then it is advisable to refer the patient for a Sacro-Occipital Technique (SOT) or cranial assessment, before any definitive dental restorative programme is initiated. The final occlusal plane should act as a 'keystone' to the body's equilibrium. Working with cranial osteopathy has immediate benefits for the holistic health plan of the modern dental practice.

# Holistic treatment

Below are some treatments that a holistic dental practice may provide for its patients. Some of the treatments will be unique, whereas others are conventional but with a different approach.

## TMJ, migraine and other head pains

General dental practitioners, such as Gelb and Siegel,[37] Smith[38] and Fonder,[39] have been early pioneers of the important role of dentistry in holistic health. They related dental imbalances to many pain symptoms of the head, neck and shoulders. They realized the importance of cranial balance and the role played by chiropractors, cranial osteopaths and dentists in reducing suffering caused by head pain. They also emphasized the importance of diet, exercise and relaxation.

Lamey et al.[40] showed that a simple TMJ-occlusal appliance can reduce migraine symptoms. The occlusal splint has become a primary tool in diagnosis and treatment of TMJ conditions. This is traditionally a removable appliance. Where major restorative changes are planned, it is sometimes easier for the patient to have the teeth built up with composite. This is a reversible and modifiable alternative to the removable acrylic splint. As it is tedious to remove the composite from teeth, the direct composite build-up alternative is better used when major restorative treatment is being considered as part of the future treatment plan. The patient must be part of the decision-making in all options of the treatment plan.

To determine the amount of occlusal opening, the practitioner can use several techniques. These range from several millimetres on empirical grounds, to using a leaf gauge between the anterior teeth to establish minimum thickness needed to 'decompress' the tissues in the TMJs. Using cranial motion, chiropractic assessments and CRA would greatly assist in assessing and achieving a good initial positioning.

It is important to give the patient advice on exercise routines, nutrition, sleeping positions, relaxation and massage to assist with the healing. Reassurance is an invaluable tool. Each patient will need a programme tailored to their individual needs. A general exercise that is attainable by most is regular walking. This needs to be brisk to achieve good aerobic levels, which will mean at least 20–30 minutes, 5 times per week.

**Orthodontics**

The holistic dentist uses orthodontic therapy to support the balance of natural function and aesthetics. The outcome of stability at the end of orthodontic treatment is best achieved by a healthy TMJ, good occlusion, a balanced cranial complex and optimum airway function. This creates facial symmetry that gives full lip support and keeps the nose from dominating the facial profile that is so often associated with the classic premolar extraction case. The trend is therefore away from extraction solutions and towards an expansion philosophy for most cases of orthodontic crowding. In addition to lateral cephalometric radiographs and study models, we should be looking to the craniofacial balance and soft-tissue form as a primary guide to orthodontic need, treatment and outcome.

Should hand-held study models be analysed, it is easy to be misled when deciding how to manage an increased overjet. It is unstable to procline lower incisors. So a common solution is to remove teeth and retract the upper anterior segment. This jams the cranium, compromises cranial movement and restricts the flow of cranial fluid. It will also move the mandible into a more distal functioning position. This potentiates TMJ instability and leads to distortion of the natural facial profile by accentuating the nose size. With the models mounted on a functional articulator, it is much easier to demonstrate that once the arches are aligned, the lower jaw can move forward into a natural relationship with the upper and reduce the overjet. Provided this treatment is done early enough, growth in the mandible will allow the condyle to achieve a physiological stable position in the glenoid fossa and the teeth to settle at the correct vertical occlusal relationship.

A good example where early intervention can benefit both orthodontic and TMJ outcome, is the use of deciduous molar build-ups. This is usually prescribed for children with early signs of class II facial profiles. These cases are classically over-closed and usually have an increased over-jet and over-bite. Other symptoms are recurrent otitis media and glue-ear complications. The latter symptoms often clear spontaneously after the molar build-ups. The build-ups are usually placed on the deciduous first and second molars. A guide plane is often built into this procedure to stimulate anterior positioning of the mandible. This allows the permanent teeth to erupt into a new and correct vertical and horizontal position, while the mandible is stimulated to grow into a better craniofacial relationship.

In the holistic model, good orthodontic treatment can do much to enhance the individual's quality of life and increase the patient's physiological capacity to accommodate disease without discomfort.

## Homoeopathy

Homoeopathy in dentistry is covered in more detail in Chapter 1. In general practice each dentist will tend to use their favourite selection of homoeopathic medicines. The following are commonly used in our practice.

*Arnica* is the best known of all the homoeopathic medicines, and perhaps the most useful in dentistry. *Arnica* given before and after a traumatic procedure, such as surgery or even an extended appointment where the patient has had their mouth open for a long time, can greatly reduce postoperative discomfort and promote healing.

After invasive procedures of the soft tissues or in cases of intra-oral abrasions or ulcers, mother tinctures of *Calendula* or *Propolis* are useful as a healing and soothing mouth wash. *Phosphorus* is useful to control haemorrhage, when there is a lot of bright red blood. *Calendula cream* is both lubricating and healing for dry or sore lips, and the patient always appreciates the consideration.

*Hepar sulph* is often considered to be homoeopathy's antibiotic. It is useful in treating the infected deciduous dentition, especially when children's co-operation is not easily won. Antibiotic use would not be in the patient's long-term interest. Yet if the body's own resources can be stimulated to live more comfortably with a diseased primary tooth, time can be won until co-operation can allow better remedial treatment. Antibiotics should be limited to rare or life-threatening situations and not used as a convenience tool.

*Chamomilla* is useful for teething pain in children and sometimes for teeth that are painful or sensitive after extensive dental work.

For an acute tooth abscess, which is swollen and throbbing, try *Belladonna*. When an abscess has started to drain, then *Silica* is recommended to assist in the drainage process. *Silica* is also useful to promote a splinter of bone or tooth to be brought to the surface.

*Homoeopathic mercury* used after extensive removal of old amalgam fillings helps the body to neutralize the toxic effect of the mercury. In a similar way, *Homoeopathic anaesthetic* mix can reduce the unpleasant effects some patients experience after local anaesthetic.

Excellent courses are run at the various homoeopathic hospitals, co-ordinated by the British Homoeopathic Dental Association. This is an essential basis for introducing homoeopathy into the dental practice.

## Mercury testing and removal

Mercury – to use or not to use? This is an important question for the holistic practice. There has been much controversy over the use of mercury amalgam restorations. It was a useful material when introduced to dentistry. It still has advantages as a restorative material, but its well-published disadvantage is its toxicity (see Chapter 7). Apart from the added responsibility of handling the raw material, before and after use,[41-43] there are issues of environmental and patient health.

When mercury was introduced to dentistry, there was little public awareness of environmental impact. Lead piping was used extensively in domestic plumbing. The impact of lead, as a heavy metal toxin, resulted in the phasing out of lead pipes in domestic plumbing over recent decades. It would appear that this was not done for any proven list of specific pathophysiological ailments, but more because of its perceived and potential risk and the availability of less toxic alternatives. Mercury in dentistry may well follow this model.

The release of mercury vapour is best tested by the use of appropriate instrumentation, such as the Jerome mercury vapour analyser, supplied by Able Instruments.[44] Galvanometer readings are useful to give an indication of the electrolytic status of the restoration. The galvanic status gives an indication of the corrosive nature of the material in the mouth. The mouth is lubricated by saliva which is an excellent electrolytic medium. It is an excellent conductor between the various metals of the dental restorations plus the metals of orthodontic and prosthetic appliances. The higher the corrosive index of the mercury amalgam restoration, the more of its contents are released into the mouth. Fillings can be removed in sequence according to this reading, from the highest to the lowest negative, then from the highest to the lowest positive.

The electrical current may in itself have an effect on human physiology, the dimension of which is still outside our present knowledge. Nerve conduction is measured in nano-amps, while the currents generated by metals in the mouth are measured in micro-amps (a thousand-fold increase). It is not difficult to understand how these currents may interfere with the body's physiology and acupuncture meridians.

Mercury released from amalgam fillings is implicated in patient sensitivity, neural toxicity and bacterial resistance.[45] Further details on this subject can be found in Chapter 7. It is important to have a balanced, pragmatic view on this issue. While there is heated debate on both sides, it is undeniable that the arguments about environmental factors and the need to reduce patient load to heavy metal exposure are ethically persuasive. It is well known that the degree of sensitivity to mercury varies widely from highly reactive to apparent indifference. Tests, such as MELISA, will help us ascertain the degree of individual sensitivity more accurately in the future.[46]

When choosing to remove mercury restorations, the patient must be well informed. There are personal, environmental, ethical and medico-legal considerations. The legal issue is comprehensively covered in Dental Protection's risk management pack on dental amalgams.[47]

The criteria range from obvious clinical signs and symptoms to the more controversial considerations such as sensitivity, aesthetics and psycho-emotional aspects. It is important, as in all areas of clinical practice, to keep excellent records of the criteria supporting such decisions. Clinical photography[48] and radiological records are very useful. Other records should include patients' comments, as well as practitioner rationale for the decision.

When removing mercury fillings, it is important to protect both the patient and the operating team. This protection should cover not only the actual removal but also the preparation before and the support after removal.

During the removal procedure, the patient should be protected by rubber dam, high-velocity suction and preferably a source of clean air. The operating team should wear disposable protective clothing and either wear special mercury-filtering face masks or have a separate source of clean air. For general protection, the room needs good ventilation, and a heavy metal air filtering system would be good practice.

The patient should be given nutritional advice and support before and after mercury removal. The operating team needs to be on a continuous anti-oxidant nutritional supplement regimen. Hal Huggins,[49] one of the early campaigners for mercury-free dentistry, gives more information in his book *It's All in Your Head*.

The majority of patients would expect the holistic practice to be mercury free. This is not unreasonable, as one would expect the health-conscious practitioner to be considering all aspects of health enhancement. This includes supporting healthy processes as well as reducing the zenobiotic exposure of the patient. This is especially relevant in the context of drugs and materials used by the practice. All materials used in contemporary restorative practice have varying degrees of disagreeable effects on human physiology. It is for this reason that care must be taken in the selection of materials used for each individual. The ideal is to preserve the body's own structure, to which end dentistry has contributed much through prevention. Work is being done to develop ways of generating natural dentine to restore damaged teeth. This will be a wonderful tool in the holistic practice of the future.

## Periodontal health: theories and therapies

Today we can say, with reasonable confidence, that most acute and chronic dental diseases are under our direct control. This is an easy concept for the modern dental practitioner to accept. He knows the powerful effect of prevention. While the reduction in sugar is of well-documented benefit to oral and general health, it is hoped that a broader knowledge of nutrition will widen the dietary advice. This is in total contrast to accepted dogma of the past, when it was thought that tooth decay and gum disease were an inevitable burden of ageing.

What of those intractable periodontal patients who do not respond to 'normal' therapies? In contrast there is the question of patients with poor oral hygiene yet little evidence of disease. The holistic dentist should look at periodontal disease with a broader view than just plaque and antibiotics.

There are many questions that arise from the literature on periodontal health. For example, why, with so much research on the bacterial theory of periodontal disease, are so many bacteria implicated? Each new paper seems to discover a new microbial combination, often accompanied by suggestions of drug therapy, over and above the usual oral hygiene protocol. The periodontal and oral medicine journals have hundreds of such references. A recent example is a paper presented by Haffajee *et al.*[50], in the *Journal of Clinical Periodontology*.

Another question is, Why do some patients present with very poor oral hygiene, but with little sign of corresponding periodontal disease? Professor A. Sheiham[51,52] has been vocal in the area of education. His research drew our attention to the epidemiological findings that poor oral hygiene does not correlate directly to periodontal disease. He drew attention to many of the factors that influence oral health, which include general health, stress, degrees of dysfunction, perception and attitude.[53]

Pasteur, accredited as the father of the microbial era, is noted for this observation on his deathbed: 'Bernard was right. The germ is nothing, the soil is everything.' This fundamental consideration is embraced in the philosophy of holistic health, whereas it is given little credit in the orthodox circles where it originated. By supporting the health of the individual holistically, the immune system is our most effective challenge to diseases of all kinds, including infection.

The story behind the birth of the germ theory and its dramatic effect on subsequent generations of scientific thought, makes for interesting reading. Dr Robert Cass[54] describes it as 'the road not taken'. In the 1870s the silk industry in France was nearly destroyed by a disease that attacked the developing silkworm. Louis Pasteur was called upon to stop the disease that he discovered was caused by a protozoan. He demonstrated that the disease could be controlled by eliminating the microbe from the silkworm nurseries.

However, Pasteur also noticed that it was not just the presence of the germ but also the physiological state of the silkworm that determined the susceptibility to infection. While his later studies with anthrax and rabies still reflected his focus on the agents of disease, he noted: 'If I were to undertake new studies on the silkworm disease, I would concern myself with the ways of increasing their general vigour. I am convinced that it would be possible to discover techniques for giving worms a higher level of robustness and thereby rendering them resistant to infection.'

In addition to his interest in the causative role of micro-organisms in disease, he was also aware of the importance of what he called the 'terrain' – the environmental factors that determined susceptibility and resistance to disease. In fact, Pasteur and his colleague and contemporary, Claude Bernard, long debated whether the disease producer, the microbe, or the body's equilibrium were more important. Pasteur sometimes reflected that 'the road not taken' may have been more beneficial and that the body's biochemical, physical and emotional state profoundly affects the course and outcome of infectious disease.

It may just have been that this period of research came at a time when superstition accredited disease to devils and demons, so to take on the 'devil–demon–germ' concept was more acceptable to contemporary thought. It is such a pity that we are still so wedded to such ideas, in what should be a more informed and scientific era.

When reviewing the periodontally diseased patient, the holistic dentist will consider the patient's general health, i.e. the patient's 'terrain', as a possible important contributing factor. They will consider nutrition and if necessary will do a dietary analysis or take the patient through the basic diet experiment. They will consider stress. Not just occlusal stress, but emotional and biochemical stress. All the influences that affect the immune system must be considered. While considering these aspects, they will also support the practice of optimum oral hygiene and high-quality restorations.

## Antibiotics

In 1994, Professor H. D. Edmonson[55] reviewed antibiotic prescribing in dental practices. He reported that over 3.2 million courses of antibiotics were prescribed by dental practitioners in England. A Scottish paper confirms that the average dentist prescribes 7 courses of antibiotics per week.[56] Details of the antimicrobials prescribed was reviewed by Lewis et al.[57] in 1989. The lay press has been concerned over growing antibiotic resistance.[58] The professional press has discussed both the opportunist invasion after antibiotic treatment, as well as antibiotic-associated colitis.[59] Little consideration is given in the majority of medical and dental practices to the effect of these antibiotics on the body's probiotic (body-friendly microbes) status. Dysbiosis (pathological imbalance in body-friendly microbes) can have far reaching health effects,[60] with the most well known to dentists being the glossitis and stomatitis associated with Candida albicans overgrowth.

Other factors play a part in the state of the body's probiotic status. These include dietary components, such as fructo-oligosaccharides (FOS) and other forms of soluble and insoluble fibre,[61] general health, pH balance at the different levels of the digestive tract and, of course, antibiotic abuses. A child born to a dysbiotic mother, even if tenderly nurtured and breast fed, is likely to start life without inheriting a probiotic inoculation. Many children are deprived in this way of an important aspect of immune defence. This can further predispose these children to oral-gastrointestinal dysfunction without having received antibiotic treatment themselves. The chances are probably in favour of them also receiving antibiotic treatment early in life. This subject has received much more attention in veterinary circles and would benefit greatly from more research in orthodox medicine. There is little reference to this problem in the medical literature. Although Walker et al.[62] discussed the drug-related superinfections in hospitalized patients in 1979, it was the Russians that devoted an entire conference to the problems of antibiotics and dysbiosis in 1987.[63]

The question the holistic practitioner asks when faced with an infection-associated challenge is; 'Has the individual sufficient immune capability to clear the challenge naturally or is there a gentle support option that can be recommended?' Such options could include a homoeopathic medicine or, where appropriate, a topical treatment such as propolis liquid. Very often just reassurance is all that is needed.

Our experience, running a holistic practice, is that fewer than a dozen courses of antibiotics need be prescribed during a full year. It is then essential to follow such prescriptions with a course of probiotic inoculate and gastrointestinal rehabilitation nutrition.

## Nutrition

It is easier to grasp the fundamentals of good nutrition when one has a better understanding of the evolution of human physiology. Homo sapiens was a hunter-gatherer until communities developed around settled agriculture some 10 000 years ago.[64] As settled communities we learnt to control food production and cook more food. In evolutionary terms our physiology is still best handling uncooked food, with a variety to supply adequate and complex nutritional needs.[65,66] Bieler[67] in his book describes Pottenger's experiments with cats. Pottenger suggests that it is unhealthy to consume cooked animal protein. In his animal study on cats, the group on the raw protein diet thrived over a 5-year period, whereas those on cooked protein became sick and developed diseases similar to those seen in human beings, including periodontal disease and loss of teeth.

The holistic dentist is concerned with a diet that will enhance normal dental arch development. The development of malocclusion is still hotly debated and probably has many causes. There is little doubt that the diet plays a major role. Those people living on less refined diets in more rural, non-deprived parts of the world, consistently suffer fewer malocclusions. Malalignment of the dental arches is the exception rather than the rule. Evidence also suggests that the hunter-gatherer suffered generally fewer diseases and attained better average heights than agricultural communities, with the exception of the wealthy Western nations.[64]

Present-day farming methods have impoverished the soil. Therefore the food harvested lacks the needed wholesomeness.[68] Organic farming is trying to redress this issue. Vitamin and mineral supplements have an important role to play therapeutically when the individual needs nutritional 'catching up'. They are also useful as additives to modern impoverished foods.

To use supplements therapeutically, the practitioner needs to assess the patient thoroughly. Apart from history-taking, CRA can be used to confirm nutritional needs. There are also many excellent functional tests, such as the 'liver challenge test', available from appropriately equipped laboratories, such as BioLab[69] and Great Smokies Diagnostic Laboratory.[70]

Water is also a much neglected nutritional component. While Dr H. G. Bieler[67] and Dr F. Batmanghelidj[71] differ in how we should offer water to our bodies, they both demonstrate how beneficial the health-restoring powers of proper hydration is to all aspects of health.

In general terms, we should advocate more water and raw, unprocessed organic food in our diets. It is also good practice to avoid zenobiotics (biological toxins), whether these are in the form of environmental toxins, a habit (e.g. smoking), food preservatives, drugs we prescribe or the restorative materials we use in our patients' mouths.

## Massage

Massage, with direct hand application, can be useful to alleviate stiffness and pain associated with TMJ or postoperative swelling, through enhancing circulation as well as the 'hands-on' emotional benefit. This last benefit can also be subtly communicated by the gentle hand on the shoulder technique, which is registered as a gesture of comfort by the majority of patients. Patient reassurance is one of the strongest tools of health care and very often, together with good hygiene, rest and time, the body will recover on its own resources.

Various portable massage 'machines' are available for those who wish to bring more technology into this area. These can be useful for the stiff neck or back, which are regions where many dentists feel a little intimidated to venture with a direct hands-on approach. This can be very useful and well appreciated by the patient after a long gruelling appointment. Massage can be good therapy for the patient and the dental team.

## Financial aspects

'God cures and the doctors send the bill' – Mark Twain.

### Fee structure

With the wider knowledge of natural medicine, we now have many more techniques to use. However, these techniques take time to learn and create financial burdens. Setting up a holistic practice can be expensive. One of the realities of day-to-day practice life is money. Dental fees are traditionally structured on a 'fee for item' basis. Some systems are based of an hourly rate, usually with a time-complexity element included, while capitation schemes are receiving greater popularity. Whichever system is used, the fee level will have to reflect the true cost of the service provided.

The fees will need to be reviewed when additional services and any other practice enhancements are made. This can be done by adjusting all fees accordingly or by adding items such as a nutritional assessment consultation to the fee scale. On the other hand, enhancements to the practice may attract new patients and being busier may reduce the need for direct fee increases. Each practitioner needs to consider his individual personal and patient needs. The holistic practitioner should be prepared to increase fees rather than reduce time with the patient. It is important to be confident of the service provided. Patients pay for outcome and comfort. Team confidence is an essential element of both.[72] Changes must always be made to the ultimate benefit of the patient.

For a new or growing practice, referrals can be an important financial consideration. The cost of new equipment, postgraduate education and learning new therapies has important financial implications. This must be met through patient fees.

### Time management

The modern patient often rejects the impersonal way they are 'time managed' under orthodox dental and medical care. This applies to general practice as well as hospital treatments. Most complementary therapies, by their nature, need longer contact with the patient. This enhances their added value for the person seeking caring health attention.

To provide the time with patients for delivering a complementary health service, and meeting the need for patients to feel unhurried, requires discipline. We have been trained to be 'efficient' with time management, but if not careful this may mean less time given to the patient. To be financially successful we need to run an efficient practice that provides time for the patient. We need to charge sensibly for that time.

## Medico-legal aspects of the complementary therapies in dentistry

Complementary therapies are no different medico-legally from other therapies that a dentist may use. Dentists must ensure that they are appropriately trained in any treatment area that they choose to provide. When groups of practitioners come together and form societies with special interests in common, it is not unusual for them to form protocols that become the benchmark for practice within that field.

Certain complementary therapies have little scientific support; therefore, practitioners working in these areas may be more vulnerable to complaints. The benchmark protocols are an important baseline from which to make decisions. The principles of risk management should apply. We are advised to keep comprehensive records, including investigations, diagnosis, treatment and discussions with the patient. Positive and negative findings should be recorded and patients should always be advised of the various alternatives of treatment available.

Well-documented records, perhaps with photographs, can be useful when writing articles for professional journals. It is these contributions that eventually lead to increasing general interest, wider research and readier acceptance of therapies in day-to-day practice.

The standard that is used in the UK is that of the Bolam test,[47] which is based on what a reasonable body of opinion would consider to be appropriate. It is therefore important to become members of recognized societies in the areas of complementary medicine that you include in your practice. The British Homoeopathic Dental Association (BHDA) and the British Dental Acupuncture Society (BDAS) are good examples. It would be useful to discuss any areas of concern with your protection society and colleagues who share your special interest.

### Conclusion

There are many useful therapies for the holistic dentist. Armed with the philosophy of natural medicine, practitioners can develop the therapies that complement their individual personalities and those of the patients they serve.

Whether we practise orthodox or natural medicine, we ultimately rely on the philosophy of holistic healing that depends on the individual's psychophysiology to do the work. We must do our utmost to support a healthy balance in our patients and prevent their equilibrium shifting too far from the centre. For this we can only use the therapies we have learnt, making sure they support rather than detract from the laws of natural healing.

I have given an overview of a practice that utilizes the therapies and concepts of natural medicine alongside orthodox dentistry. Most of the discussion has been based on practical experience. Mention has been made of tools that I have used and explored. Education, application, observation and continual evaluation are the only ways to develop professionally.

Armed with these tools we can make a meaningful contribution to the well-being of our patients, so that they feel happy and above all – **healthy**!

# References

1 Dripps R D, Eckenhoff J E, Vandam L D. *Introduction to Anaesthetics*, p 110. Philadelphia: W B Saunders Co, 1967.

2 Lee R, Hanson W A. *Protomorphology*. Milwaukee: Lee Foundation for Nutritional Research, 1947.

3 *Butterworths Medical Dictionary*. Macdonald Critchley (ed). London: Butterworths, 1990.

4 *Cassell's German Dictionary*. Betteridge H T (ed). London: Cassell Publishers, 1988

5 Erasmus U. *Fats that Heal, Fats that Kill*, p 416. Burnaby, Canada: Alive Books, 1995.

6 Vithoulkas G. *A New Model of Health and Disease*, pp 42–61. Mill Valley, Ca: Health and Habitat, 1991.

7 Gaarder J. *Sophie's World*, p 90. London: Orion Books, 1995.

8 Olsen K. *Alternative Health Care*. London: Judy Piatkus (Publishers), 1989.

9 Rossi E L. *The Psychobiology of Mind–Body Healing*. New York: W W Norton & Co, 1988.

10 Evans F. Expectancy, therapeutic instructions and the placebo response. *In* White L, Tursky B, Schwartz G (eds). *Placebo: Theory, Research and Mechanism*, pp 215–228. New York: Guilford Press, 1985.

11 Hunt R. *The Seven Keys to Colour Healing*. San Francisco: Harper & Row, 1982.

12 Moore C. Editorial. *Homoeopathy Int* 1996; **10(2)**: 5.

13 Holbeche S. *The Power of Gems and Crystals*. London: Judy Piatkus Publishers, 1989.

14 Worwood V A. *Aromantics*. London: Pan Books, 1987.

15 Tisserand R. *The Art of Aromatherapy*. Saffron Walden: C W Daniel Company, 1989.

16 Covey S R. *The Seven Habits of Highly Effective People*, pp 239–243. New York: Simon & Schuster, 1990.

17 Moss A A. Hypnodontics: hypnosis in dentistry. *In* Kroger W S (ed). *Experimental Hypnosis*, pp 321–334. Philadelphia: Lippincott Company, 1977.

18 Rossi E L. *The Psychobiology of Mind Body Healing*, revised edn., pp 229–237. New York: W W Norton & Co, 1993.

19 Kiecolt-Glaser J, Glaser R. Stress and immune function in humans. *In* Ader R, Felten D Cohen N (eds). *Psychoneuroimmunology*, 2nd edn., pp 849–868. San Diego: Academic Press, 1991.

20 Sutton M. *In Control – Power over Stress*. Albuquerque: Cooper Press, 1988.

21 Covey S R. *The Seven Habits of Highly Effective People*. New York: Simon & Schuster, 1990.

22 Holden R. *Laughter, the Best Medicine*. London: Harper Collins, 1993.

23 Willix R D. *You Can Feel Good All The Time*. London: Fleet Street Publications, 1994.

24 Hubbard L R. *The Components of Understanding*. Los Angeles: Bridge Publications, 1994.

25 Mjor I A. Problems and benefits associated with restorative materials: side-effects and long-term cost. [Review] *Adv Dent Res* 1992; **6**: 7–16.

26 Olea N, Pulgar R, Perez P *et al*. Estrogenicity of resin-based composites and sealants used in dentistry. *Environ Hlth Perspectives* 1996; **104**: 298–305.

27 Beague T P. Galvanic corrosion of Class II amalgam restorations in contact with orthodontic brackets/bands. *N Y State Dent J* 1992; **58(9)**: 48–49.

28 *Equivalent Test: Metal Specific Memory T-cell Test*. London: Charing Cross Hospital.

29 Crossner C G. Salivary lactobacillus counts in the prediction of caries activity. *Comm Dent Oral Epidemiol* 1981; **9**: 182–190.

30 Rout P G J, Rogers S N, Chapman M *et al*. A comparison of manual and automatic processing in general dental practice. *Br Dent J* 1996; **181(3)**: 99–101.

31 *Vega News*. Noma (Complex Homoe0pathy) Ltd, Unit 3, 1–16 Hollybrook Road, Upper Shirley, Southampton SO16 6RB.

32  Zoll S J. *The Bridge Between Accupunture and Modern Bio-Energetic Medicine.* Heidelberg: Kael F Haug Verlag, 1992.

33  Woolley-Hart A A. *Handbook for Low Power LASERS and their Medical Application.* London: East Asia Co, 1988.

34  Holt C R, Finney J W, Wall C L. The use of transcutaneous electrical nerve stimulation (TENS) in the treatment of facial pain. *Singapore: Ann Acad Med* 1995; **24(1):** 17–22.

35  Versendaal D A. *Contact Reflex Analysis and Designed Clinical Nutrition.* Jenison, MI: Hoezee Marketing, 1993.

36  Dollerup Fjordbo G. *On the Development of Habit - From the Viewpoint of the Alexander Technique and the Early Neuromotor Patterns of Development.* Denmark: Dollerup F G, 1993.

37  Gelb H, Siegel P. *Killing Pain Without Prescription.* New York: Harper & Row Publishers, 1980.

38  Smith G H. *Headaches Aren't Forever!* Newtown, PA: International Centre for Nutritional Research, 1986.

39  Fonder A C. The dental distress syndrome qualified. *Basal Facts,* 1987: **9**: 4.

40  Lamey P J, Steele J G, Aitchison T. Migraine: the effect of acrylic appliance design on clinical response. *Br Dent J* 1996; **180**: 4.

41  Control of Substances Hazardous to Health (COSHH), 1988. 'A Step by Step Guide to COSHH Assessment' HS(G) 97. 'EH 40/94 Occupational Exposure Limits 1994' HSE Books and Publications, P.O. Box 1999, Sudbury, Suffolk CO10 6FS.

42  British Dental Association. *Health and Safety Law for Dental Practice.* Advice Sheet A3. London: British Dental Association, 1993.

43  American Dental Association. Dental mercury hygiene. *J Am Dent Assoc* 1991; **122**: 112.

44  Able Instruments & Controls Ltd, Cutbush Park, Dane Hill, Lower Earley, Reading, Berkshire. RG6 4UT. Tel: 01734 311 188.

45  Lorscheider F L, Vimy M J. The dental amalgam mercury controversy – inorganic mercury and the CNS; genetic linkage of mercury and antibiotic resistances in intestinal bacteria. *Toxicology* 1995; **97:**19–22.

46  Stejskal V D M, Cederbrant K, Lindvall A *et al.* MELISA – an in vitro tool for the study of metal allergy. *Toxic in Vitro* 1994; **8(5):** 991–1000.

47  Dental Protection Ltd. The Safety of Amalgam Restoration. Division of Medical Protection Society, 50 Hallam Street, London W1N 6DE.

48  Wander P, Gordon P. *Dental Photography.* London: British Dental Association, 1987.

49  Huggins H A. *It's All in Your Head.* New York: Avery Publishing Group, 1993.

50  Haffajee A D, Socransky S S, Dibart S *et al.* Response to periodontal therapy in patients with high or low levels of *P.gingivalis, P.intermedia, P.nigrescens* and *B.forsythus. J Clin Periodont* 1996; **23**: 336–345.

51  Sheiham A, Croucher R. Current perspectives on improving chairside dental health education for adults. *Int Dent J* 1994; **44**: 202–206.

52  Sheiham A. A challenge for change in dental education. London: *BDA News,* April 1996: 9.

53  Sheiham A, Maizels J E, Cushings A M. The concept of need in dental care. *Int. Dent J* 1982; **32(3):** 265–270.

54  Cass R. *The Physician's Clinical Reference Manual.* 7th edn., p 12. Washington: Dr Cass, 1994.

55  Edmonson H D. Dental prescribing. *Dental Update,* **21(8):** 332–334.

56  Stephens I F D, Binnie V I, Kinane D F. Dentists, pills and pregnancies. *Br Dent J* 1996; **181(7):** 236–239.

57  Lewis M A O, Meechan C, MacFarlane T W *et al.* Presentation and antimicrobial treatment of acute orofacial infections in general dental practice. *Br Dent J* 1989; **166**: 41.

58  Begley S. Antibiotics – the end of miracle drugs? *News Week.* March 28,1994; **CXXIII(13):** 38–44.

59  Committee on Safety of Medicine. Adverse Drug Reaction Reporting Scheme. Antibiotic-associated Colitis. London: Medicines Control Agency, May 1994; **20**.

60  Chaitow L, Trenev N. *Probiotics.* London: Thorsons-Harper Collins, 1990.

61 Martin S. Intestinal permeability (leaky gut syndrome) A natural approach. *BioMed.* Newsletter May 1995; **11**.
62 Walker A M, Jick H, Porter J. Drug-related superinfection in hospitalized patients. *J Am Med Assoc* 1979; **242(12):** 1273–1275.
63 All-Union seminar devoted to the problems of antibiotics and dysbiosis. (Russian trans). *Antibiotiki I Meditsinskaia Biotekhnologiia*, 1987; **32:3**:163–235.
64 Diamond J. *The Rise and Fall of the Third Chimpanzee.* Reading: Cox & Wyman, 1991.
65 Kenton L, Kenton S. *Raw Energy.* Reading: Cox & Wyman, 1984.
66 Howell E. *Enzyme Nutrition.* New Jersey: Avery Publishing Group, 1981.
67 Bieler H G. *Food is Your Best Medicine.* New York: Ballantine Books, 1984.
68 Nichols J D. A concept of totality. *Nat Food Farm* 1992; **51:** 27–30.
69 BioLab, 9 Weymouth Street, London W1N 3FF. Tel: 0171 636 5959.
70 Great Smokies Diagnostic Laboratory. Health Interlink Ltd, Interlink House, Belswains Lane, Hemel Hempstead, Herts HP3 9HP. Tel: 01442 61333.
71 Batmanghelidj F. *Your Body's Many Cries for Water.* Falls Church, Virginia: Global Health Solutions, 1995.
72 Robbins A. *Awaken the Giant Within,* p 378. New York: Fireside, 1992.

# Bibliography

Batmanghelidj F. *Your Body's Many Cries for Water.* Falls Church, Virginia: Global Health Solutions, 1995.
Bieler H G. *Food is Your Best Medicine.* New York: Ballantine Books, 1984.
Covey S R. *The Seven Habits of Highly Effective People.* New York: Simon & Schuster, 1990.
Diamond J. *The Rise and Fall of the Third Chimpanzee.* Reading: Cox & Wyman, 1991.
Erasmus U. *Fats that Heal, Fats that Kill.* Burnaby, Canada: Alive Books, 1995.
Gaarder J. *Sophie's World.* London: Orion Books, 1995.
Gelb H, Siegel P. *Killing Pain Without Prescription.* New York: Harper & Row Publishers, 1980.
Holden R. *Laughter, the Best Medicine.* London: Harper Collins, 1993.
Howell E. *Enzyme Nutrition.* New Jersey: Avery Publishing Group, 1981.
Kenton L, Kenton S. *Raw Energy.* Reading: Cox & Wyman, 1984.
McTaggart L. *What Doctors Don't Tell You.* London: Harper Collins, 1996.
Olsen K. *Alternative Health Care.* London: Judy Piatkus (Publishers), 1989.
Pietroni P. *Alternative Health Care.* Godalming, Surrey: CLB Publishing, 1995.
Robbins A. *Awaken the Giant Within.* New York: Fireside, 1992.
Rossi E L. *The Psychobiology of Mind Body Healing,* revised edn. New York: W W Norton & Co, 1993.
Schieff M. *The Memory of Water.* London: Harper Collins, 1995.
Sharon M. *Complete Nutrition.* London: Multimedia Books, 1989.
Smith G H. *Headaches Aren't Forever!* Newtown, PA: International Centre for Nutritional Research, 1986.
Stanton H G. *The Healing Factor.* London: Macdonald, 1981.
Vithoulkas G. *A New Model of Health and Disease.* Mill Valley, Ca: Health and Habitat, 1991.

## Associations

International Society for Holistic Dentistry
Ganzheitliche Zahn-Medizin (GZM)
Seckenheimer Haupstraat, 111
D-68239 Mannheim
Germany
Tel: 00 49 621 476400
Fax: 00 49 621 473949

British Holistic Medical Association
Rowland Thomas House
Royal Shrewsbury Hospital South
Shrewsbury SY13 8XF
UK
Tel: 01743 261 155
Fax: 01734 353 637

Natural Medicine Society
Market Chambers
13A Market Place
Heanor
Derbyshire DE75 7AA
UK
Tel: 01773 710002
Fax: 01773 533855

## Courses

There are no specific courses on running a holistic dental practice other than the seminars delivered by the author. There are many courses on the various disciplines outlined in this book. Each course can be seen as a stepping stone to developing a holistic practice. Contact details of the author:

Dr Stuart Ferraris
Beaumaris Dental Health Care
6 Castle Street, Beaumaris
Anglesey LL58 8AP
UK
Tel: 01248 811041
Fax: 01248 810977

# Index

Page references to illustrations and tables are **emboldened**